MOLECULAR AND BIOLOGICAL ASPECTS OF THE ACUTE ALLERGIC REACTION

NOBEL SYMPOSIUM COMMITTEE (1976)

STIG RAMEL, *Chairman*	Executive Director, Nobel Foundation
ARNE FREDGA	Chairman, Nobel Committee for Chemistry
TIM GREVE	Director, Norwegian Nobel Institute (Peace)
BENGT GUSTAFSSON	Secretary, Nobel Committee for Medicine
LARS GYLLENSTEN	Member, Swedish Academy (Literature)
LAMEK HULTHÉN	Chairman, Nobel Committee for Physics
ERIK LUNDBERG	Chairman, Prize Committee for Economic Sciences
NILS-ERIC SVENSSON	Executive Director, Bank of Sweden Tercentenary Foundation

Nobel Symposium, 33d, Stockholm, 1976

MOLECULAR AND BIOLOGICAL ASPECTS OF THE ACUTE ALLERGIC REACTION

Edited by

S.G.O. Johansson
University Hospital
Uppsala, Sweden

and

Kjell Strandberg
and Börje Uvnäs
Karolinska Institute
Stockholm, Sweden

PLENUM PRESS □ NEW YORK AND LONDON

Library of Congress Cataloging in Publication Data

Nobel Symposium, 33d, Stockholm, 1976.
  Molecular and biological aspects of the acute allergic reaction.

  Symposium held March 2—4, 1976; sponsors: the Nobel Foundation and its Nobel
Symposium Committee.
  Includes index.
  1. Allergy—Congresses. I. Johansson, S. Gunnar O., 1938-   II. Strandberg,
Kjell. III. Uvnäs, Börje. IV. Nobelstiftelsen, Stockholm. V. Title.
QRI88.N6 1976   616.9'7   76-26677
ISBN 0-306-33703-7

Proceedings of the thirty-third Nobel Symposium on the
Molecular and Biological Aspects of the Acute Allergic Reaction
held in Stockholm, Sweden, March 2—4, 1976

ORGANIZING COMMITTEE
  PER ANDERSON, *Assistant Secretary*
  K. FRANK AUSTEN
  ELMER L. BECKER
  S. GUNNAR O. JOHANSSON
  KJELL STRANDBERG, *Secretary General*
  BÖRJE UVNÄS, *President*

EDITORIAL COMMITTEE
  S. GUNNAR O. JOHANSSON
  KJELL STRANDBERG
  BÖRJE UVNÄS

SPONSORS
  The Nobel Foundation and its Nobel Symposium Committee through
  grants from the Tercentenary Fund of the Bank of Sweden.

© 1976 Plenum Press, New York
A Division of Plenum Publishing Corporation
227 West 17th Street, New York, N.Y. 10011

EARLIER NOBEL SYMPOSIA

Symposia 1-17 and 20-22 were published by Almqvist & Wiksell, Stockholm and John Wiley & Sons, New York; Symposia 23-25 by Nobel Foundation, Stockholm and Academic Press, New York; Symposium 26 by the Norwegian Nobel Institute, Universitetsforlaget, Oslo; Symposium 27 by Nobel Foundation, Stockholm and Almqvist & Wiksell International, Stockholm; Symposium 28 to be published by Academic Press, New York; Symposium 29 by Nobel Foundation, Stockholm and Trycksaksservice AB, Stockholm; and Symposium 30 and 31 by Plenum Press, New York.

Introduction

Ladies and Gentlemen, dear guests,

It is my great pleasure and privilege to extend our heartiest welcome to you, the participants of this 33rd Nobel symposium. To
those of you who have not attended a Nobel symposium before I
would like just briefly to explain why Nobel's name is linked to
this series of symposia. Alfred Nobel, who died in San Remo in
1896, donated the main part of his fortune to the promotion of international science and culture by establishing annual prizes for
outstanding discoveries or contributions within five fields, chemistry, physics, physiology or medicine, literature and peace. The
annual awards should be distributed by five corresponding prize
committees out of which four in Stockholm and one in Oslo (at that
time Sweden and Norway were a united kingdom). The Nobel Foundation
was instituted in 1900 with the main function to administer economically the Nobel Donation. It has done so very successfully. The
Foundation has even been able to beat the inflation and the prizes
have steadily increased during the last 20 years. It might interest
you to hear that this year's prizes will amount to 681.000 Sw.
crowns each.

Due to the favourable financial development and also due to additional donations the Nobel Foundation decided to extend its interests by promoting the arrangements of symposia, lectures and
other international scientific activities. Our symposium of today
is one of the results of these increased activities and the Nobel
Foundation is the main sponsor of our meeting. Some contribution
has also been given by the Nobel Committee for Physiology or Medicine which as you might know is elected by the Medical Faculty of
the Karolinska institute. The topics chosen for symposia within the
medical field must have the approval of this Nobel Committee.

The title of the today's symposium reflects the intention of the
organizing committee to arrange a meeting on a topic within the
front line of research in experimental allergology. Immunochemistry is since some years a field of exceptionally rapid development.

Advances within this field will no doubt lead to fundamental discoveries for our understanding and therapy of various diseases due
to disturbances in our immunological mechanisms, including those
on an allergological basis. Even if the main emphasis has been
laid on various aspects of immunochemistry, also the target cells
for allergic reactions have received their share. It is the hope
of the organizing committee that the communications and discussions
during the coming three days will be profitable and enjoyable to
all of us and will enable us to return home with new knowledge
and enthusiam for additional years of successful research in experimental allergology at all levels and to allow us to meet again
within a few years for a new fruitful time together in the sign of
our patroness Minerva.

Ladies and Gentlemen, I am quite sure that Alfred Nobel should have
been very pleased to be present at a symposium of the kind we have
ventured to arrange. However, as it is you have to be content with
hearty welcome from a humble of the Nobel machinery.

Börje Uvnäs
Chairman of the organizing committee

Contents

Session IV

GENERATION OF BIOLOGICALLY ACTIVE SUBSTANCES
AND MEDIATOR – TARGET CELL INTERACTIONS

Structure of Allergens and Regulation of IgE Immune Response

COMMON CHARACTERISTICS OF MAJOR ALLERGENS

Kjell Aas

Allergy Unit, Rikshospitalet, National Hospital of
Norway, University of Oslo, and
the Allergy Institute Voksentoppen, Oslo

This discussion will be restricted to the naturally occurring
allergens that elicit immediate hypersensitivity reactions when
combining with homologous IgE antibodies in human individuals.
It is not my intention to review the literature. Comprehensive
reviews may be found elsewhere (1,2,3). I will rather focus
attention on information thought to be particularly important as
basis for future research. Allergen chemistry will only be described in detail when necessary for elucidation or illustration
of particular points of interest.

The field of allergen chemistry is a difficult one. One depends ultimately on the biological tests related to the clinical
allergy in question. This introduces many methodological problems.
Due to the extreme sensitivity of the biological systems in question (4), otherwise undetectable contaminants such as undefined
allergenic molecules, irritants or both (5), may be responsible
for the reactions recorded. Furthermore, due to manipulations
necessary for the biological tests, the material may undergo important changes with effect on the allergenic activity (aggregation,
polymerization, conformational re-organization).

All scientific data up to the present time show that natura-
ly occurring allergens are proteins. However, only a limited number of numerous proteins found in allergenic material and in allergenic extracts are important for the allergic reaction. Only one

---

This work was supported by grants from the
Norwegian Research Council for Science and the Humanities.

3

or a very few of the allergenic proteins present in a given extract act as denominator of the allergic reaction in the majority
of patients allergic to the matter. They are called "major allergens". In addition, the same extract may contain other allergenic
proteins called "minor allergens", which are important only in a
small number of the patients. Most patients reacting to any of
the minor allergens usually react also to the major allergens
present in the material, but for occasional patients the minor
allergen may be the most active one.

The question naturally arises why certain proteins such as,
for instance, antigen E in ragweed pollen (6) and allergen M in
codfish (7) act as major allergens while several other proteins
in the same material do not. Much laboratory work has been devoted to efforts to point out characteristic traits that make
allergens allergens. Progress is steadily being made in isolation
and characterization of allergenic proteins. New methods in
protein chemistry have been the most important catalysts in this
process together with refined immunological techniques.

Investigations in allergen chemistry must start with ultra-
purified and well-defined material. They must make use of methods
with extreme capacities of discrimination and with an exceptionally high degree of sensitivity. Extreme care must be taken for
the control of the specificity of biological reactions (8,9).
With this in mind, the number of allergens and allergen studies
rendering substance for this discussion is brought down to a very
few. Information derived from studies of, for instance, house
dust allergens is too confusing to be brought into a discussion
meant to be clarifying (10).

Molecular size and bridging of IgE antibodies

There is some evidence that the initiation of the allergic reaction resulting in mast cell histamine release depends on the
bridging of two IgE antibody molecules by the allergenic molecule
in question (2,11,12). Many authors have discussed the importance
of molecular size for this bridging, and several statements have
been made that a molecular size of 10.000 - 70.000 or more
restricted between 10.000 and 40.000 is a common characteristic
for major atopic allergens (1,2,3). This is substantiated by the
actual analyses of a few purified or highly purified allergens
(table I). However, if such bridging is critical, it must depend
on the number and distribution of allergen determinants accessible
on the surface of the molecule and not on the molecular size as
such.

Table 1. Range of molecular weights (m.w.)
for allergenic molecules and biologically active allergen fragments.

ALLERGEN	m.w.	ref.nr.
Ragweed pollen, E	37.800	(6)
Horse dander	34.000	(13)
Cat epithelium	32.000	(14)
Cat epithelium	55.000	(15)
Rye grass pollen, BI	27.000	(24)
Honey bee venom*	19.500	(16)
Ascaris suum	18.000	(17)
Ascaris	14.000	(18)
Allergen M, cod	12.200	(26,50)
Allergen TM I	8.490	(19,26)
Allergen TM II	3.850	(26,52)
Allergen N (4.85)	3.460	(19)
Ragweed Ra 5	5.100	(20)

* Phospholipase A

The demonstration of prominent allergenic activity of the
small fragments TM I (mw 8.492) and TM II (mw 3.854) from codfish
(19) as well as the demonstration of a high allergenic activity
in some individuals to the dialyzable polypeptide Ra 5 (mw 5.100)
isolated from ragweed pollen (20) indicate that quite low limits
must be taken into account in statements on which molecular sizes
are necessary to induce allergenicity. The upper molecular weight
limit of 40.000 or 70.000 may be due to limiting factors in mucous
membrane permeability in the allergic host.

Stanworth (2) suggests that Ra 5 and allergen M may represent
monomeric subunits which have become dissociated from a dimeric
allergen during their isolation. He suggests that bridging occurs
when these subunits reassociate under physiological conditions.
There is, however, no evidence in support of this suggestion.

Molecular charge
The net charge of a polypeptide or protein depends on the ratio
of acidic (Glu, Asp) to basic (Lys, Arg, Hist) amino acid residues, and can be estimated when the amino acid composition is
known. Isoelectro-focusing and other methods for the separation
of proteins according to the molecular isoelectric points (pi)
introduced means to define the net charge of the allergenic
molecules more precisely (table 2).

Table 2.   Differences in net charge
(iso-electric points) be-
tween various allergens.

Allergen isoelectric point

Horse dander	4.1
Codfish, M	4.75
Ascaris suum	4.8 -5.0
Ragweed pollen, E	5.0 -5.1
Rye grass pollen, BI	5.15-5.25
Ragweed, Ra 5	9.6
Phospholipase A	10.5
Detergent alkalase	basic

Most major allergens characterized with respect to pi are
distinctly anodic ones with a pi range from 2-5.5. The codfish
allergen M has its pi at 4.75, and pi of most pollen allergens
is found around 5.   The house dust allergen reported by Berrens
is claimed to have its pi at 3.1 (1). Notable exceptions are the
basic proteins from the detergent enzyme allergen alkalase with
a pi around 9, and the basic allergens of cotton seed and castor
beans (22), as well as the minor allergens Ra 3 with pi 8.5 and
Ra 5 with pi 9.6 from ragweed pollen (20.23).

However, one may assume that it is not the net charge but
the charges of the limited combining sites of the molecules that
are significant for the binding to the complementary combining
site of the IgE antibody.

Iso-allergens
The term "iso-allergens" was introduced by Johnson and Marsh
(24) for two major allergens (alpha and beta) found in rye grass
pollen. The two allergens were homogeneous and immunologically
identical. They were also almost identical in molecular weight,
amino acid composition, carbohydrate composition and peptide
fingerprints, but differed slightly in their amide content. Similar observations were made by Tangen and Nilsson in studies
of timothy pollen allergens (25). Identical allergenic activity
was found in codfish proteins with distinct isoelectric-focusing
mobilities in acrylamide gels (26). They were considered to be
iso-allergens, being proteins with identical allergenic activities, but differing in amino acid composition and net charges
with pi 4.75 and 4.85, respectively.

Antigen E appears to be present in ragweed pollen extract
in four chemical forms. Two major forms designated as B and C
are immunologically identical and have identical amino acid compositions but differ slightly in isoelectric points (27).
Similarly, allergenic activity was found in several fractions of
house dust mites separated by liquid isoelectric focusing. A
high degree of cross-reactivity was found between fractions having
very dissimilar pi, varying from 3.0 to 6.4 (28).

The results of the latter studies strongly suggest that the
extract contains one or only a few main allergens existing in
multiple molecular forms rather than several distinct allergens.
Multiple molecular forms may arise during extraction and during
fractionation manipulations with changes of the immediate environment of the molecules, or they may exist in the original form of
the proteins. Effects of this kind may be important also for the
occurrence of IgE-binding antigens with distinct mobilities which
can be demonstrated in cross-radio immunoelectrophoresis of allergenic material (29). Following investigations making use of such
techniques, Weeke and co-workers (29) stated that timothy pollen
extracts contain at least 11 distinct allergens. It remains
to be shown whether some of them are iso-allergens or not.

Stability and structure
Many allergens are remarkably stable to chemical denaturation, but this is not a common trait and marked differences are
found in susceptibility to different agents (table 3). Pepsin
digestion does not impair the activity of rye grass (Lolium
perenne) pollen (3), but readily destroys the allergenic activity
of antigen E from short ragweed pollen (30). The codfish allergen is also inactivated by hydrolysis with pepsin as well as with
trypsin, but the time needed for complete inactivation was found
to be 2-3 hours in standard experiments (7). Hydrolysis for
shorter periods resulted in products still active. Reactivity
decreased with length of the hydrolysis. Allergenicity and antigenicity in immunodiffusion with homologous rabbit antisera disappeared simultaneously.

Antigen E is readily inactivated also by other denaturing processes such as heat, whereas the rye pollen major allergen, group
I, resists boiling for 30 minutes, changes in pH and treatment
with 8M urea (3). The major allergens in birch pollen also resist heating for a prolonged time (31). In contrast to antigen E,
the codfish allergen is remarkably stable to prolonged heating,
to pH changes and to denaturing agents such as 8M urea. The codfish allergen differs also from other allergens as regards susceptibility to physiochemical degradation. Whereas group I allergen from rye grass pollen loses most of its allergenic activity
following mild formalin treatment (32), the allergenic activity of
codfish was retained unaltered or only slightly reduced following

Table 3. Differences in allergen resistance to denaturing
agents as illustrated by three allergens.

IMMUNOCHEMICAL CHARACTERISTICS OF MAJOR ALLERGENS

	Allergen M (cod)	Antigen E (ragweed pollen)	Allergen IB (rye pollen)
Stability to			
heat	+	–	+
freeze-drying	+	(+)	+
freeze and storing at -20°C	+	–	+
acids	+	–	+
tryptic digestion	(+)	(+)	(+)
peptic digestion	(+)	–	(+)
formalin treatment	+	–	–

identical treatment.

Structure
Differences in stability may reflect differences in structure. Antigen E is composed of two polypeptide chains (alpha: mw 21.800, and beta: mw 15.700). These are held together by non-covalent forces (33). A cat epithelium allergen isolated by Stokes and Turner (15) is reported to be a tetramer of units of mw 13.000 held together by disulfide bonds. The codfish allergen is a one chain polypeptide. Structural data are scarce for allergens. The conformation of allergen A from Ascaris suum has been studied by circular dichroism and infra-red spectroscopy. The native allergen has an alpha-helical content of over 50 percent, and the high proportion of ordered structure is thought to account for its resistance to chemical and enzyme attack (34). The tertiary structure of allergens has not yet been resolved by x-ray crystallography at the atomic level (35). However, since there is a biological cross-reactivity between the codfish allergen and a parvalbumin fraction from carp muscle (36,37) the data from x-ray defraction determination of the latter may prove useful. The molecule is generally spherical with all of the polar side chains at the surface (38).

However, even when the tertiary structure of the protein is determined, it is only a picture of the most probable conformation in the crystal. It remains to know how far this structure represents that of the molecule in solution and when reacting in vivo with the particular antibody (39).

Antigenicity
It has been stated that allergens are weak antigens with reference to their ability to react with antibodies raised in animals immunized with the allergen extract in question. For allergenic molecules with relatively low molecular weights this would not be surprising since large molecules are known to be better antigens than small ones. Nevertheless, the codfish allergen was shown to be a quite good antigen, at least in a number of the rabbits immunized. This shows that the antigenicity as much depends on the immune responsiveness of the animals used. From available data we can therefore conclude that some allergens are weak antigens while others are good antigens.

The allergenic activity of the codfish allergen was completely abolished following precipitation with homologous rabbit antisera. This indicates as well that the allergenic activity in the one immune system (human IgE) is closely associated with antigenicity in the other (rabbit IgG). This does not imply that the antigenic sites active in the two systems are identical even if they are found on the same molecule, however.

Fluorescence

It has been claimed that fluorescence is a common property among atopic allergens (1) although not very impressive in intensity. Both allergenic and non-allergenic proteins show similar fluorescence. Although the fluorescence data are interesting observations, they are difficult to interprete. In any case, UV absorption and spontaneous fluorescence indicate only outlines of one kind of protein structural characteristics, and may even change due to different degrees of energy transfer or quenching in different stages of denaturation, conformational variation and changes of environmental influences (40).

Fluorescence is mainly attributed to certain amino acid residues (tryptophane, tyrosine and - to a lesser extent - phenylalanine) and to a number of prosthetic groups. Berrens (1) has called particular attention to the effect exerted on fluorescence by N-substituted 1-amino-1-deoxy-2-ketoses. This type of configuration with an absorption maximum at approximately 305 nm is claimed by Berrens to be characteristic for allergenic proteins. This maximum is not found in the spectra of the minor ragweed allergen Ra 5 or the major allergen in Ascaris, however, and a high absorption between 300 and 320 nm in both TM 1 and TM 2 fragments of the codfish allergen excludes carbohydrate as a cause of this particular absorption since carbohydrate is lacking in TM 2.

Single residue as common denominator

A single amino acid residue or a particular prosthetic group may be of crucial importance in defining the activity even when acting only as part of a larger antigenic determinant, whereas other residues may be important only in the complementary stereological fit between antigen and antibody without taking directly part in the binding.

It has been suggested that the determining and characteristic trait of allergens is found in N-glycosidic linkages (1). Weight has been put on the observation that many allergenic fractions contain sugar residues attached to epsilon amino groups of lysine. However, all naturally occurring proteins contain carbohydrate more or less tightly bound to their amino acid side chains. Again it is not recommendable to claim importance for the allergenic activity as such of any minor constituent based on studies of material which is not completely pure and uncontaminated. This is substantiated, for example, by the recent demonstration of accidental contamination with hydrolytic enzymes of even highly purified allergenic preparations (41). Contaminants not identified, may be the constituent responsible for some or all of the biological activity found in a given fraction.

The amino terminal fragment TM 1 of allergen M contains one

carbohydrate moiety (glucose)(7). This sugar moiety cannot have
any significance for the allergenicity of allergen M, since sugar
is absent from the identically allergenic carboxyterminal polypeptide fragment TM 2 of the same molecule. Although apparently in-
significant for the specificity of allergenic activity in the codfish allergen M and in allergens from Ascaris and certain pollen
allergens (3), N-glycosidic linkages may play a role for allergenic activity of other molecules. This can, however, not be considered a common characteristic.

Some information is also available for the discussion of
the general importance of certain single residues for allergenic
activity. By comparison of available amino acid compositions of
a number of allergens, the role of a few of the single components
can be ruled out. This is, for instance, the case for neuraminic
acid, tryptophane, threonine, methionine, arginine, tyrosine,
proline, phenylalanine, cysteine and histidine. The amino residues mentioned are apparently not mandatory for the allergenic
activity in general, but any of them may contribute to the allergenic activity in some other allergens. On the other side, for
what we know, lysine or some other amino acid residue may represent an allergenic immunodominant - but only so on a speculative
basis up to the present time. Furthermore, the importance of,
for instance, Ca^{2+} and Mn^{2+} or various metal ions for the binding
capacities between allergenic and antibody molecules is not understood or even investigated. It is known that such ions have a
marked influence on both the chromatographic behaviour and the
biological activity of other proteins (42) and they may be important for the structural organization of the polypeptide chain
(43).

From the above considerations it appears that there is no
proof that any single component such as a given amino acid or
sugar derivative acts as a common denominator in allergenicity.
Allergenicity seems to be just another form of antigenicity in
general. The particular reactivity in the IgE immune system may
be due to peculiarities of the individually reacting host rather
than to the characteristics of the antigenic material as such.
This seems, at least, partly, to be genetically determined (3,44).

Antigenic and allergenic determinants
One may ask if the IgE immune system reacts selectively to
particular structural arrangements differing from those acting
as antigenic determinants in the IgG immune system. Antigenic
determinants are defined as the discrete areas of the protein surface structure that combines specifically with the complementary
discrete areas of the particular antibody.

Antigenic determinants may be so-called "sequential" or
"conformational" ones, respectively. A sequential determinant is

organized from a number of amino acid residues as found directly
in a linear sequence in a random or unfolded form of the molecule.
A conformational determinant results from the steric conformation
including amino acid residues that are remote in the unfolded polypeptide chain, but are found in juxtapositions in the native structures. Most protein determinants that interact with humoral IgG
antibodies are thought to be conformational (35), but sequence-
dependant antigenic determinants have been demonstrated for many
polypeptide and protein antigens (45,46). The antigenic reactivity of silk fibroin for instance, seems to be due to determinants
with similar structures and specificities being repeated in the
primary sequence of the molecule (47). A number of studies in-
vestigating the structure of antigenic sites due to the primary
structure of synthetic polypeptide chains have been summarized
by Gill (48).

     There is yet no available information about the composition
of an allergenic determinant, in the meaning of the antigenic
determinant that combines specifically with the complementary IgE
antibody. However, work is in progress which may elucidate this
(49). The allergenic molecules of codfish have undergone frag-
mentations of different kinds. Several fragments have been analyzed
with respect to sequence and allergenic activity. The highest
degree of allergenic activity is found in a peptide residue 20-44.
This peptide has been demonstrated to possess a high degree of
allergenic activity both in direct prick testing of codfish allergic patients, PK-transfer experiments and RAST. PK and RAST inhibition experiments have shown that the activity found in this fragment is representative for the whole allergen M molecule. Other
and smaller fragments have been shown to inhibit the PK-reaction
without being able to elicit a direct test reaction,suggesting
univalence with respect to the allergenic determinant. Synthetization of such peptides may well help the identification of the
allergenic determinant in question.

A hypothetical allergenic determinant model
     The complete amino acid sequence of a major allergen (aller-
gen M from codfish) (50-52) provides for the first time substance
to allow speculation about the nature and characteristics of the
allergenic determinants. Speculations of this kind must first
build on the data available from antigenic determinants in other
immunoglobuline systems than that of IgE. Detailed descriptions
of conformational determinants can only be derived for those proteins whose tertiary structure has been resolved, but some experiments suggest that the allergenic activity of allergen M from cod
may be represented by sequential determinants and then the above
difficulties may be circumvened (7).

     For consideration of a hypothetical model of an allergenic
determinant site, the following data from the IgG system may be

taken into consideration: each determinant site must be considered
as a specific stereochemical configuration. Their characteristics
may comprise certain chemical denominators such as one or a few
distinct amino acid residues, or it may be due to features common
for a few of the amino amid residues such as carboxylic or amide
groups. Other features may be less distinct in the chemical sense,
being of significance only as spacing elements keeping the chemical denominators at a correct distance from each other. Determinants of this kind may be found as part of the primary structure
or they may be created through the spatial folding of the molecule
- or both. Cross-reactivity may occur due to side chain similarities (48).

   Assuming that the stereochemical characteristics of the
allergenic determinant of allergen M may be made up of certain
amino acid side chains being chemical denominators, kept at a
critical distance from each other by other amino acid residues
representing only an inert frame work, the molecule contains a
total of 6 - or possibly as many as 8 - sites which theoretically
could represent repetitive allergenic determinants (figur 1).
The theoretical basis for this hypothetical allergenic determinant
is that the critical denominators are found in two closely connec-
ted carboxylic side chains (Asp + Glu or Asp + Asp) kept at a critical distance from the basic amine of Lys by an amino acid residue, the nature of which is rather indifferent.

   Such a structure is found as primary structure components
but may also result from slight conformation of the molecule
(figur 2). This would explain the demonstration in several experiments with the codfish allergen that the activity is retained in
the urea-treated randomely unfolded molecule, that the activity
is destroyed by prolonged hydrolysis affecting the Lys site, that
the molecule is more active than most other allergenic molecules
(due to many IgE binding sites on each single molecule), and that
the activity is found in even quite small fragments containing
the hypothetical determinant.

   This hypothetical model would also fit into the observations
of cross-reactions between fish-species reacting with IgE antibodies of a number of cod-allergic patients (36). The amino acid
sequence presented as a theoretical model for the allergenic
determinant of allergen M, is found also as a repetitive unit even
on surface of the carp albumin molecule cross-reacting with the
codfish allergen (38).

   The validity of this purely hypothetical model remains to be
proven or dismissed through experiments with synthesized peptides,
and such studies are in progress (53). Since aromatic amino acid
residues in combination with polar amino acid residues also appear

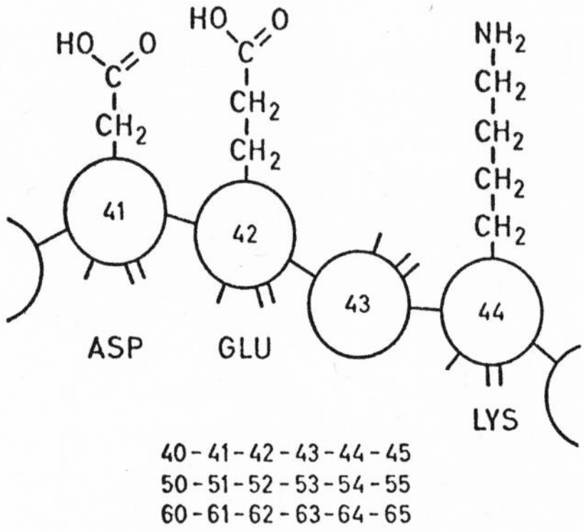

Figure 1.   A hypothetical allergenic determinant model.

to be particularly important components of antigenic determinants
in general, the frequent combination of Phe and Lys in allergen
M deserves interest as a basis for another hypothetical allergenic
determinant. This presentation of theoretical models serves,
however, only as an example of possible short-cut approaches in
future research.

Conclusion

It has not been possible to point out any physiochemical
feature that is particularly characteristic for major allergens
apart from being proteins with molecular weights below 70.000
and above 10.000 daltons, reacting with specific antibodies of

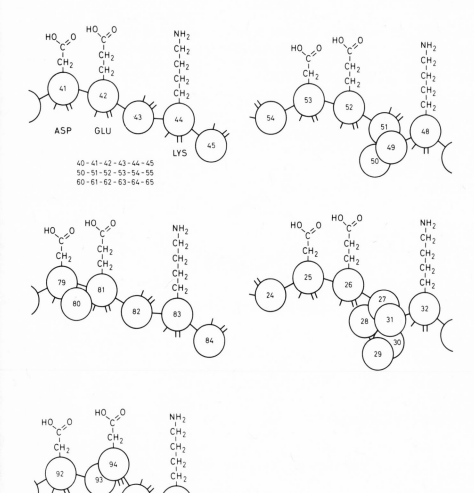

Figure 2.   A hypothetical allergenic determinant portion as
found in the codfish allergen. Sequential and
conformational variables.

the immunoglobuline E class.   Theoretically, it is possible that
there may exist physiochemical traits of crucial importance not
directly related to the allergenically active site as such.   Non-
antigenic sub-structures may, for example, be essential to the
transport through living membranes, for the passage of biochemical
barrieres or to the phagocyte presentation of the allergenic determinant to the particular immunocompetent cells of the IgE
line.

    The first steps have been taken towards elucidation of the
molecular basis of allergenicity and for the identification and
synthetization of allergenic determinants.   It is anticipated
that further achievements in this field may reveal a high order
or allergenic determinant individuality rather than common denominators in the physiochemistry of allergenic molecules.   Common
characteristics are more likely to be expressed in terms of the
allergic individuals.

References

1. BERRENS, L.: The Chemistry of Atopic Allergens,
    Karger, Basel, New York, (1971).

2. STANWORTH, D.R.: Immediate Hypersensitivity.
    North-Holland Publ., Amsterdam, (1973).

3. MARSH, D.G.: in M.Sela (ed) The Antigens, vol 3,
    Academic Press, New York, (1975) (p. 271).

4. AAS,K.: The Biochemical and Immunological Basis of
    Bronchial Asthma, Thomas, Springfield, (1972) (p. 68).

5. AAS, K.: The Bronchial Provocation Test, Thomas,
    Springfield, (1975) (p. 11).

6. KING, T.P., NORMAN, P.S. and CONNELL, J.T.,
    Biochemistry, 3, 458 (1964).

7. AAS, K., and ELSAYED, S., Develop. biol. Standard,
    29, 90 (1975).

8. AAS, K., and BELIN, L., Acta Allerg., 27, 439 (1972).

9. AAS, K., Ped. Clin. North. Amer., 22, 33 (1975).

10. AAS, K.: in Segal and Weiss (eds) Bronchial Asthma,
    Little, Borwn and Co., Boston (1976).

11. OVARY, Z., and TARANTA, A., Science, 140, 193 (1963).

12. ISHIZAKA, K.: in M. Sela (ed) The Antigens, vol 1,
    Academic Press, New York, (1973) (p. 479).

13. STANWORTH, D.R., Biochem. J., 65, 582 (1957).

14. BRANDT, R., PONTERIUS, G., and YMAN, L., Int. Arch.
    Allergy Appl. Immunol., 45, 447 (1973).

15. STOKES, C.R., and TURNER, M.W., Clin. Allergy, 5,
    241 (1975).

16. SHIPOLINI, R.A., CALLEWART, G.L., COTTRELL, R.C.,
    DOOMAN, S., VERNON, C.A., and BANKS, B.E.C., Eur. J.
    Biochem., 20, 459 (1971).

17. HUSSAIN, R., BRADBURY, S.M., and STREJAN, G., J. Immunol.,
    111, 260 (1973).

18. AMBLER, J., MILLER, J.N., JOHNSON, P., and ORR, T.S.C.,
    Immunochemistry, 10, 815 (1973).

19. ELSAYED, S., AAS, K., SLETTEN, K., and JOHANSSON, S.G.O.,
    Immunochemistry, 9, 647 (1972).

20. LAPKOFF, C.B., and GOODFRIEND, L., Int. Arch. Allergy
    Appl. Immunol., 46, 215 (1974).

21. BELIN, L., FALSEN, E., HOBORN, J., and ANDRÉ, J.,
     Lancet ii, 1153 (1970).

22. SPIES, J.R. and COULSON, E.J., J. amer. chem. Soc.,
     65, 1720 (1943).

23. UNDERDOWN, B.J., and GOODFRIEND, L., Biochemistry,
     8, 980 (1969).

24. JOHNSON, P., and MARSH, D.G., Immunochemistry, 3,
     91 (1966).

25. TANGEN, O., and NILSSON, B.E., Develop. biol. Standard,
     29, 175 (1975).

26. ELSAYED, S., AAS, K., and CHRISTENSEN, T., Int. arch.
     Allergy Appl. Immunol., 40, 439 (1971).

27. KING, T.P., Biochemistry, 11, 367 (1972).

28. ROMAGNANI, S., BOCCACCINI, P., AMADORI, A., and RICCI, M.,
     Int. Arch. Allergy appl. Immunol., in press.

29. WEEKE, B., LØWENSTEIN, H., and NIELSEN, L.,
     Acta Allerg., 29, 402 (1974).

30. KING, T.P., and NORMAN, P.S., Biochemistry, 1, 709
     (1962).

31. BELIN, L., Int. Arch. Allergy Appl. Immunol., 42,
     300 (1972).

32. ELSAYED, S., and AAS, K., unpublished material.

33. KING, T.P., NORMAN, P.S., and TAO, N., Immunochemistry,
     11, 83 (1974).

34. AMBLER, J., MILLER, J.N., and ORR, T.S.C., Immunochemistry,
     11, 309 (1974).

35. CRUMPTON, M.J.: in M. Sela (ed) The Antigens, vol 2,
     Academic Press, New York, (1974) (p. 1).

36. AAS, K.: Int. Arch. Allergy Appl. Immunol., 30, 257
     (1966).

37. AAS, K.: unpublished material.

38. KRETSINGER, R.H., and NOCKOLDS, C.E., J. Biol.
     Chemistry, 248, 3313 (1973).

39. HARTLEY, B.S., Biochem. J., 119, 805 (1970).

40. UDENFRIEND, S.: Fluorescence Assay in Biology and
     Medicine, Academic Press, New York, (1969).

41. BERRENS, L., and RIJSWIJK-VERBEEK, J. van., Int.
     Arch. Allergy Appl. Immunol., 49, 632 (1975).

42.   LIS, H., and SHARON, N., Ann. Rev. Biochemistry,
      42, 541 (1973).

43.   HASELKORN, R., and ROTHMAN-DENES, L.B., Ann. Rev.
      Biochemistry, 42, 397 (1973).

44.   AAS, K.: in M.A. Ganderton and A.W. Frankland (eds)
      Allergy '74', Pitman Medical, London (1975).

45.   BENJAMINI, E., SCIBIENSKI, R.J., and THOMPSON, K.:
      in F.P. Inman (ed) Contemporary Topics in Immuno-
      chemistry, vol 1, Plenum Press, New York, (1972)
      (p. 1).

46.   GOODMAN, J.W.: in M. Sela (ed) The Antigens, vol 3,
      Academic Press, New York, (1975) (p. 127).

47.   CEBRA,J.J.: J. Immunology, 86, 205 (1961).

48.   GILL, T.J.: in Specific Receptors of Antibodies,
      Antigens and Cells, Third. Int. Convoc. Immunology,
      Karger, Basel (1972) (p.136).

49.   ELSAYED, S., APOLD, J., AAS, K., and BENNICH, H.:
      In manuscript.

50.   ELSAYED, S., SLETTEN, K., and AAS, K.: Immunochemistry,
      10, 701 (1973).

51.   ELSAYED, S., BAHR-LINDSTRØM, H. von, and BENNICH, H.,
      Scand. J. Immunol., 3, 683 (1974).

52.   ELSAYED, S., and BENNICH, H., Scand. J. Immunol., 4,
      203 (1975).

53.   AAS, K., NILSSON, C., and CARLSSON, L.: To be published
      (1976).

DISCUSSION

ISHIZAKA, K.: Do you believe that IgE antibody combines
with the same antigenic determinant as IgG antibody?

AAS: The allergenic determinant in my presentation is defined as the antigenic determinant reacting with the IgE antibody. It may or may not be identical with antigenic determinants in other Ig systems such as that of IgG. There is some
evidence that the antigenicity in the IgE and IgG systems,
respectively, may be separate, but this cannot be confirmed
or dismissed before the antigenic sites have been defined.

MARSH: I think that one should view the idea that allergens may have some unique structure in the light of the historical concept from which allergy research has developed.
While von Piquet's original separation of immunological phenomena into "immunity" and "hypersensitivity" represented a

major breakthrough at the time, unfortunately this distinction tended to set allergy apart from the main stream of immunological thinking. In particular, the idea grew up that
allergens represent a unique subset of antigens. This view
was fostered by Coca and Grove's definition of atopic allergens as "agents which induce a strange deviation from the original state", from the Greek words atopia (strange) and allos
("other", and hence a deviation from the original state of von
Pirquet). Now that we know a lot more about the immunology of
IgE, the genetics of immune response, and the structure of
allergens, it is of doubtful value to search for special unique features of allergens suggested by these old definitions.
Instead, we have to look more toward the genetics of immune
response in the hosts themselves in order to explain IgE responses to antigens.

AAS: This is in accordance with my own view and I would
like to emphasize that the genetic influence on the expressivity of allergy is not only found in the particular immune
responsiveness but also in non-immunological characteristics
which may comprise several enzyme systems and pure immunochemical phenomena.

LICHTENSTEIN: Gleich and Adkinson (separately) have shown
that 10-30% of total IgE may be directed against a single antigen (even a hapten - BPO-HSA) while if all IgG molecules are
antibody it is clear that less than 0.1% are directed against
a single antigen. It follows, therefore, that the IgG system
must recognize far more antigens than the IgE system.

AAS: Up to the present time there is no confirmed evidence pointing to traits that make allergens - in the IgE system. There may be such traits, however. I would like to speculate that the hypothetical determinants of the allergenic molecule may be found more narrowly spaced than what is considered usual for antigen determinants in the IgG system. In the
IgG system there is rarely more than 1 antigenic determinant per
unit corresponding to 5 000 dalton in size. The antigenicity
in the IgE system may, theoretically, be characterized by presence of antigenic determinants with shorter interspaces than
found on other protein molecules. It may also be that allergenic molecules are more resistant to some biological denaturing
processes than other protein molecules. The point at the present time is that we cannot answer this question yet.

COCHRANE: Are data available on IgE versus IgG responses
following routine immunizations of man with such immunogens as
typhoid or influenza or even horse serum (as given with anti-
toxins)?

AAS: It seems to me that studies at the present time can
only partly answere this question since the antigenic materials used are so heterogenous. The antibody responses in the
two Ig systems may be directed towards different molecules
present in the solution. Furthermore, the results may be

affected by previous, unrecognized sensitization.

MARSH: We studied the responses of non-allergic individuals to relatively high doses (100 g + alumina gel) of the
rye grass group I (Rye I) and formaldehyde-modified Rye I
preparations ("allergoids"; Marsh et al. Immunology 22, 1013,
1972). In all nine cases studied, specific IgE responses were
observed, as measured by skin test, histamine release and,
more recently, by RAST (unpublished). It was interesting to
find the people immunized with allergoid became more sensitive to the native allergen than to the allergoid used for
immunization. This suggests that such people, in which neither IgE nor IgG antibodies against Rye I could be measured before immunization, had been subliminally immunized to native
Rye I by natural exposure to pollen. Other workers have immunized both non-allergic and allergic people with relatively
high doses of a wide variety of antigens, and in many cases
IgE responses are observed (see Immunology 22, 1013, 1972 for
refs.). The common features of these experiments are that
high, non-immunologally limiting antigen dosages are used.
Certain adjuvants such as alumina also greatly favor the induction of IgE responses.

COCHRANE: I brought up the question of generality of an
IgE response to an immunogen to support the final remarks of
Dr. Aas. When rabbits are injected with a variety of protein
antigens, they commonly, although not in every case, respond
with some IgE antibody. The variability of the IgE response
is not dissimilar to that of IgG response. This has been observed in rabbits injected with several different protein
antigens to induce serum sickness. This suggests that the ability to yield an IgE response is not limited to the few, but
is quite common and that Dr. Aas' comments on the way various
immunogens are presented to the host may be more important in
determining whether an IgE response will occur than a particular molecular structure of the immunogen.

JOHANSSON: The allergen structure is probably of importance also for triggering of the IgE mast cell reaction. Have
you calculated the distance in Ångström between the postulated, repetetive allergenic structures in relation to the size
of IgE and especially the distance between the Fab(ε) parts?

AAS: I hope you will allow me to refrain from answering
that question until our experiments with synthetic peptides
to test the hypothesis on possible allergenic determinants
have been completed.

TADA: I think that the ability to induce reagins is related to at least two distinct immunogenic structures which stimulate T and B cells. In our hands, none of the T cell independent antigens so far tested could induce IgE antibody in
the mouse and rat. Do you have any comment on the structural
characteristics of allergens which preferentially stimulate
certain population of T cells?

AAS: No

ISHIZAKA, K.: Ragweed antigen E as well as the major ascaris antigen, Asc 1, are potent immunogens for IgE antibody response in various animal species. It is also known that they are good carriers for anti-hapten IgE antibody response in experimental animals. I am wondering whether the cod fish allergens which Dr. Aas discussed, are also potent immunogens in experimental animals for the IgE antibody response. If so, I wonder whether they are good carriers for anti-hapten IgE antibody response.

AAS: We have no data as to this.

JANEWAY (Uppsala): Since most immunogens can induce IgE antibody, it is possible that the common feature of allergens is not related to antigenic characteristics but rather to their presence in the environment, route of entry or ability to resist degradation and to cross mucous membranes?

AAS: The allergenicity may comprise non-immunological traits which determine the fate of the molecule on its route to the immunocompetent cells. In this connection I'd like to emphasize that the codfish allergen acts as much as an inhalant allergen as a food allergen – and it seems to be particularly resistant to effects exerted on it within the host. A breast-fed infant suffered from severe immediate hypersensitivity reactions when being nursed shortly after the mother had eaten fish. The particular allergen thus remained active even after passage through two digestive systems and through several membranes. Such a molecule would be well suited for isolation and characterization studies – admitting that we treat the protein molecules rather roughly in the chemical laboratory. The presence of the allergen in the environment is critical. That is why we have codfish allergy in Norway but rarely so in Texas.

ALLERGY : A MODEL FOR STUDYING THE GENETICS OF HUMAN IMMUNE RESPONSE

David G. Marsh

Division of Clinical Immunology, The Good Samaritan
Hospital, Baltimore, Maryland 21239, U.S.A.*

INTRODUCTION

Natural Selection of IgE Production and Immune Response

In the economically well-developed nations, IgE-mediated
atopic allergy tends to be regarded as a nuisance disease, which
causes widespread morbidity in about 20% of the adult population
(1), but low mortality. Conversely, in under-developed cultures,
allergy is known to occur quite infrequently (e.g. 2-4), usually
in well under 10% of the population. In the developed world, IgE
seems to serve a detrimental rather than a useful purpose, but in
more primitive societies it seems to be playing a vital, although
not yet clearly defined, role in conferring resistance to parasitic
infestations, especially helminths. The latter assumption is
based on the widespread elevation in total serum IgE levels in
people living in areas where parasitic diseases are endemic (5),
as well as on several animal experiments which suggest a direct or
indirect protective role for IgE (6-9). In a bizarre human
"experiment" a small group of Canadian students were purposely
infested with ascaris by a disturbed roommate. The ones who
responded with the highest IgE levels had the least worms (10).

---

*Currently on sabbatical at the National Institute of Medical
Research, Mill Hill, London NW7 1AA, England.

Studies of total serum IgE levels and allergy in racially different populations raised in <u>similar environments</u> provide indirect evidence regarding the possible protective role of IgE. For example, U.S.-born Phillipino children had a three-fold higher geometric mean IgE level and a two-fold higher incidence of allergy than a matched group of U.S.-born Caucasian children (11).* In other studies, U.S. Negroes were found to have a significantly higher geometric mean IgE than U.S. Caucasians (12), and childhood asthma was shown to be significantly more common in British-born Negroes as compared with British-born Caucasians(4). Since there is now good evidence that total serum IgE level is in large part genetically determined (13, 14), I would argue that such racial differences reflect different frequencies of gene(s) controlling IgE antibody production in different races. On this basis, it seems reasonable to hypothesize that genetically determined high IgE responsiveness (reflected in high total serum IgE level) may well have been a selective advantage in primitive societies where parasitic diseases were endemic (e.g. in the recent tribal cultures in the Phillipines). Conversely, a genetic capacity towards high IgE responsiveness and concomitant high incidence of allergy (<u>cf</u> 5, 15) probably became a selective disadvantage in European Caucasians since Neolithic times, as parasitic disease became an increasingly less severe problem. Since there is unlikely to be any strong selective disadvantage against allergy, we are left with a relatively high incidence of this disease in modern Caucasian populations of European origin.

Let us now consider genetic factors governing <u>specific</u> immune response. In modern man, the main selective pressure on specific response has almost certainly been infectious disease. Several authors (16-19) have convincingly argued that many of today's common infectious diseases probably evolved only in the last 5000 or 6000 years, when the development of agriculture and towns provided the required size and density of population for survival of the respective pathogens. The staggering selective pressures of disease are apparent from the recorded effects of smallpox throughout the years and from the successive waves of bubonic plague which swept through Europe during the Middle Ages; in both

*Differences were statistically significant

cases, population mortalities of 50-90% were quite common (17).
More insidiously, the common childhood diseases such as measles,
polio and scarlet fever probably took an even greater toll over
the years. While a disease like measles may seem relatively
innocuous to modern man, who has been selected for resistance
over many generations, measles proved to be devastating when
primitive cultures were first exposed - for example, the Pacific
Islanders and South American Indians (17). Therefore, in modern
Caucasian populations, one might expect to find a high genetic
capacity to respond to those pathogens which have wreaked so much
havoc over the past few thousand years, perhaps within the
timespan of just 200-250 generations.

Genetics of the HLA System

        This brings us to a discussion of man's major histocompatibility
(HLA) gene complex and postulated linked immune response (Ir)
genes. By analogy with animal studies (20,21), it seems likely
that man possesses specific Ir genes linked to HLA, and that the
same genes control specific IgE antibody responses as other types
of specific immune response (22). I should, however, emphasize
that there is still no __hard__ genetic evidence for Ir genes in man
including those presumed to be linked to HLA (23-25).

        The HLA system (Fig. 1) consists of three serologically defined
loci, A, B and C, and two regions responsible for the mixed
lymphocyte reaction (MLR). Several other genes associated with
immune function, including complement levels, are also found within
this interesting complex (26). The well-defined A and B loci
(formerly known as LA and FOUR) are routinely studied in most
tissue typing laboratories. About 17 alleles of the A locus and

HLA GENE COMPLEX

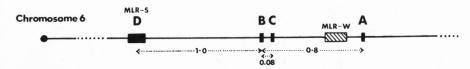

Fig. 1. The human major histocompatibility complex, HLA. Map
distances are expressed in terms of percentage recombination of
frequencies

20 of the B locus are currently recognized in this highly
polymorphic system. Due to their close genetic linkage, a pair of
A and B alleles are usually inherited as a unit, or "haplotype"
(27). Particular A and B alleles are <u>not</u> randomly assorted in the
haplotypes of a particular population, but tend to occur in
specific pairs due to the <u>linkage disequilibrium</u> of genes within
the HLA complex (28, 29). For example, the haplotype pairs A1,B8
and A2,B12 are much more common in Caucasian populations than
would be predicted from the frequencies of the respective A and B
alleles.

In order to account for some quite remarkable associations
between susceptibility to certain malignant and arthritic diseases
and specific HLA phenotypes, it has been postulated that "disease
susceptibility (DS)" loci are also in linkage disequilibrium with
HLA (28). The diseases which have been found to be associated with
HLA usually affect older people and, therefore, carry little
selective disadvantage. It has been proposed that the "DS genes"
have probably been inherited on the same chromosome as beneficial
Ir genes which confer resistance to those infectious disease agents
which evolved as man became more civilized (29). The main
selective pressures have been to keep the beneficial Ir genes, but
linked A, B, Ir and DS loci were usually inherited as well, due to
the low recombination frequencies between loci of the HLA system.
Also, functional interaction between the products of linked loci
which improved immune function would also have selected against
recombination (24). In general, the lower the recombination
frequency, the greater is the linkage disequilibrium observed.
Thus, the disequilibria between certain B and C locus antigens are
even greater than the highest disequilibria observed between A and
B locus antigens after correction is made for the haplotype
frequency (30).

What relevance do these theoretical discussions have to
genetic studies of atopic allergy? In Caucasian populations, the
frequencies of gene(s) controlling the overall capacity to
synthesize IgE as a class have probably been determined mainly by
the strong selective pressures which have operated through hundreds
of thousands of years until relatively recent times. In this case,
people having heightened overall IgE responsiveness would probably
have had a selective advantage in resisting parasitic infestation.

On the other hand, <u>specific</u> immune responsiveness (including production of IgE antibody) would have been largely determined by a need to combat more recently evolved pathogens. It seems reasonable to predict that those HLA-linked Ir genes which provided optimal responsiveness to pathogens (such as those discussed above) would have been selectively favoured during the recent evolution of man's immune system.

Thus, our present study of specific IgE responses to inhaled pollen allergens in Caucasian populations provides a way of understanding the genetics of IgE production and specific antibody response, not as a laboratory model, but within the context of powerful evolutionary forces which have shaped these systems. On the one hand, we can study the genetic control and interrelationship of IgE production and specific immune response. This is relevant not only to understanding atopic allergy, but also provides a model for studying the mechanism of gene interaction in human immune response. On the other hand, because (unlike inbred mouse experiments) we are studying a natural evolutionary process, we can eventually hope to gain insight into the allelic fine structure of human Ir genes as they relate to the selective pressures which have moulded them. Such studies will be of particular relevance to understanding human susceptibility to disease.

Allergy as a Model for the Study of Human Immune Response

The allergy model offers a number of advantages which we have discussed in detail elsewhere (24, 31). First, there is nothing physicochemically distinct about allergens which might suggest that they are a unique subset of antigens (24, 32). The dosages of most naturally inhaled allergens are extremely low -- generally under 1 µg/year (24). It is reasonable to expect that such doses are immunogenically limiting.* Second, because of the wide variety of physico-chemical structures found in common allergenic complexes, the allergy model provides a way of

*An analogy can be drawn between a person's capacity to respond effectively to such exquisitely low doses of allergens, and the selective advantage of responding well to the low doses of pathogenic antigens which are characteristic of the early stages of infection.

"fingerprinting" human immune responsiveness toward a large
representative sample of antigenic macromolecules. Finally, the
availability of several highly purified allergens and large
numbers of allergic patients facilitates these studies.

We can postulate some of the factors involved in human
allergy from studies which have been performed in animals and man.
Genetic factors may be divided into antigen specific and non-
antigen specific (Table I). According to animal studies, the
postulated HLA-linked Ir genes probably control recognition of

Table I. Controls of IgE Antibody Response

Genetic

Antigen-specific:

Interaction of antigen with T cells
Interaction of antigen with B cells
Cell-cell cooperation processes

Non-antigen-specific:

Mucosal membrane permeability
Hyperresponsiveness to foreign macromolecules
Overall regulation of IgE biosynthesis
Immunopharmacologic expressivity

Non-genetic

Antigenic Exposure:

Time of year
Geographic location

Socioeconomic factors and lifestyle:

Diet
Amount of outdoor activity

Immunotherapy

Age

specific antigenic determinants at the T-cell level as well as
cell-cell interactions involving T cells (20, 21, 33, 34). Other
non-HLA-linked genes probably play important roles in B-cell
responsiveness and other cellular events determining antigenic
recognition and processing (21).

Among the non-specific factors, it now seems unlikely that
allergic and non-allergic people differ significantly in terms of
mucosal membrane permeability (35), which was one of the early
hypotheses. We should, however, consider the possibility that
allergic subjects tend to be immunological hyperresponders -- i.e.
as a group, they tend to respond better than non-allergic people
to any foreign macromolecule (cf mouse data of Biozzi and
associates (36)). But, perhaps most important, the overall
regulation of IgE biosynthesis is likely to be of considerable
relevance in determining the expression of specific allergies.
Further genes are almost certainly important in determining the
immunopharmacologic expression of atopic allergies, including
atopic asthma and eczema (24, 37, 38).

Beside these genetic influences, several non-genetic factors
are important determinants of the initial sensitization and the
subsequent maintainance of IgE response. In summary, these
include the well-documented effects of antigenic exposure,
socioeconomic factors, immunotherapy and age (Table I). The
effect of socioeconomic and geographic environment can be quite
dramatic as shown by the epidemiologic studies of Smith (4) in
Britain and Godfrey (3) in Africa. For example, Smith showed that
the incidence of childhood atopic asthma and eczema is much higher
in West Indian or Asian school children born in England than those
born in their native land. Diet, especially in babies and young
children, is also probably important. In white Caucasian school
children born in England, the incidence of atopic asthma has
increased by 3.6 fold (from 1.76% to 6.32%) between 1956 and 1974
(4), possibly due to a decrease in breast-feeding and other
non-genetic factors (39). In terms of IgE production, sex does
not seem to be important (5, 15), but further work is necessary
to determine possible sex-associated genetic and non-genetic
factors which may influence IgE responses and expression of some
types of allergy such as childhood asthma (4).

RESULTS AND DISCUSSION

Genetic Determination of Basal IgE Levels

    The twin studies of Hamburger and associates (13, 14) showed
that total basal IgE level in serum is strongly influenced by
genetic factors; this encouraged us to study the genetic
determination of basal IgE in families (40). Preliminary studies
in a few families suggested that a major IgE-regulating gene
might be involved. For further analysis of this possibility, it
was necessary to define a cut-off point between "high" and "low"
IgE level and to assume that the two phenotypes, thus generated,
could be accounted for by a single gene locus. Since the
distributions of total serum IgE in allergic and non-allergic
Caucasian populations showed no obvious modality (Fig. 2), our
rationale was to determine the point at which there was "minimal
total misclassification" of the two populations based on IgE level

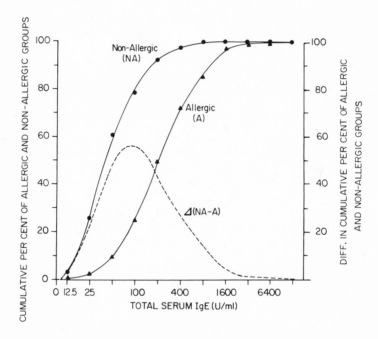

Fig. 2. Cumulative distribution frequencies for basal total serum
IgE levels for Caucasian populations of 106 unrelated non-allergic
and 205 unrelated allergic individuals living in the Baltimore
area. The dashed line is a difference curve for these two
populations. (From: Marsh et al., (40).).

Table II. Analysis for Recessive Inheritance of Total Serum IgE Levels in Caucasian Families

IgE Mating Type	No. of Fams.	No. of Offspring	No. of offspring with high IgE	
			Observed	Expected ($\pm$SD)
Low X Low (Rr X Rr)	10	41	18	15.3 $\pm$ 2.2
Low X High (Rr X rr)	11	41	26	22.6 $\pm$ 4.0
High X High (rr X rr)	5	25	25	25.0 $\pm$ 0.0
Low X Low *	1	2	0	--
Low X High *	3	9	0	--
Totals:	30	118	64	62.9 $\pm$ 3.6

*Families not analyzed by "Bias of Ascertainment" method since all offspring had low IgE Levels.

From Marsh et al., (40) and unpublished data on two further families.

-- i.e. where the cumulative proportion of non-allergic people
with atypically high IgE level plus the cumulative proportion of
allergics with atypically low IgE was minimized. On this basis,
the cut-off was found to be at 95 ±5 U/ml. However, due to seasonal
IgE variations[*], we took the cut-off to be 121 U/ml in allergic
family members, as discussed in detail elsewhere (40).

We then studied the basal IgE levels in 30 allergic families
representing 5 different IgE mating types (Table II). Only the
first three types, comprised of families where at least one
offspring has a high IgE level, were analyzed by the "Bias of
Ascertainment" method. This corresponds to situations where the
low IgE parents are presumed to be heterozygotes of an IgE-
regulating gene, R/r . In such cases, the numbers of children
with high IgE agrees closely with the theoretically predicted
values for recessive inheritance of high IgE level (see ref. 40
for further discussion). It should, however, be pointed out that
the data are also compatible with a more complex polygenic model.

We next asked the question: Which type of genetic influence
exerts the predominant effect on specific IgE responses to highly
purified allergens, postulated HLA-linked Ir genes or genetic
regulation of basal IgE level? If the former were true (as might
be implied from two recent publications (41, 42)), HLA-identical
allergic siblings should be more concordant in their patterns of
specific sensitivity than allergic siblings who differ in their
HLA genotypes. Conversely, if IgE regulation were more important,
allergic siblings with similar high IgE levels should be more
concordant than allergic siblings differing markedly in IgE level.
To test these possibilities we performed quantitative intradermal
skin test titrations with 8 immunochemically distinct allergens
isolated from grass and ragweed pollens (Table III).

Data on one particularly informative family is presented in
Figure 3. While the parents are not allergic, their five eldest
children have marked hay fever symptoms. Siblings Nos. 1 and 4
inherited the same two HLA haplotypes, A and D, from the parents,
while Nos. 2, 3 and 5 have the alternate haplotypes, B and C.

*In this and subsequent studies, serum samples were usually
collected when they were likely to have their lowest (basal) IgE
levels (40).

Table III. Molecular Weights of Highly Purified Allergens

GRASS POLLEN		RAGWEED POLLEN	
Lolium perenne		Ambrosia elatior	
Rye 1	27,000	AgE	37,800
Rye II	11,000	Ra3	11,000
Rye III	11,000	Ra5	5,000
Rye IV	55,000*		
Phleum pratense			
Timothy AgB	10,500		

*Approx. mol. wt. Not a single component.
See refs. 24 and 32 for reviews of physico-chemical properties.

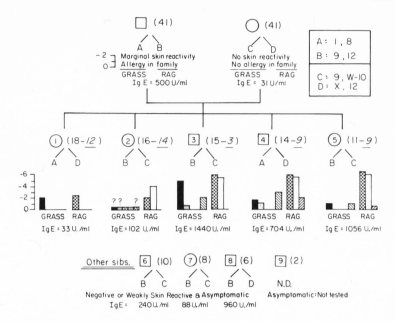

Fig. 3. Specific IgE-mediated skin sensitivities, HLA genotypes
and total serum IgE levels in a Baltimore family. Offspring are
numbered 1 through 9. Ages and ages of onset of allergic rhinitis
in allergic members (italicized) are given in parentheses. Vertical
bars represent quantitative skin sensitivities $[\log_{10}$ (allergen
concentration in µg/ml)$]$ which elicit 2-plus (0.8-1.0 cm wheal)
reactions. Designations of the allergens are as follows:
■ Rye I, ▨ Rye II, ▧ Rye III, ⦚ Rye IV, ▨ AgB, ▨ AgE,
□ Ra3, and ▨ Ra5. (From:Marsh et al (40)).

Whereas some HLA-identical sib pairs (e.g. Nos. 1 and 4) show
marked differences in their patterns of specific sensitivity,
other HLA-distinct pairs (e.g. Nos. 4 and 5) are quite similar.
On the other hand, siblings with high IgE levels (e.g. Nos. 3, 4
and 5) show a much greater concordance in their patterns of
sensitivity than sibling pairs where one has a high and the other
a low IgE (e.g. Nos. 1 and 4).

    Analysis of all our skin test data on pairs of allergic
siblings is summarized in Tables IV and V. Tests of concordance
are shown only for cases where at least one member of the sib pair

Table IV. Concordance in Specific IgE-mediated Sensitivity in
           Allergic Siblings with the Same or Different HLA
           Haplotypes

HLA Haplotypes	Number of Pairs	Concordance in Specific Sens.
Identical	9	14/34 (41%)
One different	6	11/24 (46%)
Both different	9	19/36 (53%)

Table V. Concordance in Specific IgE-mediated Sensitivity in
          Allergic Siblings with Similar or Different IgE Levels

IgE Levels	Number of Pairs	Concordance in Specific Sens.
Low-Low	3	3/6 (50%)
Low-High	11	12/43 (28%)*
High-High	10	29/45 (64%)*

* Significantly different; p=0.001

is positive to the allergen being tested. If the other member is
similarly positive, we record a concordant response (see ref. 40
for details). The last columns in these tables give the number
of concordant responses out of the total number of comparisons.
Concordance in HLA genotype seems to exert no apparent effect
(Table IV); but pairs of siblings with similar high IgE levels are
much more concordant in their specific sensitivities than pairs of
siblings with markedly different IgE levels (Table V).

At this point, we were faced with an apparent contradiction.
On the one hand, genetically controlled basal IgE level seemed to
be of overriding importance in determining specific IgE-mediated
sensitivity to highly purified allergens, masking effects which
would be anticipated if HLA-linked Ir genes exist. On the other
hand, our previous work in unrelated allergic subjects showed a
significant association between specific IgE-mediated response to
ragweed allergen Ra5 and the possession of HLA-B7 and the B7 Cross-
reacting group (Creg) in two different populations (43-46).

We reasoned that it might be relatively easy to demonstrate
an HLA association for an allergen of simple structure like Ra5
(mol. wt. 5000 Daltons), but that this would prove to be more
difficult for allergens of greater structural complexity where
several Ir genes might permit response (44). In order to observe
HLA-Ir associations for the more complex allergens, it might be
necessary to impose an additional constraint of limiting IgE
production over and above the limiting dosage characteristic of
natural exposure. This proved to be the situation for IgE
responses to two different allergens, rye grass Group I (Rye I;
mol. wt. 27,000 Daltons) and ragweed Ra3 (mol. wt. 11,000 Daltons).

Ragweed Allergen Ra3

I would first like to describe the Ra3 experiment in detail.
Here we found interrelations between serum IgE level and the
frequencies of HLA-A2 and the HLA-A2,B12 phenotype in people who
are sensitive to Ra3 (31, 47). The allergens used for this study
were antigen E (AgE; ref. 48) and Ra3 (49), both of which were
isolated in highly purified form from short ragweed pollen. The
AgE preparation obtained from the NIH was further purified in our
laboratory, and the sample of Ra3 was kindly supplied by Dr.
Goodfriend.

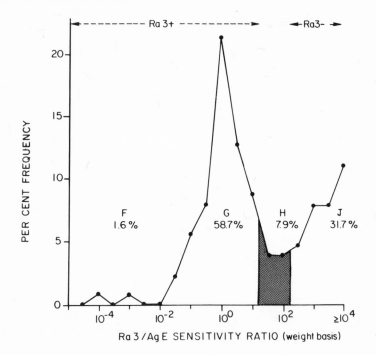

Fig. 4. Distribution frequency of Ra3/AgE skin sensitivity ratios
in 126 Caucasians who are highly allergic to ragweed pollen

     Figure 4 shows the distribution of Ra3 sensitivity in our
patient population of 126 Caucasians. A number of points deserve
to be stressed. Our population consists only of clinically
ragweed-allergic individuals. This ensures sufficient exposure to
ragweed pollen and the presence of other genetic and non-genetic
factors required for the overall expression of allergy.
Immunoglobulin E-mediated sensitivity to allergens Ra3 and AgE
were quantitatively determined by skin test titration (43).
Patients' IgE-mediated sensitivity ratios, Ra3/AgE, could then be
calculated with a maximum error of about one $\log_{10}$ (45, 47).
Almost all individuals who are allergic to ragweed are sensitive
to AgE, and no HLA associations are apparent with this allergen
(50). Sensitivity to AgE has, therefore, been used as a common
denominator to minimize the variations in Ra3 sensitivity which
arise from variable allergenic exposure and from differences in
the degree of allergic expressivity in different people (24, 50).

Table VI   Comparisons of HLA Frequencies for Ra3 Positive versus
           Ra3 Negative Subjects*

HLA	Ra3+ Groups(F+G) (N = 76)	Ra3- Group J (N = 40)	RELATIVE HLA INCIDENCES (Ra3+/Ra3-)	p VALUES† Ra3+ vs Ra3-
A2	42 (55%)	14 (35%)	1.6	0.04
A3	16 (21%)	16 (40%)	0.53	-0.03
B12	32 (42%)	10 (25%)	1.7	0.07
A2,B12 (phenotype)	21 (28%)	5 (12%)	2.2	0.06

* Comparisons restricted to Caucasians
† Chi-squared analysis where $p < 0.1$.

     Our patient population fell essentially into two allergy
phenotypes: Ra3 positive (Ra3+) and Ra3 negative (Ra3-). The HLA
phenotypes were determined on all individuals and the frequencies
of each HLA antigen were compared between the Ra3+ and the Ra3-
groups by chi-squared analysis. Ten intermediate individuals were
excluded from the analysis of our data (Table VI). The only HLA
phenotype which was significantly elevated in the Ra3+ relative to
the Ra3- population was HLA-A2, although this was not very striking
($p = 0.04$). Phenotype HLA-B12, which commonly occurs in Caucasian
haplotypes with A2, and the phenotypic combination of A2 and B12,
were also similarly elevated.

     We determined the total serum IgE levels on each patient by
double antibody radioimmunoassay (40). Figure 5 shows the
distribution of total IgE levels for Ra3+, Ra3- and intermediately
sensitive individuals. The distribution of total IgE levels for
the Ra3+ population is higher than for the Ra3- group (G.M. IgE =
258 U/ml for Ra3+, 192 U/ml for Ra3-; $0.1 > p > 0.05$ for comparison
of log IgE by t-test). However, since there was no clear modality
in either of these distributions, the total population of 126
subjects was divided into quartiles based on total IgE level in

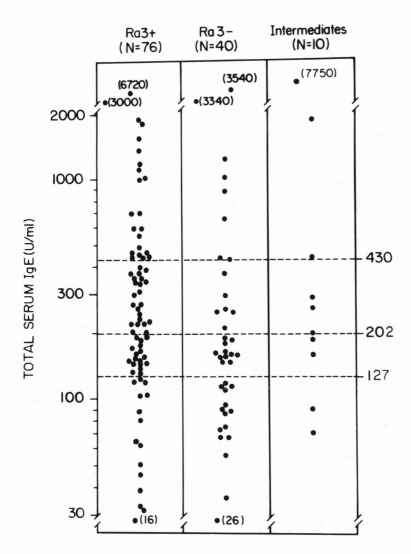

Fig. 5. Distributions of total serum IgE levels in Ra3+, Ra3-
and intermediately Ra3 sensitive people. Quartile divisions are
represented by the dashed lines. The IgE levels of people falling
outside the range of 30-2000 U/ml are given in parentheses. Most
of the IgE levels were determined on sera drawn during February –
May when IgE usually attains its lowest (basal) level (40).

order to simplify further analysis. Note that Ra3+ and Ra3-
individuals are evenly divided in the lowest IgE quartile (15
subjects each), but in the two highest quartiles there are three
times as many people in the Ra3+ than in the Ra3- group (22 versus
7 in each case). It appears that the requirement for highly
selective recognition of Ra3 becomes less stringent at high IgE
levels since a greater proportion of patients are Ra3 sensitive at
high than at low IgE.

For the Ra3+ population, the frequencies of HLA-A2, HLA-B12,
and the HLA-A2,B12 phenotype for each IgE quartile are given in
Figure 6a. The normal Caucasian population frequencies for each
of these phenotypes determined by Terasaki (27) are shown by the
dashed lines. In particular, the frequencies of HLA-A2 and the
A2,B12 phenotype are much more pronounced at low than at high
serum IgE levels. Above the first quartile, all of the phenotype
frequencies are similar to their normal Caucasian population
frequencies. The frequency of A2 in the first quartile is
significantly higher than all other quartiles (e.g. comparison of
the first versus the combined second, third and fourth quartiles
by chi-squared analysis with Yates' correction gives p = 0.003).

We now turn to analysis of Ra3+ versus Ra3- subjects,
restricted to comparisons involving Ra3+ individuals who have IgE
levels in the first quartile (Table VII). The Ra3+ patients with
low IgE represent a limiting situation for IgE response. They are
compared with Ra3- individuals in the first quartile and with all
Ra3- individuals. For both types of comparison, we see striking
elevations of HLA-A2 and the A2,B12 phenotype and some elevation
of HLA-B12 in Ra3+ versus Ra3- subjects. In the footnote to this
table, we include the normal Caucasian population frequencies of
these HLA phenotypes, all of which are well below the lower 95%
confidence limits for the frequencies of the respective phenotypes
in the Ra3+ subpopulation having low IgE.

Thus, our data show a very marked association between skin
sensitivity to Ra3 and the possession of the A locus antigen, A2,
for people with limiting low total serum IgE levels. There was
also a strong association with the A2,B12 phenotype, which
probably implies association with the A2,B12 haplotype (see later).

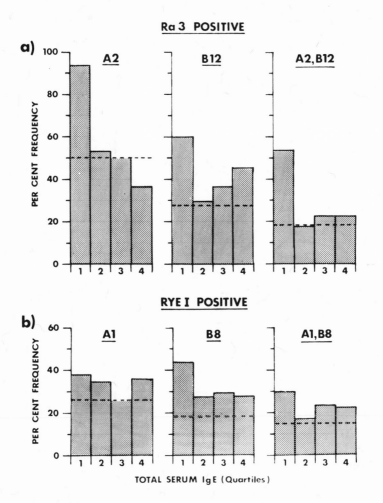

Fig. 6. a. Distribution frequencies of HLA-A2, HLA-B12 and the A2,B12 phenotype in the Ra3+ population (N = 76) subdivided according to IgE quartile (see Fig. 5)

b. Distribution frequencies of HLA-A1, HLA-B8 and the A1,B8 phenotype in a Rye I+ population (N = 136) subdivided according to IgE quartile of the entire study group (N = 214; includes Rye I- and intermediately Rye I sensitive people. Quartile divisions occur at 112, 203 and 400 U/ml.

Normal Caucasian population frequencies of each HLA phenotype (Terasaki (27)) are designated by dashed lines.

Table VII. Comparisons of HLA Frequencies for Ra3 Positive Individuals with Low Total IgE Levels versus Ra3 Negative Individuals*

HLA	Ra3 POSITIVE 1st IgE quartile (N = 15)	Ra3 NEGATIVE 1st IgE quartile (N = 15)	Ra3 NEGATIVE All IgE quartiles (N = 40)	p VALUES† Column 2 vs. Column 3	p VALUES† Column 2 vs. Column 4
A2	14 (93%)	4 (27%)	7 (29%)	0.0008	< 0.0001
B12	9 (60%)	4 (27%)	8 (33%)	0.13	0.01
A2,B12 (phenotype)	8 (53%)	1 (7%)	3 (12%)	0.015	0.0006

* Restricted to Caucasians

† Determined by chi-squared analysis with Yates' correction

	HLA-A2	HLA-B12	A2,B12 phenotype
Caucasian pop. freqs. (Terasaki (27)):	50%	27%	18%
Lower 95% confidence limits in Ra3+ pop:	81%	35%	28%

Rye Grass Group I (Rye I)

I would like, now, to review very briefly our data comparing allergic Caucasian populations who are either sensitive or insensitive to the Rye I allergen (50, 51).* Here, we found the most marked association between Rye I sensitivity and a B locus antigen, B8 (p = 0.0005), and weaker associations with A1 (p = 0.03), and the A1,B8 phenotype (p = 0.007). Like the case of Ra3, we found a marked interrelation between total IgE level and the frequency of the most commonly associated HLA antigen, i.e. for HLA-B8 in the Rye I+ population (Fig. 6b). Again, the greatest change in HLA frequency occurred between the first and second quartiles (112 U/ml in this experiment). The interrelations between IgE level and the frequencies of A1 and the A1,B8 phenotype were less pronounced than for B8.

Statistical comparisons of the frequencies of HLA-A1, HLA-B8 and the A1,B8 phenotype in Rye I+ versus Rye I- populations are presented in Table VIII. The Rye I+ subpopulation with IgE levels in the first quartile had significantly higher frequencies of B8 and the A1,B8 phenotype, and a higher frequency of A1 than either the Rye I- subpopulation with low IgE or the total population of Rye I- subjects.

ANALYSIS AND CONCLUSIONS

Genetic Regulation of IgE

There is now strong evidence that total basal serum IgE levels are, in large part, genetically determined (13, 14). The problem is to define the genetic mechanism. Based on an analysis of IgE level which allows minimal misclassification of allergic and non-allergic subjects, we found that the distribution of basal serum IgE levels in allergic families is consistent with a single major IgE-regulating gene (Fig. 2 and Table II). In this study, allergic family members were separated into two phenotypes by a cut-off point of 121 U/ml, which is very similar to the first quartile divisions of 127 and 112 U/ml in our subsequent studies

*A total of 214 patients were studied, of which 136 were classified as Rye I+ and 64 as Rye I- based on Rye I/AgE sensitivity ratios (50).

Table VIII. Comparisons of HLA Frequencies for Rye I Positive Individuals with Low Total IgE Levels versus Rye I Negative Individuals *

HLA	RYE I POSITIVE 1st IgE quartile (N = 37)	RYE I NEGATIVE 1st IgE quartile (N = 14)	RYE I NEGATIVE All IgE quartiles (N = 64)	p VALUES† Column 2 vs. Column 3	p VALUES† Column 2 vs. Column 4
A1	14 (38%)	1 (7%)	12 (19%)	0.07	0.06
B8	16 (43%)	0 (0%)	6 (9%)	0.008	0.0002
A1,B8 (phenotype)	11 (30%)	0 (0%)	5 (8%)	0.05	0.008

* Restricted to Caucasians

† Determined by chi-squared analysis with Yates' correction

of Ra3 and Rye I sensitivity in populations of unrelated individuals (Figs. 5 and 6). The common feature of all three studies is that the effects of HLA-associated specific IgE responses (presumably reflecting the effects of HLA-linked Ir genes) are masked at high IgE levels above these cut-off points. We believe that, taken together, these data strongly support the existence of two major allergy phenotypes which are characterized in large part by their different basal serum IgE levels.* In order to synthesize IgE antibody against an antigen like Ra3, people with the "low IgE" phenotype are considered to require an HLA-linked Ir gene(s) which permits antigen recognition under the most limiting conditions of antigenic exposure and IgE biosynthesis. Conversely, allergic people with the "high IgE" phenotype probably have a more permissive Ir gene requirement for specific IgE biosynthesis. In this case, the presence of any one of several different Ir gene products (which perhaps allow immune recognition under conditions of lower binding affinity between the antigen and cell receptors) will permit antigen recognition and specific IgE response. (24).

It will be impossible to define the IgE-regulating gene precisely until we find an immunological role. The present definition based on total serum IgE levels is not altogether satisfactory, since IgE levels are determined by many different genetic and non-genetic influences and vary with season. Therefore, cut-off points are chosen on a fairly arbitrary basis. We believe that a good possibility for the role of this gene is that it operates directly at the level of antigen recognition by regulating the number of different IgE antibody producing clones which respond to a limiting antigenic stimulus (52). The number of responding clones would be greater for people with high than with low IgE phenotypes. This hypothesis is completely consistent with the HLA-IgE interrelationships already discussed. It also explains why most people with genetically determined high IgE levels are allergic to many more allergens than people with low

*The corresponding genotypes would be: RR and Rr for low IgE, and rr for high IgE. The respective genotype frequencies would be approximately 0.23, 0.5 and 0.27 in Caucasian populations (40).

IgE levels (53, 54) and, conversely, why allergic people with low
IgE phenotypes are less likely to be sensitive to moderately complex
allergens like Ra3 than people with high IgE phenotypes (Fig. 5).

This hypothesis is attractive for a number of reasons. First,
the possession of a broad specificity of responsiveness within the
IgE system could well have been a useful evolutionary strategy in
protecting man against infestations by parasites. Second, our
hypothesis can be tested since it predicts that responder
individuals with low IgE phenotypes should have more homogeneous
IgE antibodies than people with high IgE phenotypes.

Estimation of the Relative Map Positions of Postulated Ir Genes
within the HLA Complex

An interesting feature of the HLA-Ir associations is that, in
people with low IgE phenotypes, sensitivities to Ra3 and Rye I are
associated with the A2,B12 and A1,B8 phenotypes, respectively.
Association is probably with the respective haplotypes, as seen by
further analysis of our data (31, 47, 50) including genotyping some
of the patients. These two haplotypes are the most common in
American and most European Caucasian populations (27) and are
thought to be associated with some selective advantage, possibly
improved immune responsiveness (29, 55).

In Ra3-sensitive people with low IgE phenotypes, the strongest
association is with an A locus HLA antigen, while our Rye I data
and previously published Ra5 data (43, 45) show strongest
associations with B locus HLA antigens. These findings are
consistent with the existence of two HLA-linked Ir regions in man,
one close to the A locus and the other close to the B locus. It
is worthwhile pointing out again that HLA-linked Ir genes are not
proved in man (23). We are presently relying on the homology
between man's HLA system and the major histocompatibility (H)
systems of several animal species where H-linked Ir genes have
been shown to exist (20, 21).

We will assume that discrete HLA-linked Ir genes, "Ir-Ra3"
and "Ir-Rye I", control IgE antibody responses to Ra3 and Rye I
in highly allergic individuals with low IgE phenotypes (first
quartile), that these are the only HLA-linked Ir genes which

permit IgE response under these limiting conditions, and that they are fully expressed. In such case, we can calculate the corresponding phenotype association disequilibria, $\triangle$, between the Ir genes and their most frequently associated A and B locus antigens (Fig. 7).

The disequilibria between Ir-Ra3 and HLA-A2 and B12 clearly show that the strongest association is with A2, and that the association between Ir-Ra3 and B12 is stronger than between A2 and B12. Conversely, the association between A1 and B8 is stronger than between Ir-Rye I and B8 which, in turn, is stronger than between Ir-Rye I and A1. Note that these associations are with HLA phenotype, not genotype. By further analysis, patient-by-patient, it should be possible to estimate the most probable genotypic associations based on the linkage disequilibria within the HLA gene complex.

To make provisional assignments of map relationships, we need to assume that phenotypic association implies genetic linkage between the respective loci and, further, that the degree of disequilibrium is directly related to the frequency of recombination (cf 29). This leads to the assignment of Ir map locations shown in Figure 7. Within the limits of the assumptions on which our analysis is based, we are confident of the location of the postulated Ir-Ra3 locus. All Ra3+ subjects with low IgE phenotypes except one have HLA-A2. The atypical person (and, also, a sibling of another patient)* have HLA-A9,B12 haplotypes which may be recombinants (31, 47). The situation with Ir-Rye I is less clear since only 43% of Rye I positives have B8 (Table VIII). This may well result from a higher recombination frequency between B8 and Ir-Rye I than between A2 and Ir-Ra3. Nevertheless, our data clearly show that the strongest association in the Rye I+

* See the responses to Ra3 in Figure 3

CALCULATION OF PHENOTYPE ASSOCIATION DISEQUILIBRIA

e.gs.

$$\triangle_{2,12} = p(A2,B12) - p(A2)p(B12)$$

$$\triangle_{2,Ir} = p(A2,Ir) - p(A2)p(Ir)$$

$$\triangle_{2-12,Ir} = p(A2,B12,Ir) - p(A2,B12)p(Ir)$$

Ir-Ra3 and HLA-A2,B12

$$\triangle_{Ir,2} > \triangle_{Ir,2-12} > \triangle_{Ir,12} > \triangle_{2,12}$$

0.167   0.117   0.083   0.040

Probable map relationships:

Ir-Rye I and HLA-A1,B8

$$\triangle_{1,8} > \triangle_{Ir,8} > \triangle_{Ir,1} \approx \triangle_{Ir,1-8}$$

0.123   0.086   0.061   0.059

Possible map relationships:

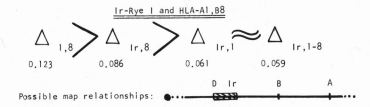

Fig. 7. Calculation of phenotype association disequilibria, $\triangle$, for (i) a hypothetical major "Ir-Ra3" gene and HLA-A2 and B12, and (ii) a hypothetical major "Ir-Rye I" gene and HLA-A1 and B8. The $\triangle$ values were calculated for people having limiting IgE levels falling within the first IgE quartiles of the Ra3 and Rye I studies respectively. Probable and possible map relationships are based on several assumptions (see text). MLR-S(D) loci and the postulated Ir-Rye I locus probably lie within the shaded area given at the bottom of the figure, but the map order is undetermined

population is with B8 and not with A1, supporting the view that Ir-Rye I is to the "left" of B8 on our gene map.†

These assignments concur with current knowledge about the genetics of HLA and its animal homologues. A region of HLA which controls alloantigens expressed on B cells has been mapped close to the D (MLR-S) region (58), and it is now thought that such B-cell specific antigens are homologues of mouse immune-associated (Ia) antigens (59). Very recently, Mann et al (60) have evidence supporting two "Ia-like" regions in the HLA complex, one associated with the A locus and the other with the B locus.

CONCLUDING REMARKS

In conclusion, we have provided good evidence for IgE-regulating and Ir genes in man; but further epidemiologic and genetic studies of populations and families will be required to prove their existence on a firm genetic basis. The allergy model provides many advantages and great scope for studying the genetics of human immune response. These studies have relevance not only to allergy, but to a broader understanding of relationships between specific immune responses and disease susceptibility in human populations.

† While our HLA map shows the centromere to be on the left (in accordance with accepted current practice), it may just as well be on the right. In such case, the human A locus would be the homologue of the mouse K locus and Ir-Ra3 could map within a human "I region" homologous to that of the mouse. Animal MLR (and probably associated I) regions located outside the chromosomal region between the main serologically defined loci exist in both rhesus monkey (56) and guinea pig (57), but have not yet been found in mouse.

ACKNOWLEDGEMENTS

I wish to thank Dr. W. B. Bias who collaborated in all the genetic experiments and Dr. K. Ishizaka who collaborated in the family study of basal IgE levels. I also greatly appreciate the materials and help given by Drs. L. Goodfriend, G. A. Chase, J. Nutter, P. S. Norman, L. M. Lichtenstein and C. A. Bruce, and the technical staff of the Divisions of Clinical Immunology and Medical Genetics of the Department of Medicine, The Johns Hopkins University School of Medicine. Ms. J. E. Marsh and Dr. T. Platts-Mills read and provided useful suggestions for improving the text. This research was funded by NIH Grants Nos. AI 09465 and Research Career Development Award No. AI 50304.

REFERENCES

1   Smith, J. Montgomery (1974), Incidence of Atopic Disease. Med. Clin. N. Amer. 58, 3.

2   Anderson, H.R. (1974), The Edpidemiological and Allergic Features of Asthma in the New Guinea Highlands. Clin. Allergy 4, 171.

3   Godfrey, R.C. (1975), Asthma and IgE Levels in Rural and Urban Communities in Gambia. Clin. Allergy 5, 201.

4   Smith, J. Morrison (1976), The Prevalence of Asthma and Wheezing in Children. Brit. J. Dis. Chest 70, in press.

5   Johansson, S.G.O., Bennich, H.H. and Berg, T. (1972), The Clinical Significance of IgE. Progr. Clin. Immunol. 1, 100.

6   Barth, E.E.E., Jarrett, W.F.H. and Urquhart, G.M. (1966), Studies on the Mechanism of the Self-Cure Reaction in Rats Infected with Nippostrongylus Brasiliensis. Immunology 10, 459.

7   Olgivie, B.M., Smithers, S.R. and Terry, R.J. (1966), Reagin-like Antibodies in Experimental Infections of Schistosoma Mansoni and the Passive Transfer of Resistance. Nature 209, 1221.

8   Capron, A., Dessaint, J.-P., Capron, M. and Bazin, H. (1975), Nature 253, 474.

9   Murrell, K.D., Vannier, W.E., Hussain, R. and Chestnut, R.
      (1975), Tenth Joint U.S.-Japan Conference on Parasitic
      Diseases, Bethesda, Maryland, p. 97.

10   Phills, J.A., Harrold, A.J., Whiteman, G.B. and Perelmutter, L.
      (1972), Pulmonary Infiltrates, Asthma and Eosinophilia Due To
      Ascaris Suum Infestation in Man. N. Eng. J. Med. 286, 965.

11   Orgel, H.A., Lenoir, M.A. and Bazaral, M. (1974), Serum IgG,
      IgA, IgM and IgE Levels and Allergy in Filipino Children In
      The United States. J. Allergy Clin. Immunol. 53, 213.

12   Grundbacher, F.J. (1975), Causes of Variation in Serum IgE
      Levels in Normal Populations. J. Allergy Clin. Immunol. 56,
      104.

13   Hamburger, R.N., Orgel, H.A. and Bazaral, M. (1973), Genetics
      of Human Serum IgE Levels. In "Mechanisms in Allergy:
      Reagin-Mediated Hypersensitivity" (L. Goodfriend, A.H. Sehon
      and R.P. Orange, eds.) Marcel Dekker, New York, p.131.

14   Bazaral, M., Orgel, H.A. and Hamburger, R.N. (1974), Genetics
      of IgE and Allergy: Serum IgE Levels in Twins. J. Allergy
      Clin. Immunol. 54, 288.

15   Gleich, G.J., Averbeck, A.K. and Swedlund, H.A. (1971),
      Measurement of IgE in Normal and Allergic Serum by
      Radioimmunoassay. J. Lab. Clin. Med. 77, 690.

16   Haldane, J.B.S. (1957), Natural Selection in Man. Acta Genet.
      6, 321.

17   Motulsky, A.G. (1960), Metabolic Polymorphisms and the Role
      of Infectious Diseases in Human Evolution. Human Biol. 32,
      28.

18   Fenner, F. (1970), in "The Impact of Civilization on the
      Biology of Man." (S.V. Boyden, ed.) University of Toronto
      Press, Toronto. p.48.

19   Black, F.L. (1975), Infectious Diseases in Primitive Societies.
      Science 187, 515.

20   Benacerraf, B. and McDevitt, H.O. (1972), Histocompatibility-
      Linked Immune Response Genes. Science 175, 273.

21 McDevitt, H.O. and Landy, M. (1972), "Genetic Control of
    Immune Responsiveness". Academic Press, New York.

22 Vaz, N.M. and Levine, B.B. (1970), Immune Responses of Inbred
    Mice to Repeated Low Doses of Antigen: Relationship to
    Histocompatibility (H-2) Type. Science 168, 852.

23 Bias, W.B. and Marsh, D.G. (1975), HL-A Linked Antigen E
    Immune Response Genes: an Unproved Hypothesis. Science 188,
    375.

24 Marsh, D.G. (1975), Allergens and the Genetics of Allergy.
    In "The Antigens", Vol. III, (ed. M. Sela), Academic Press,
    New York, p. 271.

25 Black, P.L., Marsh, D.G., Jarrett, E., Delespesse, G.J. and
    Bias, W.B. (1976), Family Studies of Association Between HLA
    and Specific Immune Responses to Highly Purified Pollen
    Allergens. Immunogenetics (in press).

26 Fu, S.M., Kunkel, H.G., Brusman, H.P., Allen, F.H. and
    Fotino, M. (1974), Evidence for Linkage Between HL-A
    Histocompatibility Genes and those Involved in the Synthesis
    of the Second Component of Complement. J. Exp. Med. 140, 1108.

27 Terasaki, P.I. (1971), HL-A Histocompatibility Determinants.
    Disease-a-Month 12, 10.

28 McDevitt, H.O. and Bodmer, W.F. (1974), HL-A, Immune-Response
    Genes and Disease. Lancet i, 1269.

29 Bodmer, W.F. (1975), Evolution of HL-A and Other Major
    Histocompatibility Systems. Symposium on Immunogenetics:
    Proc. XIII Internat. Cong. Genetics, Genetics 79, 293.

30 Nielsen, L.S., Jersild, C. Ryder, L.P. and Svejgaard, A.
    (1975), HLA Antigen, Gene and Haplotype Frequencies in
    Denmark. Tissue Antigens 6, 70.

31 Marsh, D.G. and Bias, W.B. (1976), Atopic Allergy : a Model
    for Studying the Genetics of Immune Response in Man.
    Presented at the 1975 Birth Defects Conference, Kansas City;
    National Foundation March of Dimes Publications, in press.

32 King, T.P. (1976, Chemical and Biological Properties of some
    Atopic Allergens. Adv. Immunol., in press.

33   Munro, A.J., Taussig, M.J., Campbell, R., Williams, H. and
     Lawson, Y. Antigen-Specific T-cell Factor in Cell Cooperation:
     Physical Properties and Mapping in the Left-Hand (K) Half of
     H-2. J. Exp. Med. 140, 1579.

34   Rosenthal, A.S. and Shevach, E.M. (1973), Function of
     Macrophages in Antigen Recognition by Guinea Pig T Lymphocytes.
     I. Requirement for Histocompatible Macrophages and Lymphocytes.
     J. Exp. Med. 138, 1194.

35   Kontou-Karakitsos, K.J., Mathews, K.P. and Salvaggio, J.E.
     (1975), Comparative Nasal Absorption of Allergens in Atopic
     and Non-Atopic Subjects. J. Allergy Clin. Immunol. 55, 241.

36   Stiffel, C., Mouton, D., Bouthillier, Y., Heumann, A.M.,
     Decreusefond, C., Mevel, J.C. and Biozzi, G. (1974),
     Polygenic Regulation of General Antibody Systhesis in the
     Mouse. Progr. in Immunol. II, Vol. 2 (L. Brent and
     J. Holborow eds.) No. Holland Pub. Co., Amsterdam, p. 203.

37   Bias, W.B. (1973), The Genetic Basis of Asthma. In "Asthma:
     Physiology, Immunopharmacology and Treatment" (K. F. Austen
     and L.M. Lichtenstein eds.) Academic Press. New York, p.39.

38   Black, P.L. and Marsh, D.G. (1976), The Genetics of Allergy.
     In"Bronchial Asthma : Mechanisms and Therapeutics" (M.S.
     Segal and E.B. Weiss eds.) Little, Brown & Co., Boston, Mass.
     In press.

39   Halpern S.R., Sellars, W.A., Johnson, R.B., Anderson, D.W.,
     Saperstein, S. and Reisch, J.S. (1973), Development Of
     Childhood Allergy in Infants Fed Breast, Soy or Cow Milk.
     J. Allergy Clin. Immunol. 51, 139.

40   Marsh, D.G., Bias, W.B. and Ishizaka, K. (1974), Genetic
     Control of Basal Serum Immunoglobulin E Level and its Effect
     on Specific Reaginic Sensitivity. Proc. Natl. Acad. Sci.,
     U.S.A., 71, 3588.

41   Levine, B.B., Stember, R.H. and Fotino, M. (1972), Ragweed
     Hay Fever : Genetic Control and Linkage to HL-A Haplotypes.
     Science 178, 1201.

42   Blumenthal, M.N., Amos, D.B., Noreen, H., Mendell, N.R. and
      Yunis, E.J. (1974), Genetic Mapping of Ir Locus in Man:
      Linkage to Second Locus of HL-A. Science 184, 1301.

43   Marsh, D.G., Bias, W.B., Hsu, S.H. and Goodfriend, L. (1973),
      Association of the HL-A7 Cross-Reacting Group with a Specific
      Reaginic Antibody Response in Allergic Man. Science 179, 691.

44   Marsh, D.G., Bias, W.B., Hsu, S.H. and Goodfriend, L. (1973),
      Associations between Major Histocompatibility (HL-A) Antigens
      and Specific Reaginic Antibody Responses in Allergic Man. In
      "Mechanisms of Allergy : Reagin-Mediated Hypersensitivity."
      Marcel Dekker Inc., New York, p. 113.

45   Marsh, D.G., Bias, W.B., Santilli, J., Schacter, B. and
      Goodfriend, L. (1975), Ragweed Allergen Ra5 : a New Tool in
      Understanding the Genetics and Immunochemistry of Immune
      Response in Man. Immunochem. 12, 539.

46   Santilli, J., Marsh, D.G., Bias, W.B., Schacter, B. and
      Goodfriend, L. (1975), Puncture Skin Testing with Purified
      Pollen Antigens : a Useful Tool for Genetic Studies in Atopic
      Man. J. Allergy 55, 108 (abs).

47   Marsh, D.G., Chase, G.A. and Bias, W.B. (1975), An Immune
      Response Gene for Ragweed Ra3 : Most Probable Location within
      the HL-A2,12 Haplotype. Fed. Proc. 34, 980 (abs.) Full-
      length paper submitted for publication.

48   King, T.P., Norman, P.S. and Connell, J.T. (1964), Isolation
      and Characterization of Allergens from Ragweed Pollen.II.
      Biochemistry 3, 458.

49   Underdown, B.J. and Goodfriend, L. (1969), Isolation nd
      Characterization of an Allergen from Short Ragweed Pollen.
      Biochemistry 8, 980.

50   Marsh, D.G. and Bias, W.B. (1974), Control of Specific
      Allergic Response in Man : HL-A Associated and IgE-Regulating
      Genes. Fed. Proc. 33, 774 (abs.). Full-length paper
      submitted for publication.

51   Johnson, P. and Marsh, D.G. (1966), Allergens from Common
      Rye Grass Pollen. I. Chemical Composition and Structure.
      Immunochem. 3, 91.

52   Willcox, H.N.A.and Marsh, D.G. (1976), Genetic Control Of
      Antibody Heterogeneity : its Possible Relevance to IgE and
      IgG Antibody Responses. In preparation.

53   Hoffman, D.R., Yamamoto, F.Y., Geller, B. and Haddad, Z.
      (1975), Specific IgE Antibodies in Atopic Eczema. J. Allergy
      Clin. Immunol. 55, 256.

54   Bjorksten, F. and Johansson, S.G.O. (1976), In Vitro
      Diagnosis of Atopic Allergy : the Occurrence and Clustering
      of Positive RAST Results as a Function of Age and Total IgE
      Concentration. Clin. Allergy. In press.

55   Kissmeyer-Nielsen, F. et al. (35 others). (1971),
      Scandiatransplant : Preliminary Report of a Kidney Exchange
      Program. Transpl. Proc. 3, 1019.

56   Dorf, M.E., Balner, H. and Benacerraf, B. (1975), Mapping of
      the Immune Response Genes in the Major Histocompatibility
      Complex of the Rhesus Monkey. J. Exp. Med. 142, 673.

57   De Weck, A.L. and Geczy, A.F. (1976), The Major Histocompatib-
      ility Complex of the Guinea Pig, Proc. 10th Leukocyte Culture
      Conference. Academic Press. In press.

58   Van Rood, J.J., van Leenvan, A., Keuning, J.J. and Blussé
      Van Oud Alblas, A. (1975), The Serological Recognition of
      the Human MLC Determinants using a Modified Cytotoxicity
      Technique. Tissue Antigens 5, 73.

59   Jones, E.A., Goodfellow, P.N., Bodmer, J.G. and Bodmer, W.F.
      (1975), Serological Identification of HL-A-Linked Human
      'Ia-Type' Antigens. Nature 256, 650.

60   Mann, D.L., Abelson, L., Harris, S. and Amos, D.B. (1976),
      Second Genetic Locus in the HLA Region for Human B-Cell
      Alloantigens. Nature 259, 145.

DISCUSSION

DIAMANT: If genetic factors determine the IgE production and this is of consequence for immediate type allergic diseases could you comment on why rats produce such great amounts of IgE when infested with worms but at the same time are so difficult to sensitize to produce antigen induced mast cell reactions

MARSH: Intestinal parasitic infestations induce high serum IgE levels, in part, because of the high, non-immunologically limiting dosage immunization with a complex mixture of antigens near the site of IgE producing cells.

In addition, there is potentiated IgE production as will be discussed by Dr. Jarrett. I think that she will also be able to answer the second part of your question better than I can.

I would also like to comment on the point which Dr. K. Ishizaka and Dr. Cochrane raised earlier concerning possible differences in the specificity of IgE and IgG antibodies. It seems unlikely that the gene pool of antibody variable regions is any different for IgE as compared with IgG (cf. Gally and Edelman, Nature 227, 341, 1970).

However, genetic factors controlling how many antibody producing clones are actually expressed may be different. Perhaps one may draw an analogy between the expression of IgE antibody biosynthesis in people having "high IgE phenotypes" and the expression of IgG antibody biosynthesis in most individuals.

I think that, like the high IgE producers, there is probably a greater heterogeneity of response in IgG production to a limiting antigenic stimulus in most people. This greater "permissivity" of responsiveness (arising from less stringent regulation of immune response) within the IgG producing system is also compatible with our finding that many non-allergic people make IgG but no IgE antibody to inhaled pollen allergens (Black et al, Immunogenetics, in press).

AUSTEN: Please comment on the HLA associations noted in familial allergy by Levine et al. as well as other groups. (Levine et al., Science 178, 1201, 1972; Blumenthal et al, Science 184, 1301, 1974).

MARSH: First, let me differentiate between the studies of association between immune response (Ir) and HLA which we have carried out in allergic populations, and of the studies of genetic linkage which can only be carried out on families. Proof of genetic linkage requires a very rigorous analysis which has no yet been attempted in allergy.

Dr. Bias and I have published a detailed discussion (Science 188, 375, 1975) of the papers of Levine et al. and Blumenthal et al. which suggest "genetic linkage" between IgE mediated sensitivity to ragweed antigen E and specific familial HLA haplotypes. We conclude that neither paper provides a clear indication of linkage. We have extensively studied the question of association between familial HLA haplotype and specific Ir using four different highly purified allergens (Black et al. Immunogenetics, in press). Immune function was measured by three assays: IgE-mediated skin sensitivity, serum IgG antibody and antigen induced lymphocyte proliferation in vitro. We found no evidence of association between HLA haplotype and specific Ir, measured by any one or combination of our indices of immune function. We concluded that the complexity of genetic and non-genetic factors governing Ir in natural populations like man precludes demonstration of association and genetic linkage between Ir and HLA in most families.

It is interesting to note that several of our families are quite similar to some of those of Levine and Blumenthal, if one looks just at IgE mediated responses. However, we make different interpretations. Levine suggested that Ir genes for antigen E occur with a frequency of 0.4, which gives a phenotype frequency of 0.64. He does not consider how this rather high incidence of "Ir-AgE" genes might affect his analyses, especially if they are present in non-allergic individuals (i.e. not expressed as IgE responses).

Furthermore, in the single family which he reported in detail, four of the spouses were, apparently, not studied, which further clouds any interpretation.

It is usually possible to construct hypothetical mechanisms of inheritance based on "incomplete expression" of response and "genetic recombination between HLA and hypothesized Ir genes" as Blumenthal et al. did in their study. Such analyses are, however, predicated on the assumption that singly Ir gene loci linked to HLA are proven entities, which is not permissible if that is the very hypothesis one is trying to prove.

We are in agreement with Levine and Blumenthal that HLA linked Ir genes probably exist, but we still need convincing proof.

INDUCTION AND SUPPRESSION OF IgE ANTIBODY RESPONSE [1]

Kimishige Ishizaka

The Johns Hopkins University School of Medicine at
The Good Samaritan Hospital, 5601 Loch Raven Blvd.,
Baltimore, Maryland 21239 U.S.A.

Previous studies have shown that IgE antibody is a cause of
hay fever and probably involved in other allergic diseases (1).
These findings immediately raised the possibility that prevention
or suppression of IgE antibody response may have clinical value for
hay fever patients. Our approach to this goal was to establish a
cell culture system and adoptive transfer system for the analysis
of cellular events in the IgE antibody response, and to study immunological effects of hyposensitization treatment in an animal
model. In this presentation, I would like to briefly summarize
recent progress in our approaches.

I. Generation of Helper Cells for IgE Antibody Response

It is well known that rabbit lymphoid cells primed with antigen form a large amount of IgG and IgM antibodies in vitro upon
stimulation with antigen. In view of such previous findings, we
have set up a cell culture system of rabbit lymph node cells in
which anamnestic IgE antibody response can be observed (2). This
system was useful for characterizing immunocompetent cells involved in the IgE antibody response. First of all, it was established
that anti-hapten IgE antibody response was highly T cell-dependent.
Carrier-specific helper cells were required for the anti-hapten
IgE antibody response (3,4). It was also found that B memory cells
for IgE antibody response are different from B memory cells for
IgG antibody with respect to the surface immunoglobulin (5). Our
experiments also suggested that helper cells for IgE antibody response are different from the helper cells for IgG antibody response
(4). In the experiment shown in Table I, rabbits were primed with
dinitrophenyl derivatives of Ascaris suum extract (DNP-Asc) in alum

Table I

Helper function of carrier-specific cells against primary
and secondary carriers for IgG and IgE antibody responses

Suppl. Immunization[a]	Antigen in vitro	Anti-DNP IgG[b]	IgE
		µg/ml	PCA
none	none	0.29	<2.5
	DNP-Asc	39.0	40.0
	DNP-Rag	0.35	<2.5
Ragweed ag in alum	none	0.32	<2.5
	DNP-Asc	18.5	20.0
	DNP-Rag	23.5	60.0
Ragweed Ag in CFA	none	0.40	<2.5
	DNP-Asc	40.0	40.0
	DNP-Rag	30.0	<2.5

a) Supplemental immunization was given to DNP-Asc
   primed rabbits.
b) IgG antibody was measured by radioimmunoassay.

and a portion of the primed animals received a supplemental immunization of ragweed antigen (Rag) included in either alum or complete
Freund's adjuvant (CFA). The mesenteric lymph node cells from all
the animals formed both IgG and IgE anti-hapten antibodies upon
stimulation with DNP-Asc. As expected, the lymph node cells from
the DNP-Asc primed animals failed to form anti-hapten antibodies
upon stimulation with DNP-Rag. On the other hand, the lymph node
cells of the animals which received a supplemental immunization of
alum-absorbed Rag antigen formed both IgE and IgG antibodies upon
stimulation with DNP-Rag. Comparisons between the first two groups
indicated that DNP-specific B cells which were raised by the immunization with DNP-Asc collaborated with Rag-specific helper cells
to form anti-DNP antibodies in both IgG and IgE classes. If ragweed antigen included in CFA was given to the DNP-Asc primed
animals, their mesenteric lymph node cells responded to DNP-Rag to
form IgG antibody but no IgE antibody. As the same cells responded
to DNP-Asc to form IgE antibody, the cell suspension should have
contained DNP-specific IgE-B cells. The results indicated that
Rag-specific helper cells which collaborated with DNP-specific IgG
B cells failed to collaborate with IgE-B cells and suggested the
possibility that helper cells for IgE antibody response are different from the helper cells for IgG antibody response.

Similar experiments in the mouse, however, did not reproduce
the results (6,7). In high responder strains of mouse, helper
cells for IgE antibody response were obtained by carrier immunization with either alum or CFA. In this species, priming with a

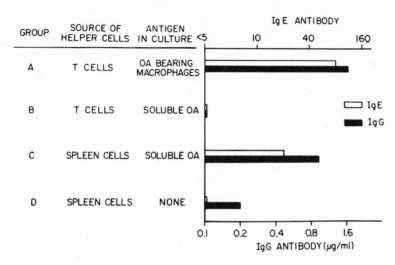

Fig. 1. Priming of T helper cells in vitro. The T cell-rich fraction of normal spleen were cultured on T cell-depleted OA-bearing
macrophages (A) or with OA (B) for 5 days and transferred into
irradiated mice together with DNP-KLH primed spleen cells for adoptive secondary response. Group C and D received cultured spleen
cells and DNP-KLH primed cells. The figure shows anti-DNP IgE and
IgG antibody titers of the recipients at the 14th day after challenge with DNP-OA.

potent immunogen without adjuvant was sufficient to generate helper
cells for IgE antibody response (6,7). In order to examine cellular requirements for T cell priming for the IgE and IgG antibody
responses, attempts were made to prime helper cells in vitro.
Normal spleen cells of BDF1 mice were cultured for 5 days on the
ovalbumin-bearing peritoneal adherent cells, or in the presence of
ovalbumin (OA), and the helper function of the cultured lymphocytes
was determined by adoptive transfer technique using DNP-KLH primed
spleen cells as a source of hapten-specific B cells. The results
clearly showed that helper function for both IgE and IgG antibody
responses was generated by the culture. The helper cells generated
in the culture were abolished by the treatment with anti-θ antiserum
and C, indicating that helper cells were θ-bearing T cells. Subsequent experiments showed that only macrophages are required for T
cell priming. In the experiments shown in Fig. 1, peritoneal cells
from normal mice were depleted of mast cells and T lymphocytes, and
the rest of the cells were incubated with ovalbumin to prepare antigen-bearing macrophages. The T cell-rich fraction of normal spleen

cells was obtained by fractionation with glass-wool column and nylon column (8), and cultured on the antigen-bearing macrophages. The cultured lymphocytes were mixed with DNP-KLH primed cells and trans- ferred into irradiated mice followed by challenge with DNP-OA. As can be seen in Figure 1, helper cells were generated by the culture. If the same T cell-rich fraction was cultured with OA in the absence of macrophages, helper cells were not obtained. An important fact was that T cells primed by the antigen-bearing macrophages had helper function for both IgE and IgG antibody responses. This find- ing eliminated the possibility that different accessory cells are involved in the priming of helper cells for IgE and IgG antibody response. These experiments, however, neither support nor exclude the possibility that helper cells for IgE antibody response are different from those for IgG antibody response.

II. Mechanisms of T-B Collaboration for IgE Antibody Response

An important finding obtained in the in vitro system was that helper function of carrier-specific cells was mediated by enhancing soluble factors (9). As suggested by Dutton et al (10), a critical experiment to demonstrate an enhancing soluble factor is to show antibody response upon stimulation of T and B cells with two inde- pendent molecules. Thus, rabbits were immunized with alum-absorbed DNP-Rag, and their mesenteric lymph node cells were incubated with a mixture of DNP-coupled to an unrelated carrier, such as DNP-KLH, and homologous carrier. Stimulation of DNP-Rag primed cells with DNP-KLH alone resulted in the formation of a small amount of anti- hapten IgG antibody and essentially no IgE antibody, but the addi- tion of free carrier definitely enhanced IgG antibody response and induced IgE antibody response. The amount of IgG and IgE antibodies formed by the mixture of DNP-KLH and Rag were 40 to 70% of those formed by the stimulation with DNP-Rag. The results suggested that soluble factor was released from carrier-specific cells and enhanced the response of DNP-specific B cells to DNP-heterologous carrier conjugate.

A definitive evidence for the hypothesis was obtained by using culture supernatant of carrier-primed lymphocytes (9). In the ex- periment shown in Fig. 2, lymph node cells of a rabbit immunized with alum-absorbed Rag were incubated with T-independent antigen such as DNP-derivative of a copolymer of d-tyrosine, glutamic acid and leucine to stimulate hapten-specific B cells. After washing to remove the DNP-conjugate, aliquots of these cells were resuspended in either fresh medium or in cell free supernatant (CFS) obtained from Rag-primed cells, and both cell suspensions were cultured. It is apparent in the figure that anti-DNP antibody responses of both IgG and IgE classes were significantly enhanced by CFS, indicating that the culture supernatant contained enhancing soluble factor. It should be noted that the factor(s) themselves do not have carrier

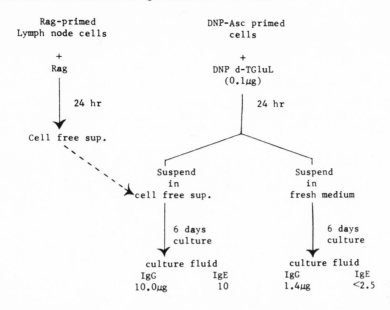

Fig. 2. Experimental design to demonstrate non-specific enhancing soluble factor for IgE and IgG antibody responses. Donors of Rag-primed cells were immunized with alum-absorbed Rag, and donors of DNP-primed cells were immunized with alum-absorbed DNP-Asc.

specificity, because the differentiation of DNP-specific cells raised by the immunization with DNP-Asc was enhanced by culture supernatant of Rag-primed cells. Thus, the factors detected in this experiment are 'non-specific' factors.

Evidence was obtained which indicated that enhancing factor for IgE antibody response is different from the factor for IgG antibody response. If the CFS preparations with enhancing activities for both IgE and IgG responses were fractionated by gel filtration or by sucrose density gradient ultracentrifugation, the IgE antibody response was enhanced by the 7S fraction, while IgG antibody response was enhanced by a fraction containing the molecules with 20,000 to 40,000 molecular weight (11). As already described, helper cells obtained by immunization with carrier in CFA enhanced the IgG antibody response but not the IgE antibody response. When the lymph node cells of the CFA immunized rabbits were incubated with carrier, CFS preparations enhanced IgG but not IgE antibody response (12). Furthermore, fractionation of such a CFS preparation by gel filration showed that the 20,000 to 40,000 MW fraction enhanced IgG antibody response but the 7S fraction did not enhance

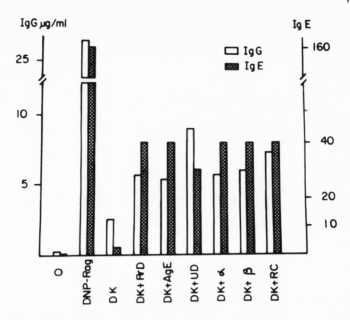

Fig. 3.   Enhancement of anti-DNP antibody response of DNP-Rag primed cells to DNP-KLH by modified antigen E.   UD and RC represented
Urea-denatured and reduced-carboxylated antigen E.   Both IgG (▭)
and IgE (▨) antibodies in the culture fluid are shown in the
figure.

the IgE antibody response (11).   The results indicated that IgE enhancing factor is distinct from IgG enhancing factor, and that failure of CFS preparations obtained from CFA-immunized rabbits to enhance IgE antibody response is due to lack of IgE enhancing factor.
The nature of the enhancing factors is unknown.   Evidence was obtained, however, that antigen is not an integral part of enhancing
factors.   It was also found that both IgE and IgG enhancing factors
lacked immunoglobulin determinants (11).

     A question arose as to whether the carrier specific helper
cells react with the same antigenic determinants as those combined
with the antibody against carrier.   As the helper cells in our
system were raised by the immunization with partially purified
ragweed antigen (Fr D by King and Norman (13)), experiments were
carried out to determine whether the helper cells are specific for
antigen E, which is the major allergen in ragweed extract.   As
shown in Fig. 3, DNP-Rag primed cells were stimulated with DNP-KLH
and the activated cells were cultured in the presence of either
Fr D or purified antigen E.   The results clearly showed that
antigen E was as effective as Fr D for the release of enhancing

factors from Rag-specific cells. This finding indicated that the
majority of helper cells are specific for antigen E.

With respect to antigen E molecules, King et al (14) have
shown that antigen is irreversibly denatured in 8 M urea because of
its dissociation into two polypeptide chains. The urea-denatured
(UD) antigen and each of the polypeptide chains, which are called
α and β chain, failed to combine with rabbit or human IgG antibody
against native antigen E or to induce erythema wheal reaction in
ragweed sensitive individuals, indicating that the major antigenic
determinants in the antigen molecules were lost by denaturation.
The denatured antigen as well as polypeptide chains, however, had
the ability to stimulate antigen E-specific T cells (15). As shown
in Fig. 3, addition of UD-antigen or polypeptide chains to the
culture enhanced both IgG and IgE antibody responses of the DNP-Rag
primed cells to DNP-KLH. On a weight basis, these modified antigens
were comparable to native antigen E with respect to the ability to
release enhancing soluble factor from Rag-specific T cells.

Evidence was obtained that these modified antigens stimulated
human T cells specific for antigen E. All of the UD antigen, α and
β chains induced DNA synthetic response of the lymphocytes from ragweed sensitive patients but failed to enhance thymidine incorporation of lymphocytes from normal individuals (15). The UD antigen
and α chain are poor immunogens in both rabbits and mice, but hyperimmunization of A/J strain of mice with these antigens included in
CFA resulted in the formation of antibodies. The antibodies are
specific for the modified antigen and did not react with the native
antigen. On the other hand, antibodies against native antigen did
not react with the modified antigens. The results indicate that B
cells specific for denatured antigen are different from those specific for native antigen (16).

In spite of different specificity at the level of B cells, both
α chain and UD antigen could prime T cells specific for the native
antigen. If one primes mice with the modified antigen prior to
immunization with native antigen E, antibody response to the native
antigen was enhanced (16). The best evidence for T cell priming
was obtained by using adoptive transfer technique (17). In the experiment shown in Fig. 4, spleen cells from mice immunized with α
chain (or UD antigen) were transferred into irradiated mice together with DNP-KLH primed cells and the recipients were challenged
with DNP-Rag. It is apparent that α chain-primed spleen cells exerted helper function for the anti-hapten antibody response and
the helper cells were abolished by the treatment with anti-θ
antiserum and C.

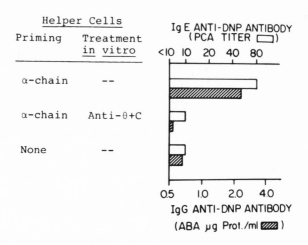

Fig. 4. Priming of antigen E specific helper cells by immunization
with α chain. Donors of helper cells were primed with 0.5 μg α
chain. 10^7 spleen cells from the donors were mixed with 10^7 DNP-
KLH primed spleen cells and transferred into each irradiated recipient. A portion of α chain-primed cells were treated with anti-θ
antiserum and C before transfer. Control group received normal
spleen cells and DNP-KLH primed cells. All recipients were challenged with DNP-Rag. Both IgE (▭) and IgG (▨) anti-DNP antibody
titers at the 10th day are shown in the figure.

III. Regulation of IgE Antibody Response

As we have obtained modified antigens which react with T cells
specific for antigen E but failed to combine with the antibody
against the same antigen, such modified antigens were employed to
analyze regulatory mechanisms for IgE antibody response. In view
of accumulated evidence which indicated a regulatory role of T
cells in the antibody response (17), we have speculated about the
possibility that stimulation of antigen-specific T cells with the
modified antigen might affect the kinetics of IgE antibody response
Thus, three groups of A/J mice were immunized with antigen E included in alum for a persistent IgE antibody response and 10 μg of
UD antigen or α chain was injected into a group once every week
(16). As shown in Fig. 5, the injections were initiated at 2 weeks
after the priming when the IgE antibody titer reached maximum. It
will be seen that IgE antibody titer began to decline after 4

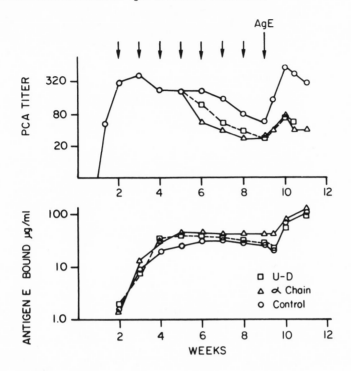

Fig. 5. Effect of weekly injections of α chain or UD antigen on the on-going IgE and IgG antibody responses to antigen E. All animals were primed with 1 µg antigen E included in alum and boosted with 10 µg antigen E in saline at week 9. Either 10 µg UD antigen or α chain were injected once a week beginning from week 2.

injections of a modified antigen. After 7 weeks treatment, all of the animals including untreated controls were boosted with 10 µg antigen E. The results showed that secondary IgE antibody response to the native antigen was suppressed in the treated animals. If the antigen E-primed animals were treated by weekly injections of 10 µg of native antigen E, IgG antibody titer increased by 10 fold but IgE antibody titer was comparable to that in untreated mice (17).

In order to learn the mechanisms for the suppression of IgE antibody formation by the treatment with UD antigen, we studied the effect of the treatment on the helper function of T cells (17). Spleen cells from the treated and untreated animals were mixed with DNP-KLH primed spleen cells and transferred into irradiated mice followed by challenge with DNP-Rag. The results showed that helper function of antigen E - primed spleen cells diminished by weekly injections of either native antigen E or modified antigen.

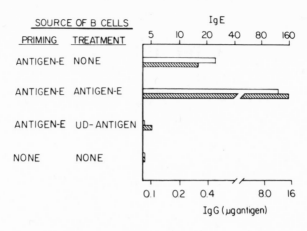

Fig. 6. Effect of weekly antigen injections of antigen E-specific
B memory cells. Ten million anti-θ treated spleen cells from untreated or treated mice, or the same number of normal B cells were
transferred together with 10^7 spleen cells from α-chain primed mice.
All of the recipients were challenged with antigen E. Both IgE
(☐) and IgG antibody titers (▨) at day 14 are shown in the
figure.

        The effect of the treatment on B cell population was also
studied by adoptive transfer technique (17) (Fig. 6). Spleen cells
from the treated and untreated animals were incubated with anti-θ
antiserum and C to remove T cells. The B cell-rich fraction from
each group was mixed with a constant number of spleen cells from
α-chain-primed animals as a source of antigen-specific T cells,
and transferred into irradiated animals. The IgE and IgG antibody
responses of the recipients to antigen E showed that both IgE-B
cells and IgG-B cells in the spleen of UD-antigen treated animals
were less than those in untreated mice. By contrast, the treatment
with antigen E increased both IgG-B cells and IgE-B cells in the
spleen. Such changes in the T cell and B cell populations partially
explain the effect of the treatment on the on-going antibody responses. A decrease of both helper function and IgE-B cells by
the treatment with modified antigen appears to be responsible for
the decline of IgE antibody formation. An increase of IgE-B cells
after the antigen E treatment might have overcome a diminished
helper function of T cells to maintain the IgE antibody level.
Similarly, a great increase of IgG-B cells, in spite of a decreased
helper function, may explain an increase of IgG antibody level in

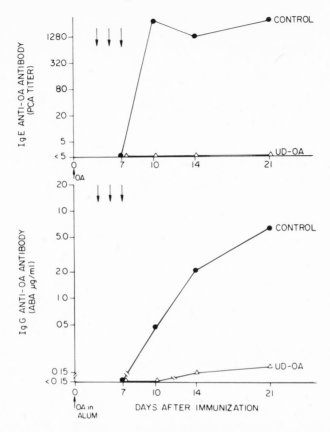

Fig. 7. Effect of urea-denatured ovalbumin on the IgE and IgG anti-body responses to ovalbumin. Two groups of mice were primed with 0.2 µg OA included in alum. One group received 100 µg UD-OA at 3, 5 and 7 days after priming.

the antigen E treated animals. Nevertheless, these experiments indicate that primary effect of the repeated injections of either modified or native antigen is depression of helper function of T cells which accounts for the suppression of secondary antibody response. As the immunotherapy for hay fever patients consisted of weekly or biweekly injections of increasing doses of allergen, one can expect that the treatment will cause depressed helper function. A gradual decline of IgE antibody titer and suppression of second-ary IgE antibody response in the treated patients after a long-term immunotherapy may be explained by the decrease of helper function.

A basic question to be asked is why helper function was de-

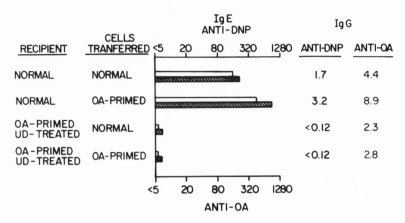

Fig. 8. Failure of OA-primed spleen cells to reconstitute suppressed
animals. Either normal or OA-primed UD-OA treated mice were sub-
stituted with 2 x 10^7 normal or OA-primed spleen cells, and then
immunized with 0.2 µg DNP-OA in alum. The figure shows both anti-
DNP (☐) and anti-OA (▨) IgE antibody titers at 14 days after
immunization.

pressed by the repeated injections of allergen or modified antigen.
In order to study the principle, we have employed a combination of
OA and BDFl mice instead of antigen E and A/J strain. In fact,
the results obtained in antigen E system was reproduced in OA
system. The major antigenic determinants in OA molecules were lost
following denaturation in 8 M urea but urea-denatured OA (UD-OA) was
capable of priming T cells specific for the native antigen (19). It
was also found that urea-denatured ovalbumin stimulated spleen cells
from OA-primed mice for DNA synthetic response, indicating that UD-
OA stimulated OA-specific T cells. Thus, we injected 100 µg of UD-
OA into OA-primed mice at 3, 5 and 7 days after the priming immunization and anti-OA antibody response was followed (Fig. 7). The
results clearly showed that both IgE and IgG antibody responses
were suppressed by the treatment (19). Spleen cells of the treated
and untreated animals were tested for their helper function and B
cell activity by adoptive transfer experiments. As expected from
the findings in antigen E system, the treatment with UD-OA suppressed the development of helper cells and B memory cells specific for
OA (19). It was also found that the OA-primed and UD-OA treated
animals did not respond to subsequent immunization with DNP-OA included in alum. In order to investigate whether the suppression of
the anti-hapten antibody response in the UD-OA treated animals is
due to "active process" or to a lack of carrier-specific immunocompetent T cells, the animals were supplemented with either normal
or OA-primed spleen cells and then immunized with DNP-OA (Fig. 8).

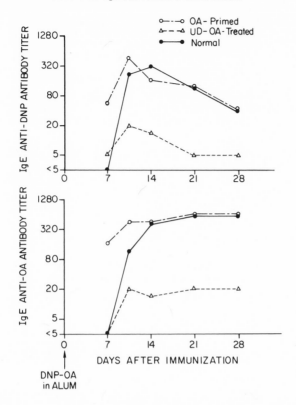

Fig. 9. Suppressive effect of splenic T cell fraction of UD-OA
treated mice. 2 x 10^7 T cells from normal (●--●), OA-primed (o--o)
or OA-primed UD-OA treated mice (Δ--Δ) were transferred into each
normal mouse and the recipients were immunized with alum-absorbed
DNP-OA. Both anti-DNP (top) and anti-OA (bottom) IgE antibody responses are shown.

Indeed, the transfer of OA-primed spleen cells into normal animals
enhanced anti-hapten antibody response of the recipients to DNP-OA.
The UD-OA treated animals, however, did not give a significant anti-
hapten antibody response and showed a meager anti-OA antibody response, even after the transfer of immune spleen cells (20). Failure of normal or immune spleen cells to reconstitute the UD-OA
treated animals suggested strongly that unresponsiveness of the
treated animals was due to active suppression. Furthermore, the
transfer of splenic T cells of the UD-OA treated animals into non-
irradiated mice diminished the antibody response of the recipients
to DNP-OA. In the experiment shown in Fig. 9, 2 x 10^7 splenic T

cells from either UD-OA treated mice or those from OA-primed mice
were transferred into normal mice and the recipients were immunized
with alum-absorbed DNP-OA. It is clear that T cells from UD-OA
treated animals suppressed both anti-hapten and anti-carrier IgE
antibody responses, whereas OA-primed cells failed to suppress the
antibody response (20). It was also found that T cells from UD-OA
treated animals suppressed not only IgE but also IgG antibody responses of both hapten and carrier specificities. An important
finding in this experiment was that the T cell preparation with
suppressive activity had very low helper function, while OA-primed
T cells which had a high helper function, failed to suppress the
antibody response. An inverse relationship between the suppressive
effect and helper function indicated that suppressor T cells are
distinct from helper T cells. In a separate experiment, it was
found that the suppressor T cells obtained by UD-OA treatment was
specific for OA. The T cell preparation failed to suppress primary
anti-DNP antibody response of normal mice to DNP-KLH. The series
of experiments therefore indicated that repeated injections of
urea-denatured antigen into high responder mice generated antigen-

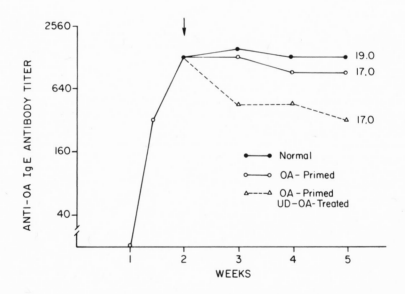

Fig. 10. Effect of suppressor T cells on the on-going IgE antibody
formation. Three groups of mice were immunized with 0.2 μg OA
included in alum. Two weeks after the immunization, each group of
mice received 2 x 10^7 splenic T cells from normal mice (●—●), OA-
primed mice (○—○) or OA-primed UD-OA treated mice(△--△). Numbers
in this figure represent IgG antibody (μg/ml).

specific suppressor T cells which regulate the IgE antibody response.
(20).

As already described, repeated injections of urea-denatured
antigen E or α polypeptide chain into antigen E-primed animals depressed the on-going IgE antibody response. Similarly, the on-
going anti-OA IgE antibody formation in BDF1 mice was depressed by
repeated injections of UD-OA (21). In order to show that the generation of suppressor T cells was responsible for the decline of the
on-going IgE antibody formation, splenic T cells from UD-OA treated
mice were transferred into OA-primed mice after immunization when
the anti-OA IgE antibody titer reached maximum. Control groups received the same number of splenic T cells from OA-primed mice or
normal T cells. (Fig. 10). The results of the experiments showed
that suppressor T cells depressed the on-going IgE antibody formation but OA-primed T cells failed to do so. It appears that depression of the on-going IgE antibody formation and suppression of
secondary IgE antibody response by repeated injections of antigen
is due to generation of suppressor T cells.

Attempts were made to increase the suppressive effect of spleen
cells which contained suppressor T cells. First of all, mice were
primed with OA and treated with UD-OA to generate suppressor T cells.
Spleen cell suspension of these mice were passed through a glass
wool column to remove macrophages, and lymphocyte suspension was
incubated at $37^{\circ}C$ for 24 hr in the presence or absence of OA.
After washing, 2×10^7 cells of each preparation or normal splenic
lymphocytes were transferred into normal recipients which were then
immunized with DNP-OA in alum. As shown in Fig. 11, lymphocytes of
the UD-OA treated mice suppressed both anti-DNP and anti-OA IgE
antibody responses. It was also found that incubation of these
cells with soluble antigen increased suppressive effect.

SUMMARY

It became clear that the IgE antibody response is highly dependent on antigen-specific T cells and that the helper function
of T cells for IgE antibody formation is mediated by soluble
factor(s). In the antibody response to ragweed antigen E and ovalbumin, evidence was obtained that determinants in the antigen
molecules for T cells are different from the antigenic determinants
for B cells. The major antigenic determinants in the antigen molecules were lost following denaturation in 8 M urea but urea-denatured antigen could prime T cells specific for the native antigen.
Repeated injections of the denatured antigen into native antigen-
primed mice depressed the on-going IgE antibody response and suppressed the secondary antibody response to the native antigen.
Analysis of the antigen-specific T cells and B cells before and
after the treatment revealed that repeated injections of either

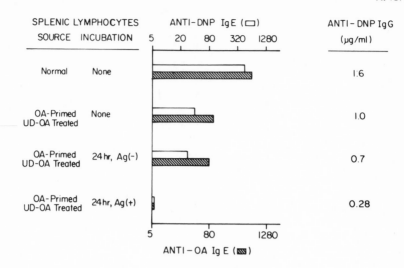

Fig. 11. Increase of suppressive effect of antigen-specific suppressor T cells by incubation with antigen. Adherent cells were
removed from spleen cells of UD-OA treated mice and splenic lymphocytes were incubated for 24 hr in the presence or absence of 100 μg/
ml of OA.   2 x 10^7 cells of each preparation or normal splenic
lymphocytes were transferred into normal mice followed by immunization with 0.2 μg DNP-OA in alum. The figure shows the IgE (☐)
and IgG (▧) antibody titer of the recipients at 10 days after
the immunization.

native or modified antigen into immunized mice diminished the helper
function of their splenic T cells. Subsequent experiments showed
that the injections of urea-denatured antigen without adjuvant
induced generation of antigen-specific suppressor T cells which
suppressed the primary antibody response of both IgE and IgG
classes. It was also found that the transfer of suppressor T cells
into antigen-primed mice depressed the on-going IgE antibody reponse. The results obtained in the experimental model suggested
strongly that gradual decline of IgE antibody titer and suppression
of secondary IgE antibody response after a long-term immunotherapy
of hay fever patients are due to the generation of suppressor T
cells.

REFERENCES

1. Ishizaka, T. and Ishizaka, K., Progress in Allergy, 19: 60, 1975.
2. Ishizaka, K. and Kishimoto, T., J. Immunol., 109: 65, 1972.
3. Kishimoto, T. and Ishizaka, K., J. Immunol., 109: 612, 1972.
4. Kishimoto, T. and Ishizaka, K., J. Immunol., 111: 720, 1973.
5. Kishimoto, T. and Ishizaka, K., J. Immunol., 109: 1163, 1972.
6. Okudaira, H. and Ishizaka, K., J. Immunol., 113: 563, 1974.
7. Hamaoka, T., Newburger, P.E., Katz, D.H. and Benacerraf, B., J. Immunol., 113: 958, 1974.
8. Julius, M.H., Simpson, E. and Herzenberg, L., Eur. J. Immunol., 3: 645, 1973.
9. Kishimoto, T. and Ishizaka, K., J. Immunol., 111: 1194, 1973.
10. Dutton, R.W., Falkoff, R., Hirst, J.A., Hoffman, M., Kappler, J.W., Kettman, J.R., Lesley, J.F. and Vann, D., Progress in Immunology, 1: 355, 1971.
11. Kishimoto, T. and Ishizaka, K., J. Immunol., 114: 1175, 1975.
12. Kishimoto, T. and Ishizaka, K., J. Immunol., 112: 1685, 1974.
13. King, T.P., and Norman P.S., Biochemistry, 1: 709, 1962.
14. King, T.P., Norman, P.S. and Tao, N., Immunochemistry, 11: 83, 1974.
15. Ishizaka, K., Kishimoto, T., Delespesse, G. and King, T.P., J. Immunol., 113: 70, 1974.
16. Ishizaka, K., Okudaira, H. and King, T.P., J. Immunol., 114: 110, 1975.
17. Takatsu, K., Ishizaka, K. and King, T.P., J. Immunol., 115: 1469, 1975.
18. Gershon, R.K., In Contemp. Topics Immunol., ed. M.D. Cooper and N. L. Warner, Vol. 3, p. 1. Plenum Press, New York 1974.
19. Takatsu, K. and Ishizaka, K., Cellular Immunol., 20: 276, 1975.
20. Takatsu, K. and Ishizaka, K., J. Immunol., in press.

↓ This work was supported by Research grants AI-11202 from U. S. Public Health Service, GB-41443 from National Science Foundation and John A. Hartford Foundation. This is publication #214 from the O'Neill Laboratories at the Good Samaritan Hospital.

DISCUSSION

TADA: Could you tell me what is the direct evidence that the target of the suppressor T cell is the helper T cell?

ISHIZAKA, K.: In the system I have discussed, we do not have any direct evidence that the target cells for the suppressor cells are the helper cells, although you may have evidence in IgG system. At this moment, our findings can be explained whether the target cells are helper cells or B memory cells.

DAVID: Would you please describe some of the characteristics of the soluble helper substance produced by T cells which help for IgE and IgG.

ISHIZAKA, K.: Enhancing soluble factors obtained from carrier primed rabbit lymph node cells are so-called "non-specific" enhancing factors. Homologous carrier was required for the release of the substance, however, the enhancing factor enhanced differentiation of B cells primed by immunization with an entirely different antigen.

The enhancing soluble factor did not contain antigen. By gel filtration through a Sephadex column and by sucrose density gradient ultracentrifugation, an enhancing factor for IgE antibody response was separated from the factor for IgG antibody response. The IgE enhancing factor was 7S, whereas the IgG enhancing factor had a molecular weight of 20,000 to 40,000. Immunoglobulin determinants (μ and γ chain determinents or light chain determinants) were not present in either of the IgE or IgG enhancing factor.

BECKER: Have you characterized the mouse suppressor T cells further, particularly in regard to its antigenic markers?

ISHIZAKA, K.: We have not studied the nature of suppressor T cells but we know that the cells bear θ antigen. We are planning to study this problem and will try to separate suppressor cells from helper cells.

JANEWAY (Uppsala): Do you have any direct evidence for the existence of helper cells specific for IgE in the mouse system?

ISHIZAKA, K.: When we have suggested the possibility that helper cells for IgE may be different from helper cells for IgG antibody response in the rabbit system, the concept of suppressor T cells was not yet established. If one considers helper cells and B cells, but no suppressor cells, there is no explanation other than to assume the presence of distinct helper cell populations for different immunoglobulin classes. However, the presence of suppressor cells raised other possibilities.

As suggested by Katz and Hamaoka, dissociation between IgE antibody response and IgG antibody response could be explained if the sensitivity of IgE B cells to suppressor and/or helper is different from the sensitivity of IgG B cells. Even if you do not make an assumption for different sensitivity for different B cells, we have to consider the fact that the number of IgE B cells is probably much less than the number of IgG B cells.

The possibility remain that the balance between helper and suppressor activity may have different effect when the number of B cell populations is different. Unless this possibility is excluded, I do not think we can make a conclusion that helper cells for IgE are actually different from the helper cells for IgG.

JANEWAY (Uppsala): You showed a rather striking effect of denatured antigen, which does not react with antibody or, presumably, B cell receptors, upon B cell activity. Could this be explained by a direct effect of suppressor T cells upon specific B cells?

ISHIZAKA, K.: The effect of the UD-OA treatment on B cell population is different depending on the time when the treatment was initiated. If one injects UD-OA on the third day after priming, or before the development of B memory cells, development of the B memory cell population was suppressed almost completely. If one begin the treatment at 2 weeks after the priming, however, not so much suppression was observed.

We have examined B memory cells at 2, 6 and 12 weeks after the priming without treatment. In this case, one can find that both IgE B cell and IgG B cell populations expand with time. When UD-OA was injected between 2 and 3 weeks, B cell activities before treatment (2 weeks) and after the treatment (6 weeks) were comparable. The B cell activity after the treatment (6 weeks) was much less than that of untreated mice at 6 weeks.

This finding indicated that the treatment suppressed maturation of B memory cells rather that diminished the memory cell population. My explanation is that helper cells were involved in the maturation of B cells and therefore that diminished helper function due to suppressor cells prevented maturation of the B cell population.

BELL (Stockholm): You mentioned that your soluble enhancing factor is not an immunoglobulin. Is it possible that it represents a fragment of an immunoglobulin and does it carry any antigenic determinants?

ISHIZAKA, K.: We used immunosorbents coated with anti-γ, anti-μ or anti-Fab antibody, but the enhancing factor was not absorbed. Therefore, our experiments do not exclude the possibility that the enhancing soluble factor may share some common structure with immunglobulin molecules. What I mentioned was that the enhancing factor does not contain either γ chain or μ

chain "class specific" determinants nor light chain determinants.

BELL (Stockholm): We are presently analyzing the molecules synthesized de novo by lymphoid cells obtained from genetically characterized rabbits and fractionated according to their membrane characteristics into T and B cells.

Since recognition structures, specified by idiotypic specificities are present both on B and T cells, one may expect certain V_H recognition structures on T cells.

Fractionated cells trypsinized or stripped of specific membrane recognition structures by the relevant antibody under co-capping, were cultured in the presence of 3H-Leucine and reanalyzed for membrane recognition structures, cytoplasmic characteristics and secreted molecules. Some recognition structures probably products of helper and suppressor T cells were identified, but the nature of these molecules with regard to C and V specificities are still equivocal.

Incidently, SDS acrylamide gel electrophoretic analysis of the T cell supernatant molecules synthesized de novo shows a distinct band corresponding to a molecular weight of 20,000 and a fainter band around 45,000-50,000, the intensity of later band varying in different preparations.

ISHIZAKA, K.: We could not obtain a soluble suppressor factor from mouse spleen cells containing suppressor T cells.

When the spleen cells were cultured in the presence or absence of antigen the cells gained suppressive activity. However, cell free supernatant did not have any suppressor effect.

T CELL-MEDIATED REGULATION OF IgE ANTIBODY PRODUCTION

Tomio Tada

Laboratories for Immunology, School of Medicine

Chiba University, Chiba, Japan

INTRODUCTION

It has been a notorious fact that reaginic antibody formation comparable to that occurring in human atopic patients is hard to induce in experimental animals. Most earlier studies expressed an awareness of the extremely transient nature of the reagin response in animals which stands in sharp contrast with the persistent and boostable reagin production in atopic diseases (1-5). This has certainly imposed strong restrictions on studying reaginic antibody response with such animal models, and thus the merit of animal experiments has sometimes been disregarded.

The reaginic antibody formation in the rat is also such an example which lasts only for a few weeks after the primary immunization even with appropriate adjuvants. The secondary reagin response is in most cases abortive. Furthermore, the reagin formation against many protein antigens is rather inconsistent, and the titer is usually very low. Thus, the reagin formation in the rat does not give by any means a good animal model system for studying the mechanism of reagin formation that actually takes place in human atopic patients.

However, such a restricted nature of reagin formation in the rat, in turn, enabled us to study the regulatory mechanisms which lead to the early termination of reagin response. Such studies would be especially pertinent for understanding why atopic patients continously produce reagins upon exposure to minute amounts of environmental allergens, against which the majority of normal people do not produce reagins. The answers for these questions will also open a vista for the future applications of immunotherapies to the clinical allergies.

I have extensively discussed these problems in a recent review article (6), and therefore I would like to present here our own experimental data which could answer some of the above questions. Utilizing the system of the short-lived reagin formation in the rat, we were able to demonstrate a regulatory function of a certain population of T cells, which was not readily observable in the persistent and boosterable reagin response in the human as well as in the mouse. The molecular mechanism of the T cell-mediated regulation with special reference to its genetic bases will also be discussed.

ENHANCEMENT OF IgE ANTIBODY RESPONSE BY
PARTIAL DIMINUTION OF T CELLS

Our studies on the T cell regulation of reaginic antibody response began with the discovery of peculiar paradoxical effects of immunosuppressive treatments on the reagin formation in the rat. We have found that various methods by which the number of T cells were relatively diminuted (such as sublethal x-irradiation, adult thymectomy and splenetomy, and treatments with certain immunosuppressive agents including anti-thymocyte serum, ATS) did not suppress, but actually enhanced the IgE antibody response (7-10). Such an enhanced reagin formation usually persisted for a much longer period of time than in normal animals.

Extreme cases were found in x-irradiation and adult thymectomy (7,8). As shown in Figure 1, the reaginic antibody formation against a dinitrophenyl derivative of *Ascaris suum* antigen (DNP-Asc) was greatly enhanced by these treatments given at appropriate times, and the high reagin titers persisted for a long period of time. This stands in a sharp contrast with the transient reagin formation in normal untreated animals induced by the same immunization regime. It was also found that such an enhanced reagin formation did not correlate with the amount of IgG antibody produced in these animals, and thus it was not due to the defective feed-back regulation by serum antibodies.

The evidence that T cells are responsible for the early termination of IgE antibody response in the rat also derives from experiments using heterologous ATS (9). It was found that a large lymphopenic dose of ATS given *before* immunization with DNP-Asc completely inhibited the reagin formation, indicating that the T cells are definitely required for the initiation of the IgE antibody response, whereas the same large dose of ATS given a few days *after* the immunization caused a marked enhancement and prolongation of the reagin formation (Figure 2). The latter finding can be explained in that the T cells are responsible for the early termination of

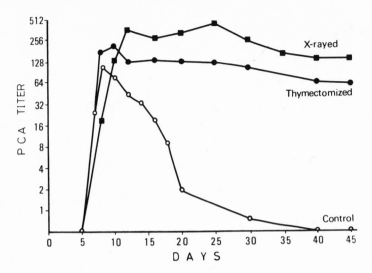

Figure 1.   Kinetics of anti-hapten reaginic antibody response
in normal (o——o)   adult thymectomized (•——•) and sublethally (400R) x-irradiated rat (■——■) immunized with DNP-Asc
plus pertussis vaccine.   Note a difinite enhancement and
prolonged production of reaginic antibody in both treated
animals as compared with the normal control.

the reagin response, and the removal of such suppressive T cells
resulted in the enhanced and prolonged reagin response.   Furthermore, if ATS was given before the secondary immunization, the animals could produce reaginic antibody even if they had been extensively immunized with the same antigen (9).   Hence, it was concluded that the regulator of reagin response is, in fact, the T cell,
and the diminution of such a regulator might have caused the enhanced and prolonged reagin response in the rat.

An important question raised at this point is as to whether
such regulation by T cells is antigen-specific or not.   It has
been known that IgE antibody response is induced via cooperative
interactions of T and B cells, in which T cells specific for carrier determinants *help* the differentiation of hapten-specific B
cells to produce anti-hapten IgE antibody (11-14).   Thus, the
principal issues to be considered are 1) whether the cells negatively regulate the anti-hapten IgE antibody response are also carrier-
specific or not ? and 2) whether the helper T cell and suppressor
T cell would belong to the same subpopulation of the T cell line-
age ?

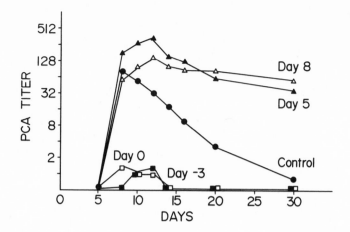

Figure 2.   Effect of anti-thymocyte serum (ATS) given at
different times before or after the immunization with DNP-
Asc plus pertussis vaccine. Note almost complete inhibition of the anti-hapten reaginic antibody response in
groups given ATS on day 0 or -3, and the enhanced and
prolonged production of reaginic antibody in groups given
ATS on day 5 or 8 at the time when reaginic antibody response was already initiated.

PROPERTIES OF THE SUPPRESSOR T CELL IN THE RAT REAGIN FORMATION

    In order to answer these questions, we have performed very
simple experiments in which T cells from various sources were
passively transferred into syngeneic rats that were producing high
anti-DNP IgE antibody by sublethal dose of x-irradiation given a
few hours before the immunization with DNP-Asc (15). The experimental protocol is shown in Figure 3. Recipient rats were x-irradiated at a dose of 400 r, followed by immunization with DNP-Asc
and *Bordetella pertussis* vaccine. Such animals mounted a high and
persistent reaginic antibody response as described above. Donor
rats were either unprimed or primed with DNP-Asc, Asc (carrier) or
DNP-bovine serum albumin (DNP-BSA) in complete Freund's adjuvant.
After three immunizations of the donor rats with these antigens,
their thymuses and spleens were removed, and single cell suspensions
were made in Eagle's minimal essential medium (MEM). Suspensions
of 10^9 cells were passively transferred into recipient rats that
had been producing high titers of anti-hapten IgE antibody.

    By this simple cell transfer technique, we were able to demon-
strate that the transfer of both thymocytes and spleen cells from

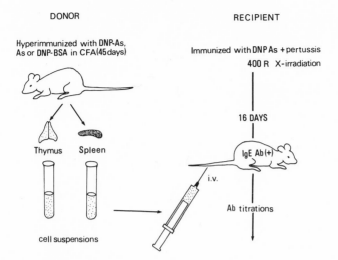

Figure 3.   Experimental procedure to test the suppressive
activity of primed T cells.   Donors were immunized with
DNP-Asc, Asc or DNP-BSA, and their thymus and spleen cell
suspensions were passively transferred into syngeneic
recipients that had been producing high and persistent
reaginic antibody against DNP-Asc by sublethal x-irradiation given before immunization.

rats that had been hyperimmunized either with DNP-Asc or Asc alone
abruptly terminated the preestablished DNP-specific IgE antibody
response.   On the other hand, both thymocytes and spleen cells from
normal rats or those primed with DNP-BSA produced no such a suppressive effect (Figure 4).   The suppressive activity of the carrier-
primed spleen cells was completely abrogated by an *in vitro* treatment of the cells with ATS and complement before the cell transfer.
Other unpublished studies indicated that the same number of lymph
node cells was ineffective, and that such a suppressive activity
was easily destroyed by 500 rads *in vitro* x-radiation.   The suppressive activity was not detectable in the spleen cells of rats
sacrificed 7 to 10 days after a single immunization.

These results now give a vague picture of the IgE suppressor
T cell.   The cells are mostly present in the thymus and spleen,
and are sensitive to x-irradiation and ATS.   The effect of the suppressor T cell was clearly carrier specific, and was generated by
intensive immunization with the carrier antigen.

The latter finding was further supported by the suppressive
effect of carrier-preimmunization (16).   Pretreatment of animals
with the carrier but not with the hapten four weeks prior to the
subsequent immunization with the hapten-carrier conjugate completely suppressed the forthcoming IgE antibody response.   As mentioned

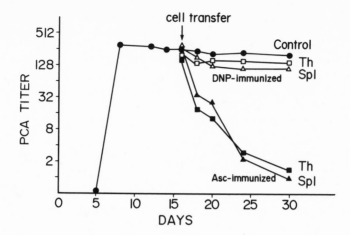

Figure 4.   Suppression of anti-hapten IgE antibody response
by passively transferred syngeneic thymocytes(Th) or spleen
cells(Spl) from donors immunized with the carrier (Asc) but
not with the hapten (DNP-BSA).   Control rats given normal
thymocytes showed no decrease in reaginic titers.

above, the treatment of such preimmunized animals with ATS before
the secondary immunization partially rescued the IgE producing
capacity (9).

     These results are in accordance with the rapidly growing know-
ledge of suppressor T cells disclosed in other experimental systems
dealing with different immunoglobulin classes (reviewed in 17).
In view of the same carrier specificity of the suppressor T cell
to the helper T cell, it should now crucially be asked whether or
not these two cell types belong to the same subpopulation of T
cells, and more specifically, whether the same or different mediators are responsible for both suppressive and cooperative effects
of T cells.   It should also reasonably be asked whether the same
or different suppressor T cells are involved in the regulation of
different classes of antibody formation.   The next section will
briefly summarize the findings we obtained on the soluble T cell
factors which mediate the suppressive and inductive cell interactions in the rat IgE antibody response in order to answer these
questions.

                SOLUBLE FACTORS FROM CARRIER-PRIMED T CELLS

     In order to delineate the mechanism of T cell mediated suppres-
sion of reaginic antibody response, we have attempted to obtain
soluble factors from the suppressor T cells which can mediate the

same effect as that of live T cells (18). We took suspensions of thymocytes and spleen cells from rats primed with DNP-Asc, Asc or DNP-BSA. Since the attempt to release the factor by a short term culture *in vitro* was unsuccessful, the cells were disrupted by freezing and thawing or by sonication, and the cell-free supernatant was obtained by ultracentrifugation at 40,000 G for 1 hr. Recipient rats were sublethally x-irradiated and immunized with DNP-Asc and pertussis vaccine so as to induce high and persistent reaginic antibody formation against DNP determinants. The cell-free supernatants were injected intravenously into recipients and the reaginic titers were closely followed.

Figure 5 shows the result of such an experiment. It was found that the injection of the extracts of both thymocytes and spleen cells obtained from donors primed with Asc or DNP-Asc produced a rapid decrease in the reaginic titer of the recipient animals, whereas those from normal as well as DNP-BSA-primed rats had no such a suppressive activity. The results indicated that a suppressive factor can be released from the cell membrane by physical disruption, and that this factor has been generated by carrier-immunization. It was also found that the suppressive T cell factor thus obtained can specifically suppress the anti-hapten antibody response provided the immunizing hapten was present on the same carrier molecule by which donor animals were immunized.

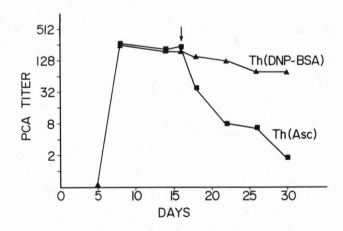

Figure 5. Suppression of anti-hapten IgE antibody response by the injection of cell-free extracts of thymocytes from Ascaris-primed donors but not from DNP-BSA-primed donors. The arrow indicates the day of injection of the extracts. The same was true for the spleen cell extracts.

The availability of such an active molecule as a soluble form enabled us to investigate the physicochemical and immunochemical properties of the suppressive T cell factor (18,19). We have characterized the suppressive T cell factor by absorption with various immunoadsorbents composed of antigens and antibodies (18). Table I summarized the results obtained by such absorption experiments. When the extracts from DNP-Asc-primed thymocytes and spleen cells were passed through a column of immunoadsorbent composed of DNP-Asc or Asc, the suppressive activity was completely abrogated, whereas the same absorption with the DNP-immunoadsorbents consistently failed to do so. Thus, the specificity of the observed suppression of IgE antibody response was found to be based on the affinity of the suppressive T cell molecule for the carrier determinants.

Table I

Properties of the rat suppressive T cell factor as revealed by absorption with antigen and antibodies

Absorption with	Loss of activity
DNP-Asc	Yes
Asc	Yes
DNP-BSA	No
Anti-Igs	No
Anti-Fab	No
Anti-μ	No
ATS	Yes
Anti-DNP-Asc	No

Since the suppressive T cell factor has specificity and affinity for the immunizing antigen (carrier), the possibility was considered as to whether the factor may be an immunoglobulin. However, this possibility was completely excluded by the fact that none of the anti-immunoglobulin antisera, i.e., polyvalent anti-Ig (including anti-γ chain), anti-Fab and anti-μ could remove the suppressive activity. On the other hand, several preparations of ATS, which had been extensively absorbed with serum proteins and bone marrow cells, could absorb the suppressor molecule, indicating that the factor is clearly originated from the T cell membrane. The possibility that the factor is of a complex form with the antigen was

also denied by the failure to remove the activity by absorption
with anti-DNP-Asc (immunizing antigen). From these results, it
was concluded that the suppressive T cell factor is a unique molecule having specificity for antigen but lacking any known immunoglobulin determinants.

It was further found that the factor was not destroyed by
digestion with ribonuclease (RNase) and deoxyribonuclease (DNase)
under an extreme condition, but easily lost its activity by digestion with trypsin and pronase. The molecular weight of the active
component was estimated to be between 35,000 and 60,000 daltons
by preparative ultracentrifugation and gel-filtration with Sephadex
G-200. The electophoretic mobility of the factor was β to α (19).

The results indicate that reaginic antibody formation in the
rat is negatively regulated by a product of T cells that were generated by hyperimmunization with antigen. The findings naturally
explain the previously noted facts that the reagin response in the
rat is terminated after a short period of time, and that the second-
ry reagin response does not occur under usual conditions of the
secondary immunization. Furthermore, the above findings are consistent with the fact that reaginic antibody formation is often
diminished by repeated immunization.

We have already reported that the induction of the reagin
response in the rat also requires a collaborative interaction between the carrier-specific helper T cell and the hapten-specific
IgE B cell (11). The question now arises as to whether this antigen-specific T cell product can assist in the induction of reaginic
antibody response under different conditions (20). In order to
answer this question, we have injected the same thymocytes and
spleen cell extracts from carrier-primed rats into syngeneic neonatally thymectomized recipients that otherwise could not produce
reaginic antibody by the same immunization regime. Simultaneously
with the injection of the extracts the animals were immunized with
DNP-Asc with pertussis vaccine. The IgE antibody response of these
rats was followed for up to 40 days after the immunization.

It was found that the same crude extracts of Asc- or DNP-Asc-
primed thymocytes and spleen cells could restore the ability of
neonatally thymectomized rats to produce reaginic and IgM antibodies
directed to haptenic determinants, whereas the extracts from DNP-
BSA-primed rats could not (Table II). The results at first glance
suggested that the suppressor molecule may act as a helper under
a condition in which T cells have been depleted by neonatal thymectomy.

However, this postulate was found to be incorrect. By absorption with anti-immunoglobulin antisera, the helper activity of the
T cell extracts was completely abrogated leaving the suppressor

activity intact. In addition,the helper activity was found to be
absorbed with monospecific anti-μ chain antibody. The molecular
weight of the helper factor was comparable to that of IgG, indicating that the activity was associated with a molecule resembling
IgT reported by Feldmann and his coworkers (21-23). This helper
activity was also removed by absorption with the immunoadsorbent
of ascaris extract, and thus the molecule is clearly carrier-specific.

Table II

Helper activity of the thymus(T) and spleen(S)
cell extracts from donors hyperimmunized with
various antigens in neonatally thymectomized rats

Donors immunized with	Maximal antibody response*	
	PCA	H A
None(T)	2	404
DNP-BSA(T)	1	279
DNP-Asc(T)	128	1,950
Asc(T)	190	3,220
Asc(S)	128	1,700

* Maximal antibody responses were obtained from
  days 8 to 12. Geometric means of 5 to 7 rats.

The results indicate that the extracts of both thymocytes and
spleen cells of carrier-primed rats contain two distinct antigen
specific molecules; one having suppressor activity with non-Ig
nature, and the other having the enhancing activity with characteristics of the monomeric IgM. Properties of these two subcellular components are listed in Table III. Although at the present
moment the origin of the IgT-like molecule in the rat is still not
determined, it is a fact that such a molecule is extractable from
carrier-primed thymocytes, and that the injection of it can reconstitute the reagin response of neonatally thymectomized rats that
otherwise cannot produce reaginic antibodies. It is still to be
determined whether such a molecule is, in fact, a T cell product
or the product of other cell types being adsorbed to T cell membrane. Our more recent observation indicated that monomeric IgM

obtained by reduction and alkylation of serum IgM antibody exerts the same enhancing effect in the neonatally thymectomized rats, whereas IgG antibody from the same specificity does not. These results do not exclude the possibility that monomeric IgM in the thymocyte extract came from B cells. Nevertheless, the induction of reagin response by carrier-specific monomeric IgM in place of live T cells provides some information on the mechanism of the triggering event of IgE B cells other than mere binding of the antigen.

Table III

Properties of suppressive and enhancing T cell components
in IgE antibody response of the rat

	Suppressor	Helper
Specificity	Carrier	Carrier
Ig determinant	-	Fab, μ
Reactivity to ATS	+	-
Molecular weight	>35,000	>100,000
	<60,000	<200,000
Electrophoretic mobility	$\beta - \alpha$	β
Chemical nature	Protein	Protein(IgT?)
Activity *in vivo*	Suppression	Enhancement

From these observations, it is apparent that reaginic antibody formation is regulated by multiple signals provided by other cell types, notably by T cells. It is at least clear at the moment that the enhancing and suppressive T cell factors are different molecules probably derived from different subsets of lymphoid cells. In addition, as has been reported by Kishimoto and Ishizaka (24, 25), antigen-nonspecific T cell factors may give some other selective pressures under certain circumstances in the rat too. In view of the selective potentiation of reagin response by helminth infections in the rat (26-28), antigen-nonspecific T cells would play an important role over the regulation of IgE synthesis, but we have no experimental data in this respect.

THE SUPPRESSIVE T CELL FACTOR IN MICE

Based on the above results obtained in the rat reagin formation, we have tried to analyse more closely the antigen-specific
suppressive T cell factor with respect to its genetic nature.
This was only possible in the mouse, since several *H-2* congeneic
lines and their recombinant strains are available for the analysis
in this species. One such approach has been made by an *in vitro*
suppression of IgG antibody synthesis (29-31), which in many respects gives several suggestions for IgE antibody response too. I
would like to show some of our recent observations which seem to
be relevant to understanding the T cell-mediated regulation in
general.

The experimental system in brief is as follows: The donor mice
of the suppressive T cell factor were immunized with two injections
of 100 µg of keyhole limpet hemocyanine (KLH) at a two-week interval, and their thymuses and spleens were obtained two weeks after
the second immunization. The cell-free extracts of primed cells
were prepared by sonication and ultracentrifugation by the similar
procedure used in the previous rat experiments. To test the suppressive activity of these extracts, a dose corresponding to 10^7
original thymocytes was added to the culture of syngeneic spleen
cells primed four weeks before with DNP-KLH. Usually 10^7 primed
spleen cells were stimulated with 0.1 µg/ml of DNP-KLH in the Mar-
brook culture bottle. DNP-specific IgG antibody forming cells
were enumerated after a 5-day culture by the hemolytic plaque forming cell (PFC) method of Cunningham and Szenberg (32) using DNP-
coated sheep erythrocytes (DNP-SRBC).

Table IV

Suppression of the *in vitro* secondary antibody response
against DNP-KLH by KLH-primed thymocyte extract

Extract added	Anti-DNP IgG PFC/culture
Control	1,799 ± 96
KLH-primed T-extract	227 ± 78
Normal T-extract	1,690 ± 197
EA-primed T-extract	1,444 ± 46
No antigen	30 ± 1

Thymocyte(T) extracts from normal or immunized mice
corresponding to 10^7 thymocytes were add to the culture
in which 10^7 DNP-KLH primed spleen cells were cultured
with 0.1 µg/ml of DNP-KLH.

Although we have not been able to induce good IgE antibody response in this *in vitro* culture technique, several important characteristics of the suppressive T cell factor have been disclosed (29). The result of one typical experiment is shown in Table IV. When DNP-KLH primed spleen cells were cultured with an appropriate amount of antigen, a good *in vitro* secondary antibody response was induced. This secondary IgG antibody response was greatly suppressed by the addition of KLH-primed thymocyte extract but not of normal or egg albumin (EA)-primed thymocyte extract. Furthermore, physicochemical and immunochemical properties of the suppressive T cell factor of the mouse were very similar to those of the suppressive T cell factor of the rat observed in the IgE antibody response (Table V). The factor was clearly antigen-specific and not of immunoglobulin nature. The molecular weight was between 35,000 and 55,000, and the activity was adsorbable with the immunoadsorbent of ATS. These properties were quite analogous to those of the rat T cell factor,which indicates that a similar mechanism may be operative in the rat IgE and the mouse *in vitro* IgG antibody responses.

Table V

Properties of the suppressive T cell factor
in the mouse

Specificity for	Carrier
Sensitivity to DNase	−
RNase	−
Pronase	+
Ig determinants	−
Molecular weight	35,000 − 55,000
H-2 barrier	+
I region gene expression	+
T cell surface antigens	+
Target	Mostly helper T cell
Release by antigen	Weak
Activity	Suppression
Possible nature	T cell receptor

By this simple experimental procedure we have been able to show some other facets of the suppressive T cell factor. The most important finding on the mouse suppressive T cell factor is that the factor is a product of a gene or genes in the major histocompatibility complex (30,31). This was demonstrated by the fact that the suppressive T cell factor was successfully removed by alloantisera reactive with the products of the H-2 complex. Using various alloantisera directed to the restricted subregions of the H-2 complex, we have succeeded in assigning the locus of the gene which codes for the suppressive T cell factor among H-2 subregions.

Table VI summarizes the representative result obtained in such an experiment, which clearly provides a logical basis for the unambigous subregion assignment of the gene coding for the suppressive T cell factor. In this experiment, the thymocyte extract of KLH-primed C3H ($H-2^k$) mice was absorbed with various alloantisera directed to restricted subregions of the H-2 complex. The absorbed materials were then tested for their residual suppressive activity by adding to the culture of syngeneic DNP-KLH-primed spleen cells with an appropriate amount of antigen. It is clearly seen that several alloantisera directed to the I region of the H-2 complex could successfully remove the suppressive activity from the thymocyte extract, whereas the antiserum reactive only with histocompatibility antigen coded by H-2K region was ineffective. By close analysis of the specificity of these antisera, it was found that the absorbing capacity was not associated with any known Ia specificities. Furthermore, it is evident that alloantisera lacking the specificity for I-A and/or I-C subregions were also effective in absorbing the suppressive T cell factor, indicating that the factor is encoded by genes present to the right of I-A and to the left of I-C subregions.

An important finding is that an alloantiserum (B10.A(18R) anti-B10.A(5R)) putatively lacking the specificity for any of the subregions of the $H-2^k$ consistently removed the suppressive T cell factor of the $H-2^k$ mice. This puzzle was recently solved by the discovery of a small subregion (I-E) between I-B and I-C in B10.A (5R) mice, which was originated from $H-2^k$ haplotype (31), and the suppressor gene is clearly located in this special 'I-E' subregion. Our more recent studies indicated EA-specific suppressor gene is also present in this subregion.

A supporting evidence for the presence of $I-E^k$ subregion in B10.A(5R) mice was obtained from a different approach to the suppressor phenomenon. We have found that there is a strict requirement for the H-2 histocompatibility to induce a suppression by the T cell factor derived from one strain of mice in the response of other strains. As summarized in Table VII, $H-2^d$ mice can only suppress the response of $H-2^d$ but not other strains such as A/J which shares only I-C, S and D regions with $H-2^d$ mice. Similarly,

Table VI

Assignment of the suppressor gene to the right of $I-C$
and to the left of $I-B$ subregion

Absorbed with*	Specificity		Anti-DNP IgG PFC/culture
	$H-2$ subregions	Ia	
Control	—	—	1,616 ± 231
Unabsorbed	—	—	150 ± 39
A.QR anti-B10.A	K	—	118 ± 18
(C3H.H-2°x129)F_1 anti-C3H	$K,I-A,I-B,I-C$	1,2	1,455 ± 115
A.TH anti-A.TL	$I-A,I-B,I-C$	1,2,3,15,7	1,458 ± 141
(B10.D2xA.TH)F_1 anti-A.TL	$I-A,I-B,I-C$	1,2,3	1,675 ± 157
(A.THxB10.HTT)F_1 anti-A.TL	$I-A,I-B$	1,2,3,15	1,540 ± 101
(B10.A(4R)x129)F_1 anti-B10.A(2R)	$I-B$	7	1,475 ± 84
B10.S(7R) anti-B10.HTT	$I-C$	7	115 ± 89
B10.A(18R) anti-B10.A(5R)	none($I-E$)	7	1,588 ± 75

* The suppressive T cell extract of $H-2^k$ mice was absorbed with immunoadsorbents of anti-Ia antisera. Note that there is no meaningful association between the absorbing capacity and Ia specificities of these antisera.

the factor from $H-2^k$ mice can suppress the responses of $H-2^k$ and $H-2^a$ mice, the latter of which share K, $I-A$ and $I-B$ subregions. Definitely no suppression was induced by the $H-2^k$ factor in the response of histoincompatible (e.g., $H-2^d$ and $H-2^s$) strains, and thus the identities among genes in the left side half (K, $I-A$, $I-B$) of the $H-2$ complex are required for the induction of suppression in cross-strain experiments.

We utilized this system to learn what subregion is responsible for the determination of the suppressive T cell factor. We took the T cell extracts of B10.A(4R) and B10.A(5R), both of which are recombinants of B10.A and B10, and tested their effect on the antibody responses of $H-2^b$, $H-2^k$ and $H-2^d$ mice. Composition of $H-2$ subregions of these mice and the identities of subregions to those of recipient strains are shown in the lower part of Table VII.

Table VII

Requirement for identities among genes in $H-2$ complex
for the suppression of antibody response

Donor of the T cell factor ($H-2$ regions)	Spleen cells from ($H-2$ haplotype)	Identities	% suppression
BALB/c	BALB/c ($H-2^d$)	K, I, S, D	86
d d d d d d	A/J ($H-2^a$)	I-C, S, D	0
	C3H ($H-2^k$)	none	0
C3H	C3H ($H-2^k$)	K, I, S, D	72
k k k k k k	CBA ($H-2^k$)	K, I, S, D	64
	A/J ($H-2^a$)	K, I-A, I-B	56
	BALB/c ($H-2^d$)	none	0
	SJL ($H-2^s$)	none	0
B10.A(4R)	C3H ($H-2^k$)	K, I-A	0
k k/b b b b	C57BL/6 ($H-2^b$)	I-B,I-C,S,D	46
B10.A(5R)	C57BL/6 ($H-2^b$)	K, I-A, I-B	0
b b b/d d d	BALB/c ($H-2^d$)	I-C, S, D	0
	C3H ($H-2^k$)	none($I-E$)	82

The results strongly supported the postulate stated above: the 4R factor could only suppress the response of $H-2^b$ mice which share $I-B$ and $I-C$ subregions but not $I-A$ subregion. The response of $H-2^k$ mice which share K and $I-A$ subregions with the donor 4R was definitely enhanced. Thus, the suppressive T cell factor is found to be determined by genes located to the right of $I-A$ subregion. The results obtained with the 5R factor were more striking. The 5R factor could suppress the response of neither $H-2^b$ nor $H-2^d$, but greatly inhibited the response of $H-2^k$ mice. The results reinforce the previous findings that 5R mice possess $I-E^k$ subregion between $I-B^b$ and $I-C^d$ subregions in the $H-2$ complex, and suppressor gene may be allocated in this $I-E$ subregion. The results obtained with other recombinant mice also support this postulate.

Another important point which was clarified in the above experimental system is that the target of the suppressive T cell factor is the helper T cell but not the B cell itself (29). This was shown by two different lines of evidence: First, the suppressive T cell factor could not affect the $in vitro$ antibody response unless the helper T cell having an identical specificity to the suppressive T cell factor coexists in the same culture. Thus for example, the KLH-specific T cell factor cannot suppress the response of DNP-EA-primed spleen cells even in the presence of the mixture of DNP-EA and DNP-KLH. In this experimental condition, DNP-specific B cells can equally bind DNP-EA and DNP-KLH, but only the EA-specific suppressive T cell factor but not the KLH-specific T cell factor could suppress the anti-DNP antibody response (29). This suggests that the factor does not directly act on B cells, but suppress the antibody response via inhibition of helper activity of T cells. Secondly, the suppressive T cell factor can be absorbed by incubation with thymocytes and splenic T cells of histocompatible strains but not with anti-θ treated spleen cells, bone marrow cells and macrophages (30). This indicates that the acceptor site for the suppressive T cell factor is present on T cells but not on B cells, and this site is also determined by genes in the $H-2$ complex.

Although these findings have so far been obtained in the $in vitro$ IgG antibody response, but certainly cast a light on the mechanism of the T cell-mediated regulation of antibody responses in general. Since the soluble factors regulating the rat IgE and mouse IgG antibody responses have sufficiently overt similarities with respect to their immunochemical and physicochemical properties, it is likely that a similar mechanism may be operative in the suppression of both responses. We are currently exploring whether the suppression of IgE antibody response could be induced by the same molecule with the nature of I region gene product in the mouse. Our recent preliminary studies suggested that this is actually true.

DISCUSSION

I have summarized our previous findings which indicate that IgE antibody formation in the rat is negatively regulated by the antigen-specific suppressor T cell. The effect of the suppressor T cell is probably mediated by a subcellular component which is extractable from thymocytes and spleen cells of hyperimmunized rats. This subcellular component, designated as the suppressive T cell factor, has specificity and affinity for the carrier part of the immunizing antigen, although no immunoglobulin determinants are detectable by absorption with various anti-immunoglobulin antisera. These results suggest that the generation of such suppressor T cells in normal immunized rats causes the early termination of IgE antibody response in the rat, and prevents the induction of secondary IgE antibody response.

However, even though various properties of the rat suppressive T cell factor have been disclosed by *in vivo* suppression studies, the exact mechanism by which the T cell factor turns off the IgE antibody response has yet not resolved. Clues for answering this question has arisen from our recent studies on the suppression of mouse IgG antibody response *in vitro* in which a similar antigen-specific T cell factor exerts the suppressive effect. The physicochemical and immunochemical properties of the mouse suppressive T cell factor are almost identical to those of the rat. By the combination of the donor of the T cell factor and the target responding cells with different *H-2* histocompatibility complex, we were able to determine that the suppressive T cell factor of the mouse is a product of a gene present in the *I* region of the *H-2* complex. It was further demonstrated that the target of the T cell factor is the helper T cell but not B cell itself.

Although it seems too early to extraporate the above findings to the regulation of IgE antibody response, a possibility should be considered that the suppressive T cell factor inactivates the helper T cell expressing the acceptor site for the T cell factor, and that such interacting cell surface molecules have stractures coded for by paired genes in the major histocompatibility complex. In view of the recent discoveries of various examples of complementation of two *I* region genes in the induction of antibody response (33-35), it is likely that the T cell-mediated suppression of IgE antibody response is also via interaction of *I* region gene products. Figure 6 is illastrated to show such a hypothesis.

There are several important problems to be solved in the future. In fact, I am aware of the sufficiently overt differences in the regulatory mechanism between IgE and IgG antibody responses as reviewed in recent articles (6,36). It is now of crucial importance to determine whether or not the same *I* region gene product observed in the mouse IgG antibody response also regulate the

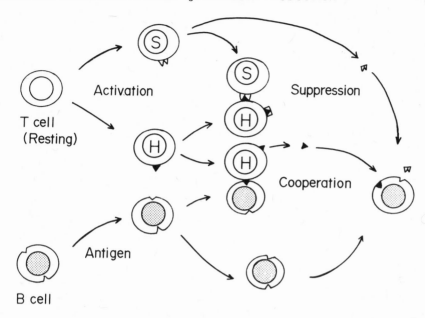

Figure 6.   A hypothetical schema of the T cell mediated suppression of antibody formation. The suppressor T cells (S)
suppress the helper T cell (H) by complementary interaction
of cell surface molecules (⛴ and ▼) both coded for by genes
in the *H-2* complex. The antigen specificity of these molecules
focuses on each other for the effective cell interaction.

IgE antibody response. Furthermore, it is known that the role of
T cells in the reaginic antibody formation is not uniform among
different animal species. As was discussed by Ishizaka (37),
antigen-nonspecific T cell factors play important roles in the
selective induction and suppression of IgE antibody response in
the mouse and rabbits. Therefore, the clarification of the interrelationship as well as of the joint actions of these multiple T
cell factors may be of great importance for the future understanding of the whole picture of the T cell-mediated regulation.

Acknowledgments: I am grateful to Drs. K. Okumura, M. Taniguchi
and T. Takemori for their collaboration in the work cited here.
Thanks are also due to Ms. Yoko Yamaguchi for her excellent secretarial help. I am also indebted to Drs. B. Benacerraf and C. S.
David for their generous supply of mouse alloantisera. This investigation has been supported by a grant in aid from the Japanese
Ministry of Education, Science and Culture.

REFERENCES

1. Mota, I., Immunology, 7:681, 1964.
2. Binaghi, R.A., Benacerraf, B., Bloch, K.J. and Kowrilsky, F.M., J. Immunol., 92:927, 1964.
3. Strejan, G. and Campbell, D.H., J. Immunol., 105:1264, 1970.
4. Mota, I., Immunology, 12:343, 1967.
5. Zvaifler, N.J. and Becker, E.L., J. Exp. Med., 123:935, 1966.
6. Tada, T., Progress in Allergy, 19:122, 1975.
7. Tada, T., Taniguchi, M. and Okumura, K., J. Immunol., 106:1012, 1971.
8. Okumura, K. and Tada, T., J. Immunol., 106:1019, 1971.
9. Okumura, K., Tada, T. and Ochiai, T., Immunology, 26:257, 1974.
10. Taniguchi, M. and Tada, T., J. Immunol., 107:579, 1971.
11. Tada, T. and Okumura, K., J. Immunol., 107:1137, 1971.
12. Hamaoka, T., Katz, D.H. and Benacerraf, B., J. Exp. Med., 138:538, 1973.
13. Kishimoto, T. and Ishizaka, K., J. Immunol., 109:612, 1972.
14. Okudaira, H. and Ishizaka, K., J. Immunol., 111:1420, 1973.
15. Okumura, K. and Tada, T., J. Immunol., 107:1682, 1971.
16. Tada, T., Okumura, K. and Taniguchi, M., J. Immunol., 108:1535, 1972.
17. Gershon, R.K., in Contemporary Topics in Immunology, 3:1, ed. Cooper, M.D. and Warner, N.L., Plenum Press, New York, 1974.
18. Tada, T., Okumura, K. and Taniguchi, M., J. Immunol., 111:952, 1973.
19. Okumura, K. and Tada, T., J. Immunol., 112:783, 1974.
20. Taniguchi, M. and Tada, T., J. Immunol., 113:1757, 1974.
21. Feldmann, M. and Basten, A., J. Exp. Med., 136:49, 1972.
22. Feldmann, M., J. Exp. Med., 136:737, 1972.
23. Felamann, M., Cone, R.E. and Marchalonis, J.J., Cell. Immunol., 9:1, 1973.
24. Kishimoto, T. and Ishizaka, K., J. Immunol., 111:1194, 1973.
25. Kishimoto, T. and Ishizaka, K., J. Immunol., 112:1685, 1974.
26. Orr, T.S.C. and Blair, A.M.J.N., Life Sci., 8:1073, 1969.
27. Orr, T.S.C., RiLey, P.A. and Doe, J.E., Immunology, 20:185, 1971.
28. Jarrett, E.E.E. and Stewart, D.C., Immunology, 23:749, 1972.
29. Taniguchi, M., Hayakawa, K. and Tada, T., J. Immunol., 116:542, 1976.
30. Taniguchi, M., Tada, T. and Tokuhisa, T., J. Exp. Med., submitted
31. Tada, T., Taniguchi, M. and David, C.S., J. Exp. Med., submitted.
32. Cunningham, A.J. and Szenberg, A., Immunology, 14:599, 1968.
33. Stimpfling, J.H. and Durham, T., J. Immunol., 108:947, 1972.
34. Munro, A.J. and Taussig, M.J., Nature, 256:103, 1975.
35. Dorf, M.E. and Benacerraf, B., Proc. Nat. Acad. Sci, USA, 72:3671, 1975.
36. Tada, T., Taniguchi, M. and Takemori, T., Transplant. Rev., 26:107, 1975.
37. Ishizaka, K., In this volume.

DISCUSSION

ISHIZAKA, K.: I would like you to clarify one point. You suggested in your early work two possible explanations for the regulation of the IgE antibody response in your rat system.

One was the suppressor cell that you mentioned to-day and the other was the possibility of too many helper cells. I understand that you dislike the latter possibility and I would like you to explain why.

TADA: When we first described the suppression of IgE antibody response by carrier specific T cells, we thought that this could be explained equally well either by suppressor T cells or by "too much help".

However, there has been accumulating evidence that the suppressor T cell belongs to a distinct subpopulation of T cells. In fact, the suppressor T cell has several characteristic features distinguishable from the helper T cell with respect to the tissue distribution, membrane markers, x-ray sensitivity and so on.

More specifically, we found that the soluble factor derived from the suppressor T cell is a molecule distinct from the factor which helps the B cell differentiation.

Therefore, it is now clear that the suppression of IgE antibody response we observed is due to the generation of suppressor T cell rather than due to "too much help"

ISHIZAKA, K.: As the on-going IgE antibody response was terminated so rapidly by thymocytes or subcellular components, you have suggested that the regulatory T cells and the suppressor substance may react with B cells or even IgE forming cells.

In the mouse IgG system, you have shown some evidence that suppressor T cells regulate helper cells rather than B cells.

I wonder whether you believe that the same mechanisms may be applied for the termination of IgE antibody formation, or do you think that the termination of the IgE antibody formation is too fast?

TADA: I think the same mechanism may be operative in the suppression of IgG and IgE antibody responses, although I do not have direct evidence for the latter.

Since the half life of IgE in the circulation is only 12 hours, the rapid decrease of IgE antibody formation after the cell transfer can naturally be explained as the consequence of the suppression of helper activity by suppressor T cells which resulted in the decreased synthesis of IgE antibody.

COCHRANE: Do you know if the T cell suppressor substance block the stimulation of B cells by T independent antigen?

TADA: We have tested whether T cell independent antigens, such as salmonella flagellin and pneumococcal polysaccharide, could generate the suppressive T cell factor in mice. But so far we have never been able to extract the factors which specifically suppress the antibody response against DNP coupled to these T cell independent carriers.

Of course, the KLH-specific factor cannot block the antibody response to unrelated antigens regardless of their T cell dependency.

MARSH: I think that there may be several regulatory mechanisms controlling IgE biosynthesis. In your system you have very nicely shown that a T cell suppressor factor is linked to the H-2 complex, but in human IgE response we find no evidence of linkage or association between total serum IgE level and HLA type.

In your experiments you are primarily studying T cell suppression of an ongoing IgE response, but we have studied regulation that seems to influence IgE antibody production de novo (i.e. whether or not a person is able to synthesize IgE antibody against a particular antigenic stimulus).

Could you comment on these apparently different regulatory controls? Possibly you have some data which suggests that regulation is really quite a complex process.

TADA: I did not have enough time to describe the complexity of the T cell regulation of antibody response. In fact, the suppressor phenomenon is controlled by at least two genes in the H-2 complex one of which determines the expression of the suppressive T cell factor, and the other the acceptor site for the T cell factor.

The expression of both genes are regulated by unknown gene or genes not linked to the H-2 complex. For example, A/J mice cannot express the suppressive T cell factor, while being able to accept the factor produced by B 10 A. On the other hand several B 10 congeneic strains can produce the factor, but are unable to accept the T cell factor of even syngeneic mice.

However, it is a general rule that only H-2 histocompatible factors can suppress the antibody response of given mouse strain Therefore, even though the suppressor phenomenon is clearly related to the H-2 complex, its expression is influenced by several factors not linked to the H-2 complex.

DAVID: What is the evidence that the soluble T cell suppressor has T cell surface antigen on it?

TADA: We have tried to absorb the suppressive T cell factor with several lots of heterologous anti-thymocyte sera, many of which could react only with T cell menbrane as revealed by immunofluorescence. The suppressive activity was invariably absorbed by those anti-thymocyte sera.

Furthermore, we have recently been able to raise antisera against the suppressive T cell factor, which could kill certain types of T cells but not B cells.

DAVID: Do you get more suppressor substance if you first incubate the cells with specific antigen? Does the factor go into the supernatant, or do you get more after extraction?

TADA: Suppressive T cell factor is hard to release by a short-term culture with antigen. However, we can extract the factor from the residual cultured cells with a yield much higher than from the original uncultured cells. This may indicate that the suppressive T cell factor is synthesized de novo during the culture period, but it is not released from the cell membrane so easily.

DAVID: It is of interest that your suppressor factor does not act across histocompatibility barriers - maybe this is because it is acting on T cell helper.

Another T cell factor - a helper factor described by Taussig and Munro which also is a product of Ir gene will act on B cells across the histocompatibility barrier. Do you believe this is due to the target cell being different in these cases.

TADA: I think that this strict histocompatibility requirement gives a strong distinction from the cooperative T cell factor of Taussig and Munro. This might be due to the difference in the structure of acceptor sites of T and B cells for the suppressor versus cooperative factors.

JARRETT: I know that you use a fairly substantial dose of antigen to immunize your rats and I should like to ask you whether you have ever tried small immunizing doses.

The reason I ask that question is because as you know we can induce booster IgE responses in Hooded Lister rats but only if these are initially immunized with a very small quantity of antigen.

I should like to know if Hooded Lister rats are really unusual in IgE production, because the other possibility is that over the years people have been studying IgE production in rats in which they have ensured that IgE production is first suppressed by injecting large doses of antigen.

TADA: In our hand, 50 to 1000 μg of antigen induced an essentially similar type of IgE antibody response in Wistar strain rats. Decreasing the dose to less than 10 μg failed to induce reagin response. However, this may depend on the strain of the rat.

I would like to mention that if we immunize rats with a single small dose of antigen, we cannot detect suppressor T cells in their spleen, and therefore the induction of suppressor T cell may perhaps be related to the dose of antigen and number of immunizations.

JANEWAY (Uppsala): Do you have direct evidence for the action of the suppressor factor upon helper T cells?

If I understand correctly, your evidence is two-fold.

First, that normal T but not normal B cells remove the factor. Second, that the specificity of the helper cells and suppressor factor are the same. But this does not seem to me adequate evidence for a direct effect on T cells, because your factor, which binds to antigen, could then ride around on carrier and affect either T or B cells with which it comes in contact.

Do you have other types of evidence, such as elimination of helper cells by suppressor factor, to show a direct action on helper cells.

TADA: At the moment, we do not have any other evidence than I have just presented. However, the factor does not act on B cells even in the presence of the corresponding antigen unless the helper T cell coexists.This would exclude the possibility that the factor directly affects the B cell.

MÜLLER-EBERHARD: Can the activity of the T cell derived regulatory molecules be detected in serum?

The reason I am asking is the recent observation by Dr. A. Grubb in Dr. Laurell's laboratory in Malmö on the occurrance of a T cell produced serum protein in man. As in the case of your suppressor factor, the T cell produced serum protein has a molecular weight if approximately 30,000, an electrophoretic mobility of $\alpha-\beta$ -globulins and, by the fluorescent antibody technique, it is found also on the surface of T cells.

TADA: It is certainly very interesting that they have found such a molecule in serum. However, we have never succeeded in suppressing the antibody response by the transfer of serum from suppressed animals.

IgE in Rats:
An Experimental Model

PRODUCTION OF IgE AND REAGINIC ANTIBODY IN RATS IN RELATION TO

WORM INFECTIONS

Ellen E.E. Jarrett

University of Glasgow, Veterinary Hospital
Wellcome Laboratories for Experimental Parasitology
Bearsden Road, Bearsden, Glasgow, G61 1QH

Natural or experimental infection with live worm parasites
is the most effective known stimulus for the production of IgE,
resulting generally in higher levels of both antibody and total
IgE than can be elicited by any other means. This general
proposition is put into perspective by adding that virtually all
animals are naturally infected with helminth parasites as are
indeed the majority of human beings. Hookworm infection alone
affects about 400 million people.

There are recent reviews which describe the occurrence and
nature of parasite specific reaginic antibody responses and
discuss the role of these antibodies in the pathogenesis of, and
the immune response in, parasitic disease (Sadun, 1972; Murray,
1972; Ogilvie & Jones, 1973; Jarrett, 1973). Here I will
describe how certain models in the rat have contributed to our
understanding of the IgE stimulating effect of helminth parasites.

IgE PRODUCTION IN Nippostrongylus brasiliensis INFECTION

The IgE response of rats infected with the nematode
Nippostrongylus brasiliensis can be resolved into three components.

First there is the parasite specific IgE response originally
described by Ogilvie (1964). This response which reaches high
levels, persists for many weeks after infection and is rapidly
boosted by reinfection (Ogilvie, 1967). In this respect alone
helminth infection is unique, contrasting with the notorious
difficulty of raising good IgE responses in rats by other stimuli.
It is for instance, still common experience that reagins to

conventional antigens can be stimulated only by injecting them
together with an adjuvant such as B. pertussis. This is true
even of antigens prepared from parasites, which although highly
allergenic, cannot be made to produce the effects so
characteristic of the live worms from which they were extracted.

Secondly, infection with N. brasiliensis can, in addition
to causing the parasite specific response, elevate IgE responses
to completely unrelated antigens. Orr & Blair (1969) found that
if they induced a reaginic antibody response in rats to egg-
albumin (EA) or conalbumin and then infected the animals with
N. brasiliensis the level of circulating EA or conalbumin
reaginic antibodies was dramatically increased, often by 100
times or more, 12 days after infection. This phenomenon which
they called the 'potentiated reagin response' was a most
significant finding, for it exposed the secret of the IgE
stimulating effects of helminth parasites. It indicated that
these creatures not only produce the potent allergen which
initiates a parasite specific IgE response but also activate in
the host a mechanism, the design of which is perhaps to augment
and maintain that response but which coincidentally influences
quite unrelated IgE production.

Finally, we have shown recently that there occurs in
infected rats a massive elevation of total serum IgE, and that
the bulk of this IgE is surplus to concentrations expected
against the two known kinds of IgE antibody response which have
been described above (Jarrett & Bazin, 1974).

FEATURES OF THE POTENTIATED REAGIN RESPONSE

The potentiated IgE response has been demonstrated to occur
in rats immunized with antigens other than EA and conalbumin
including keyhole limpet haemocyanin and house dust extract
(Jarrett & Stewart, 1972). The response can also be produced in
rats infected with another parasite, the trematode Fasciola
hepatica (Jarrett, 1972). If animals are immunized with several
antigens simultaneously, the several IgE responses which result
may be potentiated together by subsequent infection. On the
other hand, IgG antibodies directed against the same antigens,
as measured by haemagglutination (Jarrett, Henderson, Riley &
White, 1972) or more class specifically by radioimmunodiffusion
(Bloch, Ohman, Waltin & Cygan, 1973), appear to be largely
unaffected.

In the rat N. brasiliensis infection can only amplify
already existing IgE responses. In other words, the animals must
have been immunized with antigen and an adjuvant, and must be
producing a low level of IgE antibodies at the time of infection

(Orr & Blair, 1969; Jarrett et al., 1972). If the infection
occurs before immunization or too soon after, then not only does
potentiation not occur, but the IgE response to unrelated
antigen may actually be inhibited. However, once the IgE
response is established, it may be potentiated anytime thereafter
so long as it is still extant (Orr, Riley & Doe, 1972). We have
potentiated EA responses by infection as late as 80 days after
immunization which is the time when the primary IgE response in
Hooded Lister rats is about to disappear.

This requirement for prior immunization indicates that the
potentiation mechanism is exerted only on a population of cells
already programmed to produce IgE antibodies, which clearly
distinguishes the activity of parasites from that of conventional
adjuvants. The initiation of an IgE response in the rat to EA
may be accomplished by injecting antigen together with one of a
number of adjuvants including Bordetella pertussis, Freund's
complete or incomplete adjuvants and aluminium hydroxide gel
(Mota, 1964; Binaghi & Benacerraff, 1964; Jarrett et al., 1972).
The unpublished work of Orr and his colleagues and of ourselves
has shown that neither living nor dead N. brasiliensis worms,
nor any product prepared from them can substitute for these
adjuvants in the genesis of an IgE response to heterologous
antigen. Conversely the adjuvants cannot replace N. brasiliensis
in potentiating existing IgE responses, even if given daily over
the relevant period (Jarrett et al., 1972). It is wrong to
depict the two effects (i.e. initiation and potentiation) in an
all embracing statement about IgE adjuvants as some people have
done, since the mechanisms, as well as the manifestations, are
almost certainly quite different.

IgE antibody potentiation requires the presence of live
worms. Attempts to produce it with an extract prepared from
disrupted N. brasiliensis worms have been unsuccessful (Orr,
Riley & Doe, 1971). So too have been our own attempts to produce
it by injecting over several days, large quantities of the
secretory products produced by adult worms maintained in vitro.
Such culture fluid contains relatively concentrated and
uncontaminated N. brasiliensis allergen by contrast with the
mixture prepared from dead worms. Whether it also contains the
'potentiator', and indeed whether the potentiator and the
allergen are the same thing, we do not yet know.

It is entirely possible however, that the failure to mimic
the IgE stimulating effect of live worms by injecting worm
products has merely been a failure to introduce into the animals
enough of the right substance at the right time. There is
nothing to indicate that potentiation is critically dependent
on any particular physical relationship between parasite and host.
The fact that it can be achieved with helminths which parasitise

different organs, e.g. <u>N. brasiliensis</u> and <u>F. hepatica</u> suggests
that the final position of the parasite in the host is
unimportant.

However, since the immature forms of both these parasites go
through a phase in which they migrate through tissues, before
settling as adults in the lumina of the small intestine and bile
ducts respectively, the question arose whether migration through
the tissues is essential or whether a parasite whose life in the
host is restricted to the lumen of the gut could also cause
potentiation. We performed experiments in which the life cycle
of <u>N. brasiliensis</u> was restricted on the one hand to the
migrating phase by radiation-attenuation of infective larvae or
anthelmintic treatment of the host, and on the other hand to the
intestinal phase by surgical transplantation of adult worms to
the small intestine (Jarrett & Stewart, 1973a). Potentiation of
EA responses occurred in both kinds of infection, but to a far
greater extent in rats which had received adult worms. The
latter are restricted to the lumen of the small intestine and
IgE potentiation caused by them must be due to their production
of a soluble substance which is absorbed across the intestinal
epithelium. The evidence suggests that elaboration of the
potentiating substance is common to both larval and adult stages
of <u>N. brasiliensis</u> but that the adults produce more of it.
Potentiation cannot be ascribed to special effects which parasites
have by virtue of either tissue migration or of physical intimacy
with mucosae.

FEATURES OF THE TOTAL IgE RESPONSE

It could be predicted fairly confidently that the occurrence
of parasite specific and experimentally potentiated reagin
responses in infected rats would cause at least some increase in
the level of total IgE. Additionally however, it seemed likely
that naturally occurring IgE responses might also be potentiated.
If they were, then the increase in total IgE should be in excess
of that which could be accounted for by known potentiated or
parasite specific responses. In <u>N. brasiliensis</u> infection the
potentiated reagin response to unrelated antigen is transient,
lasting only a few days (Orr, Riley & Doe, 1971), whereas the
later developing parasite specific IgE response persists at high
levels for a relatively long time (Ogilvie, 1967). Another
intriguing question,therefore, was would the total IgE increase
coincide with the first or the second of these two specific IgE
responses? The discovery by Bazin and his colleagues of
immunocytomas occurring in Lou rats, and the consequent
availability of rat IgE myeloma and IgE specific antiserum
(Bazin <u>et al</u>., 1973, 1974) made it possible finally to answer
such questions.

In the meantime we had found that stimulation of the Hooded Lister rats which we used, with some conventional protein antigens, could evoke IgE responses which were quite different in duration and magnitude from those described in the literature on rat IgE. Thus, primary responses were prolonged and, provided that the animals had been immunized initially with a very small dose of antigen, could be boosted to high levels by subsequent challenge (Jarrett & Stewart, 1974). This made possible an experiment to compare total IgE levels in rats whose EA specific IgE response had been elevated on the one hand by N. brasiliensis infection, and on the other by a booster dose of antigen.

The results originally reported by Jarrett & Bazin (1974) and reproduced in Table 1, clearly showed that total serum IgE was dramatically elevated in infected rats coincident with the potentiated EA reagin response, but that this response itself, contributed only fractionally to the increase in total IgE. It was also shown that in rats which had not been previously immunized with heterologous antigen, total IgE was nevertheless raised to the same extent and at the same time after infection (i.e. day 12) before the appearance of parasite specific IgE antibodies in the serum. In these rats greatly increased levels of total IgE therefore occur in the absence of any known IgE antibody responses.

TABLE 1

Comparison of total IgE levels in rats whose primary egg-albumin (EA) IgE response has been boosted with antigen or potentiated by helminth infection.

Group	Treatment	EA PCA[++] titre	Total IgE μg/ml
1	20 normal rats	-	most rats <0.35
2	12 days after 1 μg EA + B. pertussis	92 ± 36	1.33 ± 0.25
	Rats divided into 2 groups of 10		
3	4 days after 10 ng EA	1228 ± 231	1.80 ± 0.39
4	12 days after 4000 N.brasiliensis larvae[*]	1316 ± 270	288 ± 47

* This is before parasite specific IgE is detectable in the serum.
++ Passive cutaneous anaphylaxis.

What is all this IgE? We have suggested that it comprises
in large part, the sum of numerous potentiated IgE responses
against antigens, endogenous or environmental, to which the
animal has become naturally sensitized. Otherwise, we must
assume it to be non-antibody IgE, which is not known to exist,
or alternatively anti-parasitic IgE which is for some reason not
specifically detectable.

The latter is at least theoretically possible. Although
parasite specific IgE cannot be detected in the serum until 16
days or so after infection its presence on mast cells can be
demonstrated as early as days 7 to 10, either in vitro by antigen
induced histame release (Wilson & Bloch, 1968) or in vivo through
the occurrence of immediate hypersensitivity reactions following
antigen challenge (Urquhart et al., 1965; Jarrett & Stewart,
1973b). Since distant sites, e.g. the skin, show increasing
sensitization from day 10 onwards some parasite specific IgE
must be continuously released into the circulation from its site
of production (Jarrett & Stewart, 1973b). That it cannot be
detected (by PCA) is probably because there is just not enough of
it present in the circulation at any one time. We have suggested
that the level builds up and becomes detectable later when the
reagin absorbing capacity of the body mast cells has been
satisfied. But there is another possibility, that parasite
specific reagins in the circulation are rendered undetectable in
the PCA test by complexing with antigen produced by the worms.
In this way the subsequent appearance of these antibodies might
be explained by the fact that N. brasiliensis infection is
terminated by worm expulsion from the intestine this process
being virtually complete at 16 days (reviewed by Jarrett &
Urquhart, 1971). Whether a significant proportion of the total
IgE response could represent complexed parasite specific IgE
remains to be seen.

The occurrence of elevated IgE levels in N. brasiliensis
infection has been confirmed (Carson, Metzger & Bloch, 1975;
Ishizaka et al., 1975) and has been reported also in infections
of the rat with F. hepatica (Jarrett & Bazin, 1974 and
Schistosoma mansoni (Rousseaux, Capron & Bazin, 1975).
Differences amongst various rat strains have been demonstrated:
although considerably raised IgE levels have occurred in all
strains studied, these have been much higher in Hooded Lister
than in Wistar or Fischer rats (Jarrett & Bazin, 1974; Rousseaux,
Capron & Bazin, 1975; Jarrett, Haig & Bazin, 1976).

TEMPORAL RELATIONSHIP BETWEEN PARASITE SPECIFIC,
POTENTIATED AND TOTAL IgE RESPONSES

The events after a first and second infection of Hooded

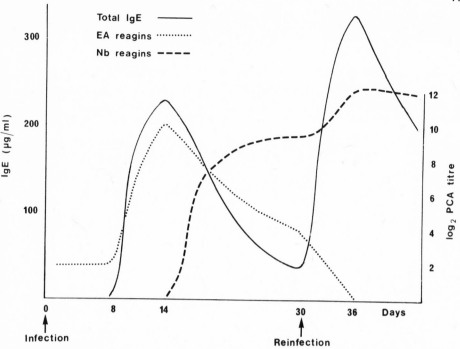

Fig. 1: Temporal relationship between total IgE and egg-albumin
(EA) and N. brasiliensis (N.b) IgE responses in a first and
second N. brasiliensis infection of Hooded Lister rats.

Lister rats with N. brasiliensis are represented in Fig. 1.

     During a first infection, the potentiated reagin response
and the elevation of total IgE occur synchronously reaching a
peak 12 to 14 days after infection, with the fastest rate of
production occurring between days 8 and 10 (Jarrett, Haig & Bazin,
1976).

     The two non-specific responses also decline together, and
during this decline, parasite specific reagins appear and rise
to a high level. The peak of the parasite specific IgE response
occurs some 2-3 weeks later, when both the potentiated and total
IgE responses have largely declined. Moderately elevated total
IgE levels persist however for a long time, being in the region
of 25 μg/ml 80 days after infection.

     The events after reinfection are different. Total IgE rises
again, often to even higher levels than in a first infection, but
this occurs by the 6th day and is synchronous with the parasite

specific secondary IgE response. On the other hand, the EA
response is not repotentiated and in fact, in our experience,
often disappears altogether after reinfection.

One important conclusion from these results is that the
potentiated reagin response and the total IgE response are almost
certainly the result of the same stimulus. The potentiated
response is in fact an indicator system within a larger phenomenon.

We do not know why the EA response is not repotentiated
following reinfection. Perhaps a suppressor mechanism is
activated or alternatively the EA specific cells involved are,
for other reasons, no longer susceptible to the stimulating effect.
The fact however that known IgE responses are not repotentiated
leaves us with the question whether the same is true of our
hypothetical potentiated IgE responses, or whether they on the
other hand are potentiated in a second as in a first infection.
If they are not, what is the antibody content of this secondary
total IgE response? It must surely be of the same nature as in
the primary total IgE response. Quantitative considerations
indicate at any rate that it is not all parasite specific since
total IgE levels rise by a far greater factor than parasite
specific IgE: also the kinetics of the decline of these two
responses are quite different. For the present the problem has
become more complicated than originally conceived.

A second conclusion regarding the mechanisms of the non-
specific IgE stimulating effect arises from the advanced
occurrence of the total IgE response in the second infection, a
matter which is discussed below.

While the ability to stimulate IgE responses non-specifically
as well as specifically could be common to most if not all
helminth parasites, we must not expect the patterns just described
to be exactly the same for each infection. Indeed, this particular
temporal relationship is probably peculiar to N. brasiliensis
infection of the rat. The time course of these events in any
other host-parasite relationship must be influenced by such
factors as the size, duration and vigour of the infection and the
occurrence of reinfections, and also by the immunological
characteristics of the host species.

There is already evidence that this is so. Potentiated
reagin responses to DNP-EA have been reported recently in
N. brasiliensis infected mice, but in this species it seems that
the parasite infection must be given 5 to 14 days before
immunization with antigen in order to have a potentiating effect
(Kojima & Ovary, 1975). Also the potentiated response occurs
much later relative to infection than in rats (i.e. around
25-35 days after infection). This is surprising, since in the

mouse, which is not a natural host for N. brasiliensis, worms are
expelled from the small intestine even earlier than they are in
the rat.   The potentiation which has been reported is then
occurring long after the worms have gone.   It would be
interesting to see what the estimation of mouse total IgE could
contribute to this picture.

In the rat the physical presence of actively secreting worms
seems important, and in rats given repeated infections with
N. brasiliensis both the potentiated (Orr, Riley & Doe, 1972) and
the total IgE responses can be to some extent prolonged.   In this
context it is notable that the immune response of the host causes
pathological structural changes to N. brasiliensis worms before
they are actually expelled (Ogilvie & Hockley, 1968).   Since such
worms cannot become re-established upon transfer to a new host
it is obvious that adverse physiological effects have also
occurred.   An interesting result is that in young rats which are
to a considerable extent immunologically unresponsive to
N. brasiliensis and in which worm expulsion is incomplete
(Jarrett, Jarrett & Urquhart, 1966, 1968) total IgE levels
nevertheless rise and fall at the same time as in adult rats
despite the continuing presence of a sizeable worm burden
(Table 2).   The conclusion from this result is that either the
worms in these unresponsive rats have ceased to secrete the IgE
stimulating factor, or alternatively that despite its continuous
secretion a regulating mechanism acts to decrease IgE production.

TABLE 2

Total IgE and worm burdens in adult and young rats
after infection with 1000 N. brasiliensis larvae

Days after infection	Adult rats		Young rats	
	µg/ml IgE	Nos. Worms	µg/ml IgE	Nos. Worms
7	2.49 ± 1.35	308 ± 66	0.98 ± 0.03	375 ± 82
14	147 ± 26	64 ± 37	91 ± 54	286 ± 84
24	53 ± 20	9 ± 4	30 ± 3.9	218 ± 65
35	34 ± 13.6	8 ± 3	33 ± 10.7	228 ± 60

Groups of 5 rats were killed on each of the days shown and the
figures represent the mean ± S.E. of total IgE and worm numbers.
The young rats were 4-5 weeks old at infection.

MECHANISMS

The evidence thus far indicates that a substance largely produced by adult N. brasiliensis worms and absorbed across the intestinal epithelium selectively but non-specifically stimulates antigen primed IgE responses. This substance must of course ultimately have its effect on IgE B cells or their plasma cell progeny, and indeed an increase in the number of the latter has been shown (Ishizaka et al., 1976), but the possibilities are that the effect is exerted either directly on these cells or indirectly through an intermediary cell or sequence of cells.

In order to find if the effect was produced through T cells we have examined IgE production in N. brasiliensis infected thymus deprived rats (Jarrett & Ferguson, 1974). In these rats an IgE response to EA was more difficult to induce in the first place, but could be achieved in 30-50% of the animals by increasing the dose of antigen thereby presumably reducing the requirement for T cell help. After infection however, potentiation of the EA response did not occur, nor as we subsequently found was the total IgE level raised by more than a small amount (Table 3). The parasite specific IgE response was also greatly reduced or absent in these animals. It seems, therefore, that T cells are essentially involved in the stimulation of both parasite specific and parasite non-specific IgE.

TABLE 3

Effect of T cell depletion on rat IgE responses in N. brasiliensis infection

	T cell depleted rats	Normal rats
Total IgE μg/ml mean ± S.E.	6.16 ± 2.32	153 ± 16.9
Egg-albumin IgE G.M.* PCA titre (range)	9.2 (4-64)	1321 (512-4096)
N. brasiliensis IgE G.M. PCA titre (range)	12.9 (2-64)	722 (256-2048)

Groups of 8 normal or T cell depleted rats producing low levels of EA reagins were infected with 2000 N. brasiliensis larvae and were bled 12 and 20 days later. The total IgE and EA specific IgE responses shown above were estimated on day 12 and the N.b IgE response on day 20 of infection.

*Geometric mean passive cutaneous anaphylaxis titre.

The next question is which T cells are involved and how might they produce the observed effects? One possibility is that the parasite derived 'potentiator' has its effect directly and non-specifically on the heterologous antigen primed T cells which control the IgE responses destined for potentiation. In thymus deprived rats these cells would of course be absent.

However, let us return to the fact that the total IgE response in a reinfection with N. brasiliensis is maximum on day 6, instead of on day 12 as in a first infection and is clearly coincident with the parasite specific booster response. This indicates either that the total IgE is all parasite specific which as far as we can see it is not, or that its production is boosted by a non-specific IgE stimulating factor released from N. brasiliensis specific T cells on reactivation by N. brasiliensis antigen. By inference, in a primary infection, the mechanism of stimulation of the total IgE response which includes the potentiated reagin response would be the same. Such antigen non-specific T cell factors which may influence antibody production are by no means unknown (reviewed by Tada, 1975) although not usually shown to such dramatic effect.

In this scheme the same or similar T cells are involved in the parasite specific IgE response through a separate specific helper function.

The same conclusions have been reached by Kojima and Ovary (1975) to account for N. brasiliensis induced potentiation in the mouse. These are based on their observations that potentiation in a first infection coincided with the generation of both EA and N. brasiliensis specific T cells and that adoptive transfer of the latter to suitably stimulated mice could confer a measure of the potentiating ability.

We have now reached full circle and are again faced with the possibilities that the effect of this 'second step' non-specific IgE stimulating factor produced by T cells could be exerted either directly on IgE B cells or again via other T cells such as the antigen primed ones mentioned above. The further mechanism has not yet been elucidated.

EFFECTS OF THE IgE RESPONSES ON THE HOST

The effects of IgE responses on the parasites, i.e. the role of IgE in immunity to helminth infection will not be discussed here. Rather I will consider the question of the 'side effects' of the production of IgE on the host.

The hypersensitivity reactions occurring as a result of

parasite specific IgE responses have been discussed in detail
before and have been reviewed extensively by Murray (1972) and
Sadun (1972). Briefly, the naturally occurring hypersensitivity
response in N. brasiliensis infection is largely expressed in
gross alterations in the small intestine, i.e. hyperaemia,
increased vascular permeability and oedema leading to a leakage
of plasma into the lumen (Barth, Jarrett & Urquhart, 1966).
Electronmicroscopic examinations using the tracer enzyme
horseradish peroxidase have shown that the structural abnormality
underlying this 'leak lesion' is a breakdown of the epithelial
cell junctions which normally act as a barrier to the egress of
macromolecules (Murray et al., 1971). This lesion is the basis
of protein-losing enteropathies of parasitic infections.
Associated with these events is a dramatic increase in the
number of mast cells in the lamina propria (Miller & Jarrett,
1971) and these have been shown to be discharging their contents
(Murray, 1972). The lesion is rapidly resolved when the worms
are expelled. Additionally, as previously mentioned
hypersensitivity can be demonstrated by the occurrence of
immediate skin reactions following intradermal, or anaphylactic
shock following intravenous injection of N. brasiliensis antigen
from as early as 10 days after infection.

What is the effect on the host of the non-specific IgE in
N. brasiliensis infection? As far as the potentiated reagin
response is concerned, very little. Hooded Lister rats develop
a high degree of hypersensitivity as a result of immunization
with EA and B. pertussis alone. The increase in titre of specific
IgE antibodies brought about by infection with N. brasiliensis has
negligible effects on the degree of hypersensitivity of the animal
(Jarrett & Stewart, 1973b).

The increase in total IgE on the other hand has very marked
effects, not on the production of hypersensitivity reactions but
in their inhibition. Infected rats become almost completely
refractory to passive sensitization with exogenous reaginic serum
for the production either of PCA reactions or anaphylactic shock
(Jarrett et al., 1971) in exactly the same way as has been
reported for human myeloma patients (Johansson, 1971; Ogawa
et al., 1971) and due presumably to the same mechanism, i.e. the
pre-emption of mast cell receptors by actively produced IgE. An
exactly comparable situation was subsequently shown in helminth
infected human beings (Bazaral, Orgel & Hamburger, 1973).
Recently, this effect has been demonstrated in vitro in both
species: mast cells removed from N. brasiliensis infected rats
will take up 90% less IgE than mast cells from uninfected animals
(Ishizaka et al., 1975) and allergic sensitization of human lung
fragments is prevented by prior incubation in the serum of
parasitised individuals (Godfrey & Gradidge, 1976).

The severity of individual hypersensitivities induced by passive sensitization is thus up to a point inversely related to the total IgE levels of the recipient. Whether the same is true of naturally occurring hypersensitivities it is too early to say, but it would seem to follow.

Could the non-specific stimulation of IgE in helminth infection in fact be designed, by providing competition for mast cell receptors, to reduce the severity of allergic reactions to the parasite allergens per se. In prolonged or heavy infections this could be an important function. Again, unrelated allergies might be coincidentally affected.

It has been noticed that clinical allergies, to pollen for instance, occur less frequently in rural Africa where parasitic infection is ubiquitous and total IgE levels are high (Godfrey, 1975). Many other factors might of course influence that situation and further careful studies will be necessary before the full effects of both helminth specific and non-specific IgE will perhaps become clear.

Meanwhile, the intriguing association between helminth infection and IgE production is drawing increasing attention from immunologists and clinicians as well as parasitologists. Hopefully this will promote a clearer understanding of the mechanism of IgE production and of its physiological as well as its pathological role.

SUMMARY

It has been shown that helminth parasites of the rat, in addition to evoking a parasite-specific IgE response have the facility, acting via T cells, to exert a profound effect on unrelated IgE production. This is manifest in the potentiation of existing IgE responses to other antigens and in a great elevation of total serum IgE. The non-specific stimulating effect of helminths, which is exerted selectively on IgE antibody responses, is mediated by a substance secreted by live worms.

From thymectomy and time course studies in rats infected with N. brasiliensis the evidence by implication is that a non-specific IgE stimulating factor is produced by parasite specific T cells following their activation by a parasite derived 'potentiating' antigen. Whether the IgE stimulating factor has its effect directly on IgE B cells or again indirectly on the antigen specific T cells controlling their responses is not yet clear.

The production of helminth specific and non-specific IgE

has particular effects on the host, quite apart from those effects which may ultimately be exerted on the parasites. Thus, the possession of helminth specific IgE leads not surprisingly to helminth specific hypersensitivity, the nature and severity of allergic reactions in any infection being dependent to a large extent on the situation and number of the parasites in the host.

The potentiation of existing individual IgE responses to unrelated antigens (by N. brasiliensis infection) appears to have negligible effects, in that the animals do not thereby become more hypersensitive to those antigens. On the other hand, the great increase in the amount of total IgE can be shown to confer an 'allergy protective effect' in that infected rats show poor passive sensitization with reaginic serum for cutaneous or systemic anaphylaxis due to the saturation of mast cell receptors by actively produced IgE. It could be that an essentially similar competitive mechanism acts in naturally infected animals to diminish the severity of parasite-specific or other acute allergic reactions.

ACKNOWLEDGEMENTS

This research was generously supported by grants from the Asthma Research Council, the Medical Research Council, the Royal Society and the Wellcome Trust.

REFERENCES

Barth, Ellen E.E., Jarrett, W.F.H. & Urquhart, G.M. (1966). Studies on the mechanism of the self-cure reaction in rats infected with N. brasiliensis. Immunology, 10, 459.

Bazaral, M., Orgel, Alice & Hamburger, R.N. (1973). The influence of serum IgE levels of selected recipients including patients with allergy, helminthiasis and tuberculosis on the apparent P-K titre of a reaginic serum. Clin. Exp. Immunol., 14, 117.

Bazin, H., Beckers, A., Deckers, C. & Moriame, M. (1973). Transplantable immunoglobulins secreting tumours in rats V. Monoclonal immunoglobulins secreted by 250 illeocaecal immunocytomas in Lou/W & LE rats. J. Natn. Cancer Inst., 51, 1351.

Bazin, H., Queringecun, P., Beckers, A., Heremans, J.F. & Dessy, F. (1974). Transplantable immunoglobulin secreting tumours in the rat IV. Sixty three IgE secreting immunocytoma tumours.

Immunology, 26, 713.

Binaghi, R.A. & Benacerraf, B. (1964). The production of
anaphylactic antibody in the rat. J. Immunol., 92, 920.

Bloch, K.J., Ohman, J.C., Waltin, J. & Cygan, R.W. (1973).
Potentiated reagin response : initiation with minute doses of
antigen and alum followed by infection with N. brasiliensis.
J. Immunol., 110, 197.

Carson, D., Metzger, H. & Bloch, K.J. (1975). Serum IgE levels
during the potentiated reagin response to egg-albumin in rats
infected with N. brasiliensis. J. Immunol., 114, 521.

Godfrey, R.C. (1975). Asthma and IgE levels in rural and urban
communities in The Gambia. Clinical Allergy, 5, 201.

Godfrey, R.C. & Gradidge, C.F. (1976). Allergic sensitization of
human lung fragments prevented by saturation of IgE binding sites.
Nature, 259, 484.

Ishizaka, Teruko, Konig, W., Kurata, M., Mauser, Linda & Ishizaka,
K. (1975). Immunologic properties of mast cells from rats
infected with N. brasiliensis. J. Immunol., 115, 1078.

Ishizaka, Teruko, Urban, J.F. & Ishizaka, K. (1976). IgE
formation in the rat following infection with N. brasiliensis.
I. Proliferation and differentiation of IgE B cells.
Cellular Immunology (in press).

Johansson, S.G.O. (1971). Personal communication.

Jarrett, Ellen, E.E. (1972). Potentiation of reaginic (IgE)
antibody to ovalbumin in the rat following sequential trematode
and nematode infections. Immunology, 22, 1099.

Jarrett, Ellen, E.E. (1973). Reaginic antibodies and helminth
infection. Vet. Rec., 93, 480.

Jarrett, Ellen & Bazin, H. (1974). Elevation of total serum IgE
in rats following helminth parasite infection. Nature, 251, 613.

Jarrett, Ellen & Ferguson, Anne (1974). Effect of T cell
depletion on the potentiated reagin response. Nature, 250, 420.

Jarrett, Ellen, E.E., Haig, D.M. & Bazin, H. (1976). Time course
studies on rat IgE production in N. brasiliensis infection.
Clin. Exp. Immunol., 24 (in press).

Jarrett, Ellen, E.E., Henderson, D., Riley, Patricia & White, R.G.

(1972). The effect of various adjuvant regimens and of nematode infection on the reaginic antibody response to ovalbumin in the rat. Int. Arch. Allergy, 42, 775.

Jarrett, Ellen, E.E., Jarrett, W.F.H. & Urquhart, G.M. (1966). Immunological unresponsiveness in adult rats to the nematode N. brasiliensis induced by infection in early life. Nature, 211, 1310.

Jarrett, Ellen, E.E., Jarrett, W.F.H. & Urquhart, G.M. (1968). Immunological unresponsiveness to helminth parasites: I. The pattern of N. brasiliensis infection in young rats. Exp. Parasit., 23, 151.

Jarrett, Ellen, E.E., Orr, T.S.C. & Riley, Patricia (1971). Inhibition of allergic reactions due to competition for mast cell sensitization sites by two reagins. Clin. Exp. Immunol., 9, 585.

Jarrett, Ellen, E.E. & Stewart, Diana (1972). Potentiation of rat reaginic (IgE) antibody by helminth infection. Simultaneous potentiation of separate reagins. Immunology, 23, 749.

Jarrett, Ellen, E.E. & Stewart, Diana C. (1973a). Potentiation of rat reaginic (IgE) antibody by N. brasiliensis infection. Effect of modification of life cycle of the parasite on the host. Clin. Exp. Immunol., 15, 79.

Jarrett, Ellen, E.E. & Stewart, Diana C. (1973b). The significance of circulating IgE. Correlation of amount of circulating reaginic antibody with cutaneous sensitivity in the rat. Immunology, 24, 37.

Jarrett, Ellen, E.E. & Stewart, Diana C. (1974). Rat IgE production. I. Effect of dose of antigen on primary and secondary reaginic antibody resonses. Immunology, 27, 365.

Jarrett, Ellen, E.E. & Urquhart, G.M. (1971). The immune response to nematode infection. International Review of Tropical Medicine, 4, 53. Academic Press.

Kojima, S. & Ovary, Z. (1975). Effect of N. brasiliensis infection on anti-hapten IgE antibody response in the mouse. II. Mechanism of potentiation of the IgE antibody response to a heterologous hapten-carrier conjugate. Cellular Immunology, 17, 383.

Miller, H.R.P. & Jarrett, W.F.H. (1971). Immune reactions in mucous membranes. I. Intestinal mast cell response during helminth expulsion in the rat. Immunology, 20, 277.

Mota, I. (1964). The mechanism of anaphylaxis. I. Production and biological properties of mast cell sensitizing antibody. Immunology, 7, 681.

Murray, M. (1972). Immediate hypersensitivity effector mechanisms. II. In vivo reactions. "Immunity to animal parasites". Ed. Soulsby, E.J.L. Academic Press, p.155.

Murray, M., Jarrett, W.F.H. & Jennings, F.W. (1971). Mast cells and the macromolecular leak in intestinal immunological reactions. Immunology, 21, 17.

Ogawa, M., McIntyre, R., Ishizaka, K., Ishizaka, T., Terry, W.D. & Waldman, T.A. (1971). Biologic properties of E. myeloma proteins. Am. J. Med., 51, 193.

Ogilvie, Bridget M. (1964). Reagin-like antibodies in animals immune to helminth parasites. Nature, 204, 91.

Ogilvie, Bridget M. (1967). Reagin-like antibodies in rats infected with the nematode parasite N. brasiliensis. Immunology, 12, 113.

Ogilvie, Bridget M. & Jones, Valerie E. (1973). Immunity in the parasitic relationship between helminths and hosts. Progress in Allergy, 17, 94. S. Karger.

Ogilvie, Bridget M. & Hockley, D.J. (1968). Effect of immunity on N. brasiliensis adult worms: reversible and unreversible changes in infectivity reproduction and morphology. J. Parasitol., 54, 1073.

Orr, T.S.C. & Blair, A.M.J.N. (1969). Potentiated reagin response to egg-albumin and conalbumin in N. brasiliensis infected rats. Life Sciences, 8, part II, 1073.

Orr, T.S.C., Riley, Patricia & Doe, J.E. (1971). Potentiated reagin response to egg-albumin in N. brasiliensis infected rats. II. Time course of the reagin response. Immunology, 20, 185.

Orr, T.S.C., Riley, Patricia A. & Doe, J.E. (1972). Potentiated reagin response to egg-albumin in N. brasiliensis infected rats. III. Further studies in the time course of the reagin response. Immunology, 22, 211.

Rousseaux, R., Capron, A. & Bazin, H. (1975). Personal communication.

Sadun, E.H. (1972). Homocytotropic antibody response to parasitic infections. "Immunity to animal parasites". Ed. Soulsby, E.J.L.

Academic Press, p.97.

Tada, T. (1975). Regulation of reaginic antibody formation in
animals. Progress in Allergy, 19, 122. S. Karger.

Urquhart, G.M., Mulligan, W., Eadie, R.M. & Jennings, F.W. (1965).
Immunological studies on N. brasiliensis in the rat: The role
of local anaphylaxis. Exp. Parasit., 16, 210.

Wilson, R.J.M. & Bloch, K.J. (1968). Homocytotropic antibody
response in rats infected with the nematode N. brasiliensis
J. Immunol., 100, 622.

DISCUSSION

ISHIZAKA, T.: We have examined the development of IgE bearing B cells and IgE plasma cells in mensenteric lymphnodes and
spleen after infection by the use of immunofluorescence and
autoradiography. Before infection the percentage of IgE bearing
cells was less than 0.5. The number of IgE B cells started to
increase 8 days after infection and reached maximum at 14 days
after infection.

When neonatally thymectomized rats were infected with larvae, IgE bearing cells appeared in both mesenteric lymphnodes
and spleen at 8 days after infection and reached maximum at 14
days. The percentage of IgE bearing cells was 3 to 4 times higher than that observed in non-thymectomized rats. However, very
low IgE levels and no IgE antibody against worm antigen was
formed in the thymectomized rats.

These results, led us to speculate that T cells are not
involved in the development of IgE B cells, but are required
for the differentiation of IgE B cells to plasma cells.

ISHIZAKA, K.: You mentioned that enhancement of IgE production is caused by a factor secreted by living adult worms.
Do you have any evidence that the factor is really secreted
from the living adult worms? I am wondering whether the factor
could be formed by inflammation.

JARRETT: The evidence that a potentiating factor is produced by live worms is circumstantial in that potentiation cannot be reproduced by the injection of dead worm extracts and
in the fact that potentiation is largely stimulated by adult
worms confined to the intestinal lumen.

It is of course possible that there is an intervening
step such as you suggest but then we would need to assume that
the inflammation of parasitic infection is quite different from
that occurring in other diseases.

ISHIZAKA, K.: I am wondering whether filtrate from cultured worms may have the activity to enhance IgE production.

Have you ever performed such an experiment?

JARRETT: Yes, but so far we had not managed to inference the IgE response by this means.

BECKER: You have failed to obtain a repotentiation where you reinfect your rat. Are you able to obtain a secondary response on injection of ovalbumin at the same time?

JARRETT: Yes. Secondary responses can be obtained when the potentiated response will no longer occur, and the converse is also true - potentiated responses occur after infection of rats in which booster responses have been inhibited because of immunization with a large dose of antigen.

MÜLLER-EBERHARD: Is the IgE that is not directed against parasitic antigens in part anti-IgE, that is an anti-antibody?

JARRETT: That is not known.

GOETZL: What is the time course of subsidence of the parasite specific IgE antibody level?

In our experience with patients with filarial infections both the total IgE and the ability to release mediators from peripheral basophils by the introduction of specific antigen are marked decreased within several weeks of successful chemotherapy eliminating the infestation.

JARRETT: The parasite specific IgE response in N. brasiliensis infection declines slowly over some months even although most of the worms are expelled by day 18-20 of the infection.

UVNÄS: Which correlation is there between IgE level in serum and the sensitivity of isolated mast cells from rats?

JARRETT: In the straight forward parasite specific situation there is no correlation between IgE level in the serum and sensitivity of mast cells. Both intact rats and their isolated mast cells become sensitive to N. brasiliensis before the appearance of parasite specific IgE in the circulation.

Increments in the sensitivity, as measured by skin test reaction diameter, can be detected in the few days preceeding the appearance of the parasite specific IgE and for a day or two thereafter. However, after day 16 or so following infection there is no further appreciable increase in the level of hypersensitivity as measured either by skin tests, or by susceptibility to systemic anaphylaxis despite the very marked increase in the level of antiparasite reagins which subsequently occurs.

The most logical explanation of this state of affairs is that once the mast cell receptors are saturated either by specific or non-specific IgE or any combination of the two further increments in circulation of specific IgE become irrelevant to mast cell sensitivity.

BAZIN: The fact that rats cannot be sensitized after a parasitic infection seems reasonable if we remember the long half life of normal IgE in the skin (Tada et al. Int. Arch. A. 1975, 48, 116). The specific receptors of the mast cells are occupied and the new IgE antibodies cannot bind until the former IgE molecules are removed.

JOHANSSON: In the light of your work with parasite infestated rats, could you, please, comment on an unusual case that we have.

Two years ago the patient was successfully treated from amoebiasis. His serum IgE level is still very high, about 500,000 kU/l. According to the work of dr. H. Bennich the IgE is monoclonal with light chains of kappa type. No amoeba antibody of IgE type can be detected in the serum.

JARRETT: I think all I can really contribute to that case is the fact that IgE levels are not usually raised in amoebiasis. Perhaps the amoebae were "red herrings".

JOHANSSON: Is your rat "nonsense-IgE" monoclonal?

JARRETT: That has not actually been determined but it is surely unlikely.

LICHTENSTEIN: I will report that man, in this circumstance behaves as the rat, e.g. if you "rush" desensitize man. The total IgE may go up 20-30 fold, but the patients sensitivity (skin test or basophil histamine release) does not change. This is not due to non-specific IgE, since as much as 50% may be specific IgE. I agree with you that it is because the mast cells are probably saturated.

This raises two points. The RAST in this case does not detect biological sensitivity in a quantitative way and in fact the IgE antibody in excess may protect the patient as if it were IgG blocking antibody.

MARSH: I believe that infestation of an animal with a second parasite can cause the expulsion of an already existing parasite. Does this mechanism relate to the potentiated IgE response which you have described?

JARRETT: What you speak of can happen by two mechanisms, occasionally there is cross reactivity and the immune response to one parasite can affect another.

The second mechanism is the one whereby the sheer physical changes induced by local anaphylactic reaction to one parasite can make life untenable for co-existing parasites in the same area. This has been demonstrated with gastrointestinal parasites of sheep. As far as I know these phenomena do not relate to the potentiated reagin response.

IgE-MYELOMAS IN RATS

Hervé Bazin and Andrée Beckers

Experimental Immunology Unit, Faculty of Medicine,
University of Louvain
Clos Chapelle-aux-champs, 30-1200 BRUSSELS-Belgium

INTRODUCTION

Monoclonal immunoglobulins synthesized by myelomas (plasmocytomas, immunocytomas) are a valuable asset in the study of
structure, synthesis and physiological properties of the immunoglobulins. This type of tumour is wellknown in man. In animals,
it has been described in mice (Dunn, 1954), dogs (Groulade,
Morel, Creyssel & Groulade, 1959), hamsters (Mohr & Dontenwill,
1964), horses (Dorrington & Rockey, 1968) and cats (Kehoe,
Hurvitz & Capra, 1972). But the very low spontaneous incidence
of this type of tumour in animals has not provided a great
variety of different monoclonal immunoglobulins. Moreover, in
most of these species, tumourtransplantation is not possible
for lack of inbred strains and therefore, the quantity of myeloma proteins available is generally restricted.

The induced plasmocytomas in the BALB/c mouse, described
by Merwin and Algire (1959) and developed by Potter and Robertson (1960) provided immunologists with an extremely important
and precious tool. However, the "BALB/c plasmocytomas" model
is limited by unique species, small-sized animals and mainly,
absence of monoclonal IgD or IgE immunoglobulins.

Obviously, experimental studies of physico-chemical or
biological properties of IgE immunoglobulins have not progres-
sed very easily. However, since IgE was first described (Ishizaka and Ishizaka, 1966), immunoglobulins analogous to human
reagins have been discovered in various animal species, largely
as a result of their biological properties, in the monkey
(Ishizaka, Ishizaka & Tada, 1969), rat (Stechschulte, Orange &

125

Austen, 1970; Jones & Edwards, 1971), rabbit (Ishizaka, Ishizaka & Hornbrook, 1970), cattle (Hammer, Kickhöfen & Schmidt, 1971), mouse (Prouvost-Danon, Binaghi, Rochas & Boussac-Aron, 1972) and dog (Halliwell, Schwartzman & Rockey, 1972). However, the serum level of the reaginic antibodies or even of the total IgE is very low in all species, and in spite of increases in certain circumstances (Johansson, 1967; Johansson, Mellbin & Vahlquist, 1968b; Gleich, Averbeck & Swedlund, 1971) the purification of this immunoglobulin is difficult. Nevertheless, Aalberse, Brummelhuis and Reerink-Brongers (1973) and Isersky, Kulczycki and Metzger (1974) succeeded in isolating human or rat polyclonal IgE with a reasonable degree of purity.

The discovery of an IgE myeloma in man (Johansson & Bennich, 1967) considerably enhanced the technical possibilities of the study of IgE in this species.

In animals, in spite of some cross reactions between human and animal IgE (monkey by Ishizaka et al., 1969; dog by Halliwell et al., 1972 and numerous species by Neoh, Jahoda, Rowe & Voller, 1973), experimental studies have been severely limited by the lack of purified IgE as well as of specific antisera to epsilon chain. The discovery of rat monoclonal IgE synthesized by transplantable tumours gave great impetus to the experimental study of IgE immunoglobulin and the antibodies in this class (Bazin, Beckers, Deckers & Moriamé, 1973; Bazin, 1974).

IMMUNOCYTOMAS OF LOU/Wsl RATS

Animals

The rats used in this study are all from the LOU/Wsl strain or from their crosses with the AUGUST/Wsl, AxC/Wsl and OKAMOTO/Wsl inbred strains. "LOU" is an abreviation of LOUVAIN, and "Wsl" is the official code for our own laboratory animals (Festing & Staats, 1973). Two substrains of LOU/Wsl rats were obtained. Thus the LOU/C/Wsl rat substrain was selected for its high incidence of immunocytomas and the LOU/M/Wsl rat substrain was chosen for its reproduction rate which, although better than that of the C substrain, is still not very high. These two substrains are mutually histocompatible, as shown by indefinite acceptance of skin grafts from LOU/C/Wsl substrain by all LOU/M/Wsl male breeders (Bazin et al., 1973). All the known details concerning the origin of these rats have already been described (Bazin, Deckers, Beckers & Heremans, 1972).

The rats were fed with commercial rat pellets (UAR-Villemoisson sur Orge-France) and had free access to tap water. They were maintained in Makrolon cages.

Ileocecal Immunocytomas

The LOU/C/Wsl rats have a high incidence of immunoglobulin-secreting tumours or immunocytomas which appear in the ileocecal lymph node, after 8 months (Bazin et al., 1972;Bazin et al., 1973). Tumours of this type were first identified in the LOU rat ancestors by Mainsin, Dunjic and Maldague in 1955, but similar tumours had apparently been sporadically seen previously in other rats (Bazin et al., 1972), the incidence varying from 0 to 3% in rats from a number inbred or outbred strains. About 20 different publications give descriptions of cases of lymphosarcoma or reticulum cell sarcoma originating in the ileocecal lymph node, but it is impossible to be sure that they are the same type of tumour, since no study of serum proteins has been performed on these animals. Fig. 1 shows the age distribution of LOU immunocytomas. The first immunocytomas make their appearence in eight to nine month-old rats. The incidence appears to be the highest at 12 to 15 months. However, some of them

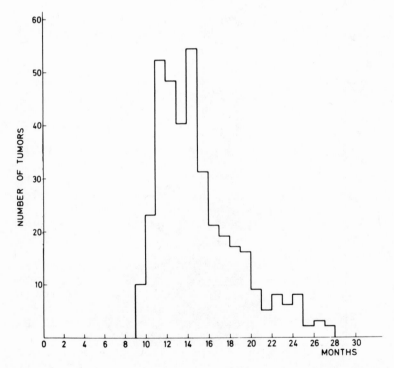

Figure 1. Age distribution of 374 spontaneous ileocecal immunocytomas in the LOU/C/Wsl rats.

may appear in twenty-seven month-old rats, the maximum age for
these animals in our laboratory. The age distribution of the
immunocytomas in LOU rats seems to be identical in males and
females (Fig. 2). By contrast, the incidence is different.
Table 1 shows the percentage of ileocecal immunocytomas in
male and female LOU/C/Wsl rats. In male rats, the tumour incidence is double that in females: 34.4 and 17 per cent respectively. By comparison, the incidence of ileocecal immunocytomas in LOU/M/Wsl is very low: 1 to 2 per cent.

Various manipulations have been tried to increase the
incidence of ileocecal LOU immunocytomas or to shorten their
latent period. These consisted of monthly intraperitoneal injections of 1 ml 3 Pristane   (Aldrich, USA) from the age of 2.5
months; similar injections of complete Freund adjuvant (DIFCO);
a single dose of irradiation of 300 or 500 rads, or divided

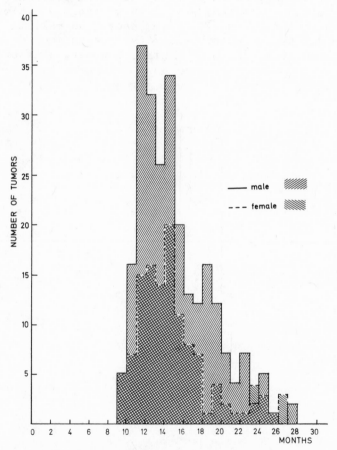

Figure 2. Age of incidence in male and female of 374 LOU spontaneous ileocecal immunocytomas.

doses (3x150 rads) at monthly intervals on the whole body or
the ileocecal area only, and the administration of an acellu-
lar extract of immunocytomas to new born LOU/C/Wsl rats. None
of these attempts significantly increased the incidence or
shortened the latent period of LOU/C/Wsl rat immunocytomas.

Macroscopic and Microscopic Descriptions of the Immunocytomas

The site of origin of the immunoglobulin-secreting tumours
developed by the LOU rats and their crosses with some inbred
strains appears to be the ileocecal lymph node. The tumours
make their appearance in the rat peritoneal cavity in the form
of solid masses. They are mobile under the fingers and easy
to detect by palpation of the abdomen. They grow fast and the
tumour-carriers generally die within one month, after the tumour has become palpable. At autopsy, the primitive tumour nearly always presents as one or more nodules in the ileocecal region. In some cases, when the tumour has evolved, all the ab-
dominal viscera are infiltrated with metastases. The tumours
are always highly vascularized and necrotic in places. Ascitic
fluid is present sometimes and can be helpful in detecting the
primitive tumour. Metastases are observed in the mediastinal
lymph node as well as in the pleural cavity.

The histological appearence of these tumours in LOU ancestors was described by Maisin et al., (1955). In most of the
cases, proliferating cells cannot be described as plasma cells.
They are poorly differentiated. The secreting tumour cells
exhibit a marked uniformity in size a fine granular nucleus

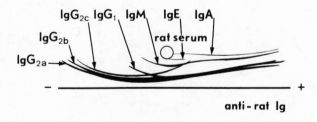

Figure 3. Schematic representation of combined immunoelectrophoretic pattern in agarose gel of the seven rat immunoglobulin
classes and subclasses.

Table 1. Incidence of ileocecal immunocytomas in LOU rats and their crosses and backcrosses with the AUGUST/Wsl, A x C/Wsl and OKAMOTO/Wsl rats.

	Number of immunocytomas/number of rats under observation and percentage.			
	male		female	
LOU/C/Wsl	145/422	(34.4%)	72/424	(17%)
LOU/M/Wsl	1/138	(0.7%)	7/328	(2.1%)
(LOU/C/Wsl ♀ x AUGUST/Wsl ♂)F1*	10/72	(14.0%)	5/77	(6.5%)
(LOU/C/Wsl ♀ x AxC/Wsl ♂)F1*	8/65	(12.3%)	7/78	(9.0%)
(LOU/C/Wsl ♀ x OKAMOTO/Wsl ♂)F1	0/61	(.0%)	0/57	(.0%)
LOU/C/IH(OKA)/Wsl (N3)	8/94	(8.5%)	3/73	(4.1%)

* Animals still under observation. The percentages given are a minimum evaluation of the incidence which will probably be higher.

with relatively small nucleoli and a rim of deeply basophilic
and pyroninophilic cytoplasm. In the electron microscope, this
type of cell displays a well-developed endoplasmic reticulum.
The cells of the non-secreting tumours are polymorphic with
respect to form and size. Their nuclei are grossly granular
with very large nucleoli. Their cytoplasm are poorly basophilic and their endoplasmic reticulum is underdeveloped, although
ribosomes may still occur in large numbers.

Etiology of LOU Rat Immunocytomas

The etiology is unknown. LOU immunocytomas possibly have
a viral origin and develop only on favourable genetic background. Table 1 shows that in both histocompatible rat strains,
LOU/M/Wsl and LOU/C/Wsl, there is a very different incidence
of tumours. Crosses between LOU/C/Wsl females and AUGUST/Wsl
or AxC/Wsl males produce F1 hybrids with a tumour incidence
less than that of the LOU/C/Wsl rats, but higher than the LOU/
M/Wsl incidence. In contrast, LOU/C/Wsl female rats crossed with
OKAMOTO/Wsl male rats give hybrids in which no tumours develop.

Therefore, one or more dominant loci of resistance to the
tumour incidence could exist in the OKAMOTO/Wsl strain. The
tumour incidence of LOU/C/IH(OKA)/Wsl (N3) rats, i.e. rats
approximately congenic to LOU/C rats and having the loci of
the OKAMOTO/Wsl heavy chains, has been studied. These rats
were derived from F1 hybrids backcrossed twice to female LOU/
C/Wsl rats, then crossed with each other and selected according
to their homozygozity for loci of the OKAMOTO/Wsl heavy chains
and their histocompatibility with LOU/C/Wsl rats. Their tumour
incidence is less than that of the F1 hybrids (LOU/C/Wsl x AU-
GUST/Wsl) or (LOU/C/Wsl x AxC/Wsl) although they possess about
80% of the LOU/C/Wsl rat genome.

Biosynthesis of Immunoglobulins

C. Deckers (1963) was the first to observe myeloma-like
proteins in the serum of LOU/C/Wsl rat ancestors, which were
carrying primitive or transplanted ileocecal tumours. A further
study showed that some of the LOU rat immunocytomas could also
secrete Bence Jones proteins, which were found in large quantities in their urine (Bazin & Beckers, unpublished results).
Now, seven classes or subclasses of immunoglobulins have been
described in rats (Bazin, Beckers & Querinjean, 1974a). Fig. 3
is a schematic representation of immunoelectrophoretic analysis
in agarose of immune rat serum, using an antiserum against various rat immunoglobulin (sub)-classes. Table 2 give the distribution of serum monoclonal immunoglobulins and Bence Jones

Table 2. Distribution of the monoclonal immunoglobulins
          synthesized by 250 consecutive LOU/C/Wsl ileo-
          cecal immunocytomas.

	secreting tumours	monoclonal Ig with or without Bence Jones proteins	Bence Jones proteins only
number of tumours	185	159	26
absolute percentage	74	64	10
percentage of secreting tumours	100	86	14

proteins synthesized by 250 LOU immunocytomas, which appeared
consecutively in our breeding colony. As can be seen, the percentage of secreting tumours in the LOU rat model is high and
comparable to that of the BALB/c induced plasmocytoma. The
class distribution of LOU monoclonal immunoglobulins is given
in Tables 3 and 5. The distribution is quite similar in different LOU substrains and LOU/C F1 hybrids: the most frequent
monoclonal proteins are the IgE class, closely followed by IgG1,
IgG2a and IgG2c, then the IgM and IgA, and finally IgG2b. The
IgE myeloma proteins always represent the highest percentage
(Table 4). IgE serum levels of LOU/C/Wsl rats carrying a primitive immunocytoma when sacrified are given in Fig. 4.

All the Bence Jones proteins secreted by LOU rat immunocytomas and studied so far have proved to be of Kappa type
(Querinjean, Bazin, Beckers, Deckers, Heremans & Milstein, 1972;
Wang, Fudenberg & Bazin, 1975; Wang, Fudenberg & Bazin, in
press). Only two light chains of LOU rat monoclonal immunoglobulins (IgG1 class) have been found to be of Lambda type (Querinjean, Bazin, Starace, Beckers, Deckers & Heremans, 1973).

However, most of the light chains of myeloma immunoglobulins and Bence Jones proteins produced by LOU rat immunocytomas
have not yet been studied. Percentages of Kappa and Lambda type
light chains of the LOU immunocytomas will probably be quite
similar to the non-myeloma rat light chains, i.e. about 95%
Kappa chain and 5% Lambda chain (Hood, Gray, Sanders & Dreyer,
1967).

Table 3. Class distribution of complete monoclonal immunoglobulins synthesized by immunocytomas from various crosses and backcrosses of LOU rats with different inbred strains.

	number of immunocytomas	number of Ig-secreting immunocytomas	IgM	IgA	IgE	IgG1	IgG2a	IgG2b	IgG2c	ND*
LOU/C/Wsl	612	383	11	12	160	150	23	3	20	4
LOU/M/Wsl	8	4	1	-	2	1	-	-	-	-
(LOU/C/Wsl ♀ xAUGUST/Wsl ♂)F1	15	9	-	-	8	1	-	-	-	-
(LOU/C/Wsl ♀ x AxC/Wsl ♂)F1	15	11	-	-	5	5	1	-	-	-
(LOU/C/Wsl ♀ x OKAMOTO/Wsl ♂)F1	0	-	-	-	-	-	-	-	-	-
LOU/C/IH(OKA)/Wsl (N3)**	11	7	1	-	4	1	1	-	-	-
Total	662	414	13	12	179	158	25	3	20	4

* not determined.

** F1 hybrids between LOU/C/Wsl and OKAMOTO/Wsl rats backcrossed twice with LOU/C/Wsl female rats and crossed between themselves afterwards. These rats carry the immunoglobulin heavy chain loci of OKAMOTO rats in a predominantly LOU/C/Wsl background.

Table 4. Number and percentage of IgE monoclonal proteins synthesized by LOU immunocytomas

	secreting immunocytomas	IgE monoclonal proteins	percentage
LOU/C/Wsl	383	160	41.8
LOU/M/Wsl	8	2	25.0
(LOU/C/Wsl ♀ x AUGUST/Wsl ♂)F1	15	8	53.4
(LOU/C/Wsl ♀ x AxC/Wsl ♂)F1	15	5	33.3
(LOU/C/Wsl ♀ x OKAMOTO/Wsl ♂)F1	0	–	–
LOU/C/IH(OKA)/Wsl (N3)	11	4	36.4
Total	414	179	43.2

Production of Monoclonal IgE

About 90% of primitive and spontaneous LOU immunocytomas
can be transplanted in LOU/C/Wsl, LOU/M/Wsl or their F1 hybrids. The tumours are removed under sterile conditions and
teased in a Petri dish. The tumour tissue is minced until it
can be aspirated through a 19-gauge needle into a syringe.
Approximately 0.1 to 0.2 ml is injected subcutaneously into
one side of the breast. This tumour tissue can also be inoculated into the peritoneal cavity. In this case, an ascitic
tumour can be obtained after few passages with most of the
immunocytomas. The ascitic tumour can be transplanted by ino-
culating recipient rats intraperitoneally with 0.2 to 0.5 ml
ascitic fluid.

After subcutaneous transplantation, the first palpable
nodules appear from one week to one month after inoculation.
In some cases, delays can be much longer, up to one month for
tumour appearence and three months for host death. The latent
periods of LOU immunocytomas are generally shortened as soon
as their ascitic form is obtained, i.e. after some transfers
by the intraperitoneal route.

The immunoglobulin secreting properties of LOU immunocytomas are quite variable. Generally, most of the tumours maintain
their ability to produce monoclonal proteins through a large
number of in vivo passages. For example, IgG1 and IgG2a secreting tumours have been transplanted for three years without any
change in production of monoclonal proteins. In some other cases,
the secreting properties decreased more or less rapidly. The IgE
producing tumours seem to be more prone to lose their secreting
properties. In most of the IgE myelomas, tumour production is
considerably reduced after one or two transplantations, and
disappears completely after some more passages. Few IgE immunocytomas have kept their monoclonal immunoglobulin synthesis for
a long time. IR2, IR162, IR183, IR331 and IR637 are the best
producers up to now. Monoclonal IgE serum levels from 10 to
20 mg/ml can normally be obtained with these tumour lines. A
great help in preserving LOU immunocytomas is storing them in
liquid nitrogen. The technique used has been described previously (Bazin et al., 1972). Periods of storage up to three years
left the malignant potential of the immunocytomas and their
secreting properties unaffected. Thus, it is possible to regain
production of IgE monoclonal proteins by returning to the first
tumour passages, when a line under exploitation has lost most
of its secreting properties.

Another possible method of producing IgE monoclonal proteins is to propagate the tumour in vitro as continuous lines.
The technique used for the first studies has been described by

Table 5.   Percentage of monoclonal immunoglobulins synthesized by 614 LOU
           immunocytomas and 472 BALB/c plasmocytomas

	IgM	IgA	IgE	IgG1	IgG2a	IgG2b	IgG2c IgG3	ND
LOU	3.1	3.1	41.9	39.0	6.2	0.8	4.9	1.0
BALB/c*	0.5	73.7	.0	10.2	6.9	8.4	0.3	-

* Potter , 1972.

Burtonboy, Bazin, Deckers, Beckers, Lamy & Heremans, (1973).
Various IgE immunocytomas have already been adapted to in vitro
cultures by Bennich (IR2-IR162), Metzger (IR162) and Krembel,
Savage and Samaille (IR331) (personal communication). These in
vitro continuous cell lines can be transferred into LOU/C/Wsl
rats and produce immunocytomas which cannot be distinguished
from the original tumours, at least after short periods of
culture.

PHYSICO-CHEMICAL PROPERTIES OF RAT MONOCLONAL IgE

Purification of IgE Monoclonal Protein

     Serum or ascitic fluid collected from rats bearing IgE im-
munocytomas is diluted twice in saline and precipitated by ammonium sulfate at 50 per cent final concentration (Carson, Metzger & Bazin, 1975). The precipitate is washed with 50 percent
saturated ammonium sulfate, resuspended in saline and dialyzed
against 0.05 M tris-HCl buffer, pH 8.0. This fraction is applied to a DEAE-cellulose column and eluted with a convex gradient. The starting buffer is 0.05 M tris-HCl, pH 8.0; and the

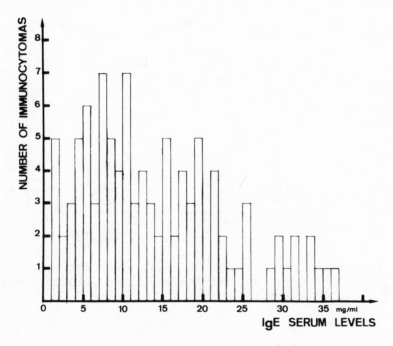

Figure 4. IgE serum concentration of LOU/C/Wsl rats bearing
a primitive IgE secreting immunocytoma when killed.

limit buffer 0.10 M tris-HCl, 0.40 NaCl, pH 8.0. The monoclonal
IgE is concentrated by ultrafiltration, dialyzed against 0.10
M tris-HCl, 0.15 M NaCl, 1 percent sodium azide pH 8.0 and applied to a AcA 34 (LKB Sweden) column. The elution pattern obtained gives three peaks, the first is monoclonal IgE, the
second, IgG immunoglobulins, and the third, transferrin. The
purity of the IgE monoclonal protein is good, as assessed by
immunoelectrophoresis and Ouchterlony tests. For example, 30
ml of serum from rats carrying the IR162 immunocytoma have been
precipitated by ammonium sulphate dialyzed and applied on a
DEAE-cellulose (DE-32-Whatman) column (diameter 3 cm - length
30 cm). Figure 5 gives the elution pattern obtained. Peak 2 was
applied on a AcA 34 column (diameter 2.5 cm - length 200 cm).

Figure 6 shows the elution pattern where peak 1 represents
the purified IR162 protein. Figure 7 is an agarose gel electrophoresis showing the fraction 2 of the DEAE chromatography, the
fractions 1, 2 and 3 of the AcA 34 gel filtration, as compared
to a normal rat serum and a serum from rat bearing the IR162
immunocytoma. The extinction coefficient of the myeloma IR162
IgE was given as 13.6 at 280 nm for a solution containing 1%
protein (Kulczycki & Metzger, 1974).

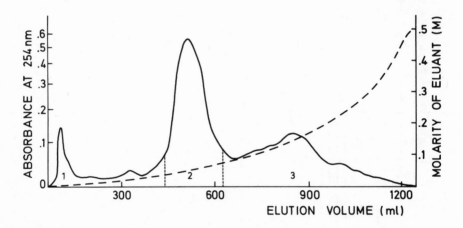

Figure 5. Elution pattern of a DEAE-cellulose chromatography
of serum proteins from rat carrying the IR162 immunocytoma,
salted out by 50% ammonium sulphate.

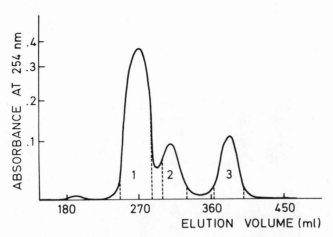

Figure 6. Gel filtration on AcA34 of the fraction 2 DEAE-
chromatography of rat serum bearing the IR162 immunocytoma.

Electrophoretic Mobility

In 1% agarose gel, at pH 8.6, most of the rat IgE myeloma
proteins were found to migrate as relatively homogenous components, although their bands were never as sharp as those of
monoclonal proteins from other classes. Nearly all of them are
situated in the $\gamma 2$ (or else the $\gamma 1$) range.

Heat Lability of IgE Myeloma Protein

Rat monoclonal IgE proteins, as normal rat IgE, are no
longer precipitated by specific antisera upon heating (Bazin,
Querinjean, Beckers, Heremans & Dessy, 1974b).

Molecular Weight

On Sephadex G200 (Pharmacia-Sweden), IgE monoclonal proteins are eluted with the first part of the second peak. On a
calibrated column of sephadex G200, the IR162 myeloma protein
gave a molecular weight estimate of 198,000 ($\pm$ 10.000) Daltons.
The purified IR2 protein sedimented as a homogenous peak in the
ultracentrifuge with a sedimentation coefficient ($S^0_{20,w}$) of

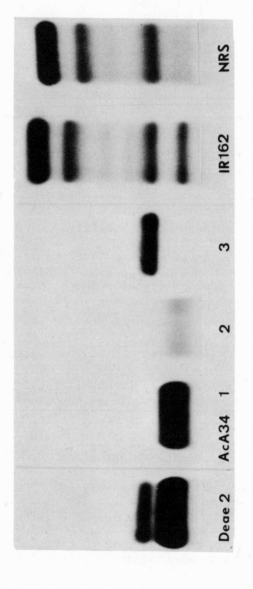

Figure 7. Agarose gel electrophoresis of DEAE-chromatography fraction 2, AcA34 gel filtration fractions 1,2 and 3, as compared to a serum of rat carrying the IR162 immunocytoma and a normal rat serum.

Table 6. Molecular weight of rat monoclonal immunoglobulins
         from different classes, as determined by gel filtra-
         tion on G200 Sephadex, SDS polyacrylamide gel electro-
         phoresis and ultracentrifugation.

Classes	Proteins studied	Gel filtration	Acrylamide electro-phoresis	Ultra-centrifugation
IgA	IR22	-	163 000	-
IgE	IR2-IR16-IR162	198 000	183 000	179 000
IgG1	IR27	150 000	157 000	157 000
IgG2a	IR25-IR33	150 000	155 000	148 000
IgG2c	IR64	150 000	155 000	155 000

7.6S, as compared to 6.4S and 6.8S for IgG2a (IR33) and IgG1
(IR27) immunoglobulins respectively analyzed under the same
conditions. The average value of molecular weight of three IgE
myeloma proteins (IR2, IR16, IR162) appeared to be 183,000 ±
8,000 when examined by SDS polyacrylamide gel electrophoresis.
Table 6 summarizes these data and compares them with the values
obtained for monoclonal immunoglobulins from other classes.

    The molecular size of heavy chains of different rat mono-
clonal immunoglobulin classes was estimated by SDS-7 percent
acrylamide gel electrophoresis and found to be 68,000 for the
IgE class (IR162), 58,000 for the IgA class (IR22) and 54 to
55,000 for the IgG class (IR27, IR25, IR64) (Bazin et al.,
1974 a and b.).

BIOLOGICAL PROPERTIES OF RAT MONOCLONAL IgE

Antigenic Determinants of IgE Monoclonal Proteins

    Immunization with class specific antigenic determinants
of rat IgE monoclonal proteins resulted in the production of
antiserum which abolished the PCA activity of rat serum containing antibodies to Nippostrongylus brasiliensis (Bazin et
al., 1974b). The same antiserum reacted with natural reaginic
IgE antibodies fixed on the mast cells in the normal rat skin,

as demonstrated by reverse cutaneous anaphylaxis and also rosette experiments (Bazin et al., 1974b). Therefore, rat monoclonal IgE carries some or all the antigenic determinants specific to normal rat IgE. Idiotypic determinants were found in
all the monoclonal IgE studied up to now (Tada, Okumura, Platteau, Beckers & Bazin, 1975). Allotypic determinants have not
been discovered so far in the epsilon chain of rat. But rat
IgE molecules carry Kappa chains where an allotype has been
described (Beckers, Querinjean & Bazin, 1974).

Antigenic relationships between human and rat normal IgE
immunoglobulins detected by their reaginic properties have been
described (Kanyeresi, Jaton & Bloch, 1971; Liacopoulou & Perelmutter, 1971). Neoh, Jahoda, Rowe and Voller (1973) have not been
able to demonstrate an IgE homologue in sera of normal or Nippostrongylus brasiliensis infected rats with chicken or sheep
anti-human epsilon chain sera (PS myeloma protein). We were also
unable to detect any common antigenic identity between human and
rat myeloma IgE by using passive hemagglutination of sheep red
blood cells covered with rat monoclonal IgE and several anti-
human epsilon chain antisera. Passive hemagglutination of these
same sheep red blood cells by a rabbit anti-rat epsilon chain
serum has not been inhibited by human myeloma IgE.

Strong arguments have been adduced by Prouvost-Danon,
Wyczilkowska, Binaghi and Abadie (1975) suggesting that structural similarities exist between rat and mouse IgE molecules.
In particular, a goat anti-rat epsilon chain serum (raised by
inoculation of purified IR2 monoclonal rat IgE) was able to
neutralize the reaginic activity of mouse anti-ovalbumin serum.

IgE Serum Level in Rat Bearing an Immunocytoma

In human serum, the normal IgE concentration has been
determined to be about 0.3 µg/ml (Johansson, Bennich and Wide,
1968). In animals, its serum concentration is also extremely
low as compared to the other immunoglobulin classes. With the
help of IgE myeloma proteins, serum concentrations of IgE have
been measured in a number of different strains of rats. Results
have been found to vary between 4 ng and 16 µg/ml, which does
not represent a variation greater than that observed in man
(Bazin et al., 1974a; Jarrett & Bazin, 1974; Capron, Dessaint,
Capron & Bazin, 1975; Bennich, personal communication). In rats
infected with Nippostrongylus brasiliensis or Schistosoma mansoni values up to 400 µg/ml have been described (Jarrett &
Bazin, 1974; Capron et al., 1975; Ishizaka, König, Kurata,
Mauser & Ishizaka, 1975; Rousseaux, personal communication).

A group of LOU/C/Wsl rats were bled every month of their

life. In rats which grew primitive tumours other than IgE tumours (whether or not these are secreting), IgE serum levels
were identical to those of rats without tumours. In rats producing IgE myeloma, IgE serum levels rose extremely rapidly
during the month of tumour appearance.

IgE Synthesizing Cells

In normal rats, the number of cells synthesizing IgE
immunoglobulins seems to be very small, whether in the intestinal or pulmonary mucosae or in the lymph node or splenic
tissues. After parasitic infection, numerous IgE plasma-cells
were found in the mesenteric lymph node. Few or none of these
same cells synthesizing IgE were disclosed in the spleen, intestinal mucosa or bronchial lymph nodes (Mayhofer, Bazin & Gowans,
in preparation).

In rats bearing an immunocytoma, the myeloma IgE synthesis
seems to be actually monoclonal, as some tumours are now transplanted in vivo or in vitro over years without any change in the
electrophoretic mobility and class-specific or idiotypic antigenic determinants of their secretion products.

Catabolism of Normal and Monoclonal IgE

Tada et al., (1975) described the half life of normal rat
IgE as 12.0 hours and 7.40 ± 0.89 days in serum and skin respectively as measured by reaginic activity. Studies on the serum
half lives of IR2, IR16 and IR162 monoclonal IgE proteins gave
values of 12.0 ± 2.1 hours as determined by radioactivity or by
quantitation of their idiotypic determinants. Since it is known
that the catabolic rate of mouse IgG subclass in serum is influenced by their concentration (Fahey & Robinson, 1963) the
same IR2 IgE myeloma protein was injected intravenously to three
groups of rats, which were given 2 ml normal serum, 2 ml serum
of rat bearing the IR162 immunocytoma (40 mg monoclonal IgE) or
2 ml serum of rat carrying the IR230 immunocytoma (30 mg IgG2a
monoclonal protein), 24 hours earlier. Results showed that the
IgE half life is independent of its own serum level and of the
concentration of the different IgG classes (Tada et al., 1975;
Bazin, Beckers, Moriamé, Platteau, Naze-De Mets & Kints, 1975).

Antigen Binding Properties of Rat IgE Myeloma Proteins

No antigen binding capacities of the different IgE monoclonal proteins studied up to now have yet been found. In particular, we have checked, without success, the common antigens

found to be able of binding to BALB/c monoclonal proteins,
with the help of Dr. M. Potter (N.I.H., Bethesda, U.S.A.).

Binding of Rat Myeloma IgE on Mast Cells

Addition of purified IR2 monoclonal IgE protein to a
Nippostrongylus brasiliensis serum clearly inhibited its reaginic properties as judged by PCA test. This competition between the IR2 protein and anti-Nippostrongylus antibodies for
binding sites in the skin strongly suggested that rat myeloma
IgE binds to mast cells (Bazin et al., 1974b).

We also have tested anti-ovalbumin serum raised in Hooded
Lister rats on LOU/M/Wsl with or without immunocytomas. The
presence in urine and serum of large quantities of monoclonal
immunoglobulins has been confirmed in all the rats bearing tumours. As seen in Table 7, only those rats bearing immunocytomas secreting myeloma IgE could not be sensitized for PCA reactions. The somewhat lower PCA titres observed in rats bearing
IgG2a immunocytomas is not lower than that obtained in rats
carrying IgA tumours. It is unlikely therefore to be the result
of competition between IgG2a and IgE molecules for mast cell
receptors. More direct evidence of the binding of rat IgE myeloma

Table 7. PCA titres of an anti-ovalbumin Hooded Lister rat serum
         tested in (OKAMOTO x LOU/M) F1 rats bearing or not a
         LOU/C immunocytoma.

Rats bearing an immunocytoma secreting	Code number of the tumour	PCA titres (in three different rats).		
[*]	-	512[**]	512	512
Kappa Bence Jones protein	IR102	256	512	512
IgM	IR202	256	256	512
IgA	IR22	128	128	128
IgE	IR162	Nil	Nil	Nil
IgG1	IR595	256	512	512
IgG2a	IR418	128	128	128
IgG2c	IR304	512	512	512

[*]   not inoculated with a tumour.

[**] reciprocal of the highest dilution of the antiserum resul-
      ting from a 5 mm diametre reaction.

protein on normal or tumoral rat mast cells was given by the studies using iodinated IR162 myeloma IgE (Kulczycki & Metzger, 1974; Conrad, Bazin, Sehon & Froese, 1974; Ishizaka et al., 1975). The binding characteristics were similar for normal or myeloma rat IgE.

CONCLUSION

The LOU rat immunocytoma model provides an appreciable number of new possibilities for experimental research in immunology and especially in allergy. Among these, the possibility of an almost unlimited quantity of monoclonal IgE freely available from a relatively well-known animal species is obviously the most useful. Moreover, the characteristics of these rat myeloma IgE seem to be similar to those of the natural IgE from the same species, in particular the class antigenicity and binding properties on mast cells.

Yet, most of the problems raised by the LOU model have not been solved up to now. Our knowledge is still limited in different fields such as the incidental genetics of these tumours, an explanation of their appearance in the ileocecal lymph node, the abnormally high proportion of IgE class monoclonal proteins and the possible antigens which these could be capable of binding...

Hopefully, this experimental model will provide the opportunity to increase our understanding of the role of IgE antibodies in normal and pathological states.

ACKNOWLEDGEMENTS

We wish to thank our colleagues: G. Burtonboy, C. Deckers, F. Dessy, P. Querinjean, J. Rhodain, R. Rousseaux for their help and especially Dr. E. Jarrett (University of Glasgow, Great Britain) for reviewing the manuscript. We are indebted to J. Naze-De Mets, B. Platteau and J.P. Kints for their excellent technical assistance. We gratefully thank D. Amthor for her great help in preparing the manuscript.

This work was supported by the "Fonds Cancérologigue de la Caisse Générale d'Epargne et de Retraite", Brussels, the DGRST, France, contract N° 74.7.0491, the National Institutes of Health, U.S.A., contract N° RO1.AI.12840.

We also thank Professor G. Biserte (Institut du cancer, Lille, France) and Professor J. Samaille (Institut Pasteur, Lille, France) for kindly allowing us to keep part of our LOU

rat colony in their animal house, and Dr. M. Potter for his
kind gift of antigens.

H. Bazin is staff member of the European Communities,
Biology Division, publication N° 1307. A. Beckers is in receipt
of a fellowship from the "Fonds Cancérologique de la Caisse
Générale d'Epargne et de Retraite", Brussels.

BIBLIOGRAPHY

AALBERSE R.C., BRUMMELHUIS G.H.J. & REERINK-BRONGERS E.E.
The purification of human polyclonal IgE by immuno-
absorption. Immunochemistry 10 : 295, 1973.

BAZIN H. Tumeurs secrétant des immunoglobulines chez le
rat LOU/Wsl : étude portant sur 200 immunocytomes.
Ann. Immunol. (Institut Pasteur) 125c : 277, 1974.

BAZIN H., BECKERS A., DECKERS C. & HEREMANS J.F.
Transplantable immunoglobulin secreting tumours in rats.
I.General features of LOU/Wsl strain rat immunocytomas
and their monoclonal proteins . Eur. J. Cancer 10:568,197

BAZIN H., BECKERS A., DECKERS C. & MORIAME M.
Transplantable immunoglobulin-secreting tumours in rats.
V. Monoclonal immunoglobulins secreted by 250 ileocecal
immunocytomas in LOU/Wsl rats. J. Nat. Cancer Inst.51:
1359, 1973.

BAZIN H., BECKERS A. & QUERINJEAN P.
Three classes and four subclasses of rat immunoglobulins:
IgM, IgA, IgE and IgG1, IgG2a, IgG2b , IgG2c.
Eur. J.Immunol. 4 : 44, 1974a.

BAZIN H., QUERINJEAN P., BECKERS A., HEREMANS J.F. &
DESSY F. Transplantable immunoglobulin-secreting tumours
in rats. IV. Sixty-three IgE-secreting immunocytoma
tumours. Immunology 26 : 713, 1974b.

BAZIN H., BECKERS A., MORIAME M., PLATTEAU B., NAZE-DE MET
J. & KINTS J.P.   LOU/C/Wsl rat monoclonal immunoglobulins
1975 FEBS meeting-AKAMEMIA KIADO-Budapest, 36:123, 1975.

BECKERS A., QUERINJEAN P. & BAZIN H.
Allotypes of rat immunoglobulins.II. Distribution of the
allotypes of Kappa and Alpha chain loci in different
inbred strains of rats. Immunochemistry 11 : 605, 1974.

BURTONBOY G., BAZIN H., DECKERS C., BECKERS A., LAMY M.
& HEREMANS J.F. Transplantable immunoglobulin-secreting
tumours in rats. III. Establishment of immunoglobulin-
secreting cell lines from LOU/Wsl strain rats.
Eur.J.Cancer 9 : 259, 1973.

CAPRON A., DESSAINT J.P., CAPRON M. & BAZIN H.,
Specific IgE antibodies in immune adherence of normal
macrophages to Schistosoma mansoni schistosomules.
Nature (London) 253 : 474, 1975.

CARSON D., METZGER H. & BAZIN H.
A simple radioimmunoassay for the measurement of human
and rat IgE levels by ammonium sulfate precipitation.
J.Immunol. 115 : 561 , 1975

CONRAD D.H., BAZIN H., SEHON A.H. & FROESE A.
Binding parameters of the interaction between rat IgE and
rat mast cell receptors.
J.Immunol. 114: 1688, 1974.

DECKERS C. Etude éléctrophorétique et immunoélectro-
phorétique des protéines du rat atteint de leucosarcome.
Protides Biol. Fluids . 11 : 105, 1963.

DORRINGTON K.J. & ROCKEY J.H.
Studies on the conformation of purified human and canine
gamma A-globulins and equine gamma T-globulins by the
optical rotary dispersion.
J.Biol. Chem. 243 : 6511, 1968.

DUNN T.B. Transplantable plasma cell neoplasm in strain
C3H mice . Proc. Am. Assoc. Cancer Res. 1 : 13, 1954.

FAHEY J.L. & ROBINSON A.G.
Factors controlling serum gamma-globulin concentration.
J.Exp. Med. 118 : 845, 1963.

FESTING M. & STAATS J.
Standardized nomenclature for inbred strains of rats.
Transplantation 16 : 221, 1973.

GLEICH G.J., AVERBECK A.K. & SWEDLUND H.A.
Measurement of IgE in normal and allergic sera by radioimmunoassay. J.Lab. Clin. Med. 77 : 690, 1971.

GROULADE J., MOREL P., CREYSSEL R. & GROULADE P.
Un des cas de paraglobulinémie chez le chien.
Bull. Acad. Vét. France 6 : 354, 1959.

HALLIWELL R.E.W., SCHWARTZMAN R.M. & ROCKEY J.H.
Antigenic relationship between human IgE and canine IgE.
Clin. Exp. Immunol. 10 : 399, 1972.

HAMMER P.K., KICKHÖFEN B. & SCHMIDT T.
Detection of homocytotropic antibody associated with a
unique immunoglobulin class in the bovine species.
Eur.J.Immunol. 1 : 249, 1971.

HOOD L., GRAY W.R., SANDERS B.G. & DREYER W.J.
Light chains evolution.
Cold Spring Harbor Symp. Quant.Biol. 32 : 133, 1967.

ISERSKY C., KULCZYCKI A. & METZGER H.
Isolation of IgE from reaginic rat serum.
J.Immunol. 112 : 1909, 1974.

ISHIZAKA K. & ISHIZAKA T.
Physicochemical properties of human reaginic antibody.
I. Association of reaginic activity with an immunoglobulin
other than gamma A-or gamma G-globulin.
J.Allergy 37 : 169, 1966.

ISHIZAKA K., ISHIZAKA T.& TADA T.
Immunoglobulin E in the monkey.
J.Immunol. 103 : 445, 1969.

ISHIZAKA K., ISHIZAKA T. & HORNBROOK M.M.
A unique rabbit immunoglobulin having homocytotropic
antibody activity.
Immunochemistry 7 : 515, 1970.

ISHIZAKA T., KÖNIG W., KURATA M., MAUSER L. & ISHIZAKA K.
Immunologic properties of mast cells from rat infected
with Nippostrongylus brasiliensis.
J.Immunol. 115 : 1078, 1975.

JARRETT E.E.E. & BAZIN H.
Elevation of total serum IgE in rats, following Helminth
parasite infection.
Nature 251 : 613, 1974.

JOHANSSON G.O. Raised levels of a new immunoglobulin
class (IgND) in asthma.
Lancet 1967, ii, 951.

JOHANSSON G.O. & BENNICH H.
Immunological studies of an atypical(myeloma) immunoglo-
bulin.
Immunology 13 : 381, 1967.

JOHANSSON G.O., BENNICH H. & WIDE L.
A new class of immunoglobulin in human serum.
Immunology 14 : 265, 1968a.

JOHANSSON G.O., MELLBIN T. & VAHLQUIST B.
Immunoglobulin levels inEthiopian preschool children with
special reference to high concentrations of immunoglobulin
E (IgND).
Lancet i, 118, 1968b.

JONES V.E. & EDWARDS A.J.
Preparation of an antiserum specific for rat reagin
(rat gamma E ?)
Immunology 21 : 383, 1971.

KANYERESI B., JATON J.C. & BLOCH K.J.
Human and rat gamma E : serologic evidence of homology.
J.Immunol. 106 : 1411, 1971.

KEHOE J.M., HURVITZ A.L. & CAPRA J.D.
Characterization of three homogenous feline immuno-
globulins.
J.Immunol. 109 : 511, 1972.

KULCZYCKI A.& METZGER H.
The interaction of IgE with rat basophilic leukemia
cells. II. Quantitative aspects of the binding reaction.
J.Exp. Med. 140 : 1676, 1974.

LIACOPOULOU A. & PERELMUTTER L.
Antigenic relationship between IgE immunoglobulin and
rat homocytotropic antibody.
J.Immunol. 107 : 131, 1971.

MAISIN J., MAISIN H., DUNJIC A. & MALDAGUE P.
La radiobiologie comme méthode de travail en physio-
pathologie et en cancérologie expérimentale.
Bull. Acad. Suisse Sci. Med. 11 : 247, 1955.

MAYHOFER G., BAZIN H. & GOWANS J.L.
The distribution and nature of cells binding anti-IgE
in the organs of normal rats and in rats immunised with
Nippostrongylus brasiliensis (in preparation).

MERWIN R.M. & ALGIRE G.H.
Induction of plasma-cell neoplasms and fibrosarcomas in
BALB/c mice carrying diffusion chambers.
Proc. Soc. Exp. Biol. Med. 101 : 437, 1959.

MOHR U. & DONTENWILL W.
Organ-und Blutveränderungen beim KG-13-Plasmocytom des
Goldhamster.
Z. Krebsforsch 66 : 29, 1964.

NEOH S.H., JAHODA D.M., ROWE D.S. & VOLLER A.
Immunoglobulin classes in mammalian species identified by
cross-reactivity with antisera to human immunoglobulin.
Immunochemistry 10 : 805, 1973.

POTTER M.   Immunoglobulin-producing tumours and myeloma
proteins of mice.
Phys. Rev. 52 : 631, 1972.

POTTER M. & ROBERTSON C.L.
Development of plasma cell neoplasms in BALB/c mice
after intraperitoneal injection of paraffinoil adjuvant
heat-killed staphylococcus mixtures.
J.Nat. Cancer Inst. 25 : 847, 1960.

PROUVOST-DANON A., BINAGHI R., ROCHAS S. & BOUSSAC-ARON Y
Immunochemical identification of mouse IgE.
Immunol. 23 : 481, 1972.

PROUVOST-DANON A., WYCZILKOWSKA J., BINAGHI R. & ABADIE A
Mouse and rat IgE. Cross-sensitization of mast cells and
antigenic relationship.
Immunol. 29 : 151, 1975.

QUERINJEAN P., BAZIN H., BECKERS A., DECKERS C., HEREMANS
J.F. & MILSTEIN C. Transplantable immunoglobulin-secreti
tumours in rats. II. Purification and chemical characteri
zation of four Kappa chains from LOU/Wsl rats.
Eur.J.Biochem. 31 354, 1972.

QUERINJEAN P., BAZIN H., STARACE V., BECKERS A., DECKERS
& HEREMANS J.F.   Lambda light chains in rat immunoglobul
Immunochemistry 10 : 653, 1973.

STECHSCHULTE D.J., ORANGE R.P. & AUSTEN K.F.
Immunochemical and biologic properties of rat IgE. I.Immu
chemical identification of rat IgE.
J. Immunol. 105 : 1082, 1970.

TADA T., OKUMURA K., PLATTEAU B., BECKERS A. & BAZIN H.
Half-lives of two types of rat homocytotropic antibodies
in the circulation and in the skin.
Int. Arch. Allergy, 48 : 116, 1975.

WANG A.C., FUDENBERG H.H. & BAZIN H.
The nature of "species-specific" aminoacid residues.
Immunochemistry 12 : 505, 1975.

WANG A.C., FUDENBERG H.H. & BAZIN H.
Partial aminoacid sequences of Kappa chains of rat
immunoglobulins : genetic and evolutionary immplications.
Biochemical genetics (in press).

DISCUSSION

LICHTENSTEIN: Perhaps the experts in the audience can
settle the question of the relation between human and rat IgE.
As you know two groups in North America have been able to
passively sensitize rat mast cells with human IgE for degranulation and histamine release. Drs. Plout, Bloch and I have
failed to show any receptor competition going both ways - human
IgE sensitization or competition with rat IgE on rat mast cells
or the revers with no success.
I thought the issue was dead but apparently not. Thus,
Dr. Prouvost-Danon recently demonstrated with, I believe, mouse
mast cells passive sensitization with human IgE. What is the
experience of the group?
BAZIN: One must consider the two problems separately. On
one hand a possible antigenic relationship between human and
rat IgE and on the other hand a possible homology of the part
of their structure which bind to the membrane receptors of the
mast cells.
We have not been able to demonstrate an antigenic relationship between human and rat IgE, but a negative result is
never a definitive result. It might be possible to raise another antiserum to human or rat epsilon chain which can be used
to demonstrate a cross reactivity. At present it is only possible to state that the antigenic relationship between human
and rat IgE is certainly a small one if it exists.
I have no personal experience of the binding of human
IgE to rat mast cells.
DIAMANT: It seems that the world is divided in two groups,
one succeed to sensitize rat mast cells passively with human
IgE, the other does not succeed. I belong to the latter group
in spite of 5-6 serious trials at different times during the
last two years.
We have failed even after having obtained detailed descriptions from the groups that claim to be successful. The only
thing we have noticed is nonspecific histamine release from
rat mast cells when exposed to human serum of too strong concentrations.
BENNICH: The reaction between rat IgE and antisera to rat
IgE is not inhibited by human IgE and rat IgE does not inhibit

the corresponding reaction between antihuman IgE and human IgE. Furthermore human IgE (radiolabelled) does not bind to rat mast cells.

AUSTEN: Please comment on competition between IgG_{2a} and IgE in PCA studies. We were able to show competition in vitro with rat mast cells. However, while IgE bound firmly to the cell, IgG_{2a} did not.

BAZIN: In vitro and in vivo experiments could give different results. In our experiment, the injection of antigen was done 72 hours after the injection of reaginic serum. With such an experimental protocol, the competition between IgG_{2a} and IgE for the mast cell receptors seems to be very small.

MÜLLER-EBERHARD: Some human myeloma proteins have antibody activity. Have you been able to find among the many rat IgE myeloma proteins any with reaginic activity?

BAZIN: Unfortunately, we have not succeed in such a search although we have tried different antigens and, in particular, those known to bind to the BALB/c myeloma proteins.

MACROPHAGE CYTOTOXICITY MEDIATED BY IgE ANTIBODY

In vitro study on S. mansoni schistosomules

A. Capron, J.P. Dessaint, M. Joseph, R. Rousseaux
and H. Bazin*

Institut Pasteur de Lille (France)
*Faculté de Médecine de Louvain (Belgium)

Metazoal parasite infections offer valuable models for the
investigation of the role of IgE, since one of the pre-eminent features of worm infections is the production of large amounts of
this immunoglobulin in humans (1) and in animals (2). Although
the only identified function of IgE is the mediation of immediate
type hypersensitivity reactions (3), a protective role of IgE has
been considered in various host-parasite models : in rats infected
by Nippostrongylus brasiliensis, in guinea pigs infected by Tri-
chinella spiralis and in rats experimentally infected by Schistosoma mansoni.

In these various models, evidence suggesting a protective
role of IgE is supported by experiments which have shown a positive
correlation between resistance to infection and production of reagin-like antibodies.

In schistosome infections a parallel can be drawn between the
degree of resistance to S. mansoni or S. haematobium infection and
the ability of the host to produce reagins (4).

In rats infected by S. mansoni, recent experiments (5) have
indicated that specific IgE antibodies appear to have a remarkable
activity in mediating in vitro killing of schistosomules by normal
macrophages.

This mechanism, which apparently represents a new function for IgE molecules, distinct from their role in immediate type
hypersensitivity, will be related and discussed in the present
paper.

MODELS

The in vivo Model

Rats provide a unique model for the study of immunity to
schistosomes. Indeed after percutaneous infection by S. mansoni
cercariae, the rat allows the normal development of worm population during the first 3 weeks of infection. Between day 21 and 27
following primary infection and according to the various stains
used (Sprague Dawley, Wistar, Fisher, Hooded Lister), most of the
schistosomes are expelled from the host (6, 7, 8, 9, 10). The exact
immune mechanism responsible for worm expulsion is still unclear
but this phenomenon is followed by the acquisition of an important
but transient degree of resistance to reinfection. In vitro studies
have indicated the existence of cytotoxic complement dependent IgG
antibodies (9, 11) and the possible interaction of antibodies with
various cells including neutrophils (12), eosinophils (13) or macrophages (5).

Direct cytotoxicity by sensitized cells from immune donors
has never been observed and so far attempts to transfer immunity
either by cells (14) and/or by serum (7, 14) have led only to partial success.

The in vitro Model

Syngeneic Fisher rats were used throughout our experiments.
Serum samples were obtained by bleeding infected rats at various
intervals after exposure to 400 cercariae of S. mansoni. Uninfected
rats were used as controls.

Normal syngeneic Fisher rat macrophages were collected by
peritoneal washing with Eagle's MEM and plated in Falcon dishes.
Non-adherent cells were washed off after 3 hours incubation. The
adherent population was incubated at 37°C in MEM containing 20 % of
either infected or normal rat serum. Adherent cells were not washed
after incubation.

Approximately 200 S. mansoni schistosomules recovered according
to the technique described by CLEGG and SMITHERS (16) were added.

Macrophage adherence was estimated after a 3 hours contact.
Cytotoxic effect on schistosomules was estimated by microsco-
pical examination, dye exclusion test and by ^{51}Cr release according to BUTTERWORTH et al. (13).

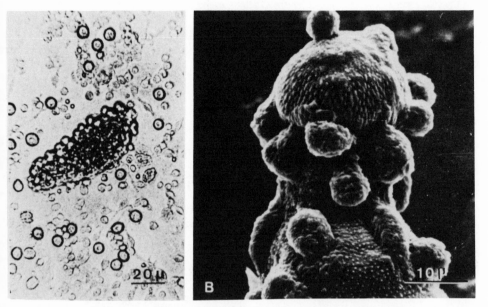

Fig. 1 : Immune adherence of normal Fisher rat macrophages to
S. mansoni schistosomules mediated by S. mansoni infected syngeneic
rat serum.
- right : macrophage-coated schistosomule under phase contrast
         microscope
- left : scanning electron microscopy.

RESULTS

     When incubated in the serum of Fisher rats immune to Schisto-
soma mansoni, the peritoneal adherent cells of normal inbred Fisher
rats are strongly adherent to S. mansoni schistosomules (fig. 1). A
highly significant correlation was obtained between the percentage
of macrophage-coated schistosomules and the time elapsed since infection (r = 0.562 ; n = 80 ; p < 0.001) (5). After 50 days of infection, the mean percentage of macrophage-coated schistosomules
was significantly higher than in controls (88.4 % and 29.8 % respectively ; p < 0.001).

Identification of Effector Cells

     Cells adhering to schistosomules were identified as macropha-
ges according to the following criteria : 85 percent of adherent

cells were shown to phagocyte latex particles or neutral red. Ultra-
structural studies have shown that these adherent mononuclear cells
exhibited all the known morphological characters of peritoneal macrophages. Less than 5 percent of the adherent cells were identified
as mastocytes.

Effect on Schistosomules

After seven hours of contact with immune serum-incubated macrophages, important ultrastructural changes occur in the schistosomule
(fig.2). After 20 hours, a highly significant release of ^{51}Cr is
observed, while microscopic observation shows an important mortality
of schistosomules and pictures of phagocytosis by macrophages
(fig. 2), differing from complement-dependent lesions obtained with
IgG antibody (9).

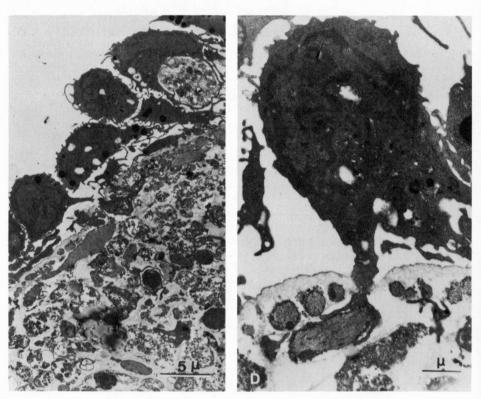

Fig. 2 : Ultrastructural study of infected serum mediated macrophage adherence to S. mansoni schistosomules.

Table 1 : 16 hours percentage chromium release (mean ± S.D.) from labelled Schistosoma mansoni larvae cultured with normal Fisher rat peritoneal macrophages in various sera. Spontaneous chromium release is given for each serum, without macrophages.

* IgE level : 1.5 µg/ml
** IgE level : 0.05 µg/ml

	Normal serum	50 days immune serum*	Heat-inac- tived immune serum	Idem + guinea pig serum	Anti-IgE absorbed immune serum**	Foetal calf serum
Normal rat macrophages	33.95 % ± 2.84	62.61 % ± 1.68	35.53 % ± 5.83	37.71 % ± 1.64	37.64 % ± 3.09	27.47 % ± 3.70
Medium without macrophages	31.26 % ± 3.02	40.74 % ± 2.15	36.20 % ± 3.27	37.84 % ± 1.89	38.20 % ± 2.55	25.30 % ± 1.21

Identification of Serum Factors

Adherence and cytotoxicity of immune serum-incubated macrophages was inhibited by heating the serum for periods of 30 - 180 min. (5). Adherence was not restored by addition of fresh guinea-pig serum and macrophage cytotoxicity was not increased significantly (Table 1). Moreover, macrophage adherence was unaffected by EDTA (0.002 M).

Absorption of S. mansoni immune rat sera by increased quantities of anti-rat IgE goat serum specific for ε chain or $F(ab')_2$ of the same antiserum led to a progressive decrease of the macrophage adherence which was reduced to 50 % with 1.5 mg/ml of anti-IgE goat antibody (5). Similar experiments with anti-rat IgG (IgG, IgG_{2a}, IgG_{2b}) IgM and IgA did not exhibit any significant decrease.

To avoid possible interference of soluble IgE-anti-IgE complexes and excess of anti-IgE antibodies, the same absorption experiment was carried out in solid phase using goat IgG anti-rat IgE linked to Cyanogen Bromide activated Sepharose 4B. In these experimental conditions a highly significant decrease of macrophage-coated schistosomules was observed and the disappearance of IgE was controlled by radio-immunoassay (Table 2). Macrophage cytotoxicity was also significantly reduced (Table 1).

A comparative study of IgE level in serum and macrophage adherence to schistosomules during the course of infection of rats by S. mansoni has shown a closely parallel evolution (fig. 3).

Table 2 : Absorption experiment by anti-ε immunosorbent.

Serum batches		IgE level μg/ml	Percentage of macrophage coated schistosomules	Significance
unabsorbed	a	9.70 ± 0.47	86.25 ± 6.02	
	b	10.20 ± 0.44	92.25 ± 5.06	$p < 0.001$
absorbed	a	1.31 ± 0.32	4.80 ± 3.56	
	b	0.01 ± 0.40	12.2 ± 9.70	

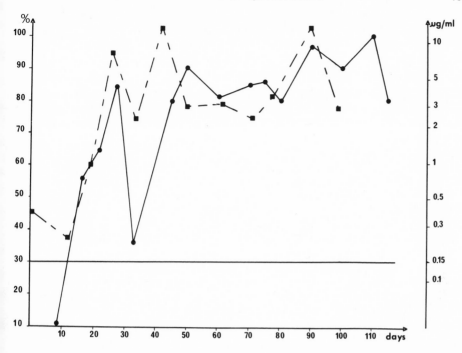

Fig. 3 : Serum IgE level measured by radioimmunoassay (μg/ml) and serum mediated macrophage adherence (percentage of macrophage coated schistosomules, dotted line) at various times after infection of Fisher rats by 400 S. mansoni cercariae (horizontal line shows upper values in uninfected rats).

SPECIFICITY AND MECHANISMS

The involvement of IgE molecules in macrophage adherence and cytotoxicity being inferred from the above experiments, the possible mechanism and its specificity calls for discussion.

Specificity controls were performed with IgE myeloma serum (IR 162) and with sera containing unrelated reaginic anti-ragweed, anti-ovalbumin, anti BGG-DNP and anti-Nippostrongylus brasiliensis antibodies with respective homologous PCA titres of 1/256 to 1/512 according to the technique of JARRETT and FERGUSON (17). None of these sera elicited any significant adherence of macrophages to schistosomules. On the other hand macrophages incubated with immune rat serum did not exhibit any cytotoxic activity on cell line culture of 8629 T_1C_5, using Cr^{51} release.

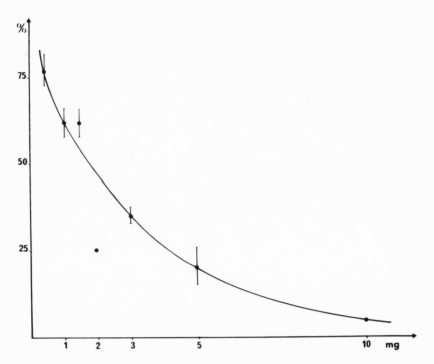

Fig. 4 : Percentage of macrophage-coated schistosomules obtained
after incubation with supernatants of infected rat serum incubated
with increased amounts of S. mansoni saline extract and then centri
fuged.

Absorption of rat immune sera by soluble S. mansoni antigens
before incubation was shown to significantly decrease the adherence
of macrophages to the schistosomules (fig. 4). On the other hand,
absorption of rat immune serum by increased quantities of anti-
S. mansoni rabbit IgG led also to a progressive decrease of macrophage adherence (fig. 5).

The same absorption experiment was carried out in solid phase
using anti-S. mansoni rabbit IgG linked to cyanogen bromide activated Sepharose 4B. In these experimental conditions a highly signi-

ficant decrease of macrophage adherence was observed (table 3).
Absorption of anti-S. mansoni rabbit IgG with host antigens prior
to linkage to Sepharose led to identical results.

From the above experiments it can be suggested that either
unbound anti-S. mansoni IgE antibody or IgE immune complexes are
involved in the adherence of macrophages to schistosomules.

Five to 8 % of the total IgE level was found to be specific
IgE antibodies (fig. 6) isolated by means of S. mansoni immunosorbent.

The existence of circulating antigens in the serum of infected
rats was investigated at various times after infection.

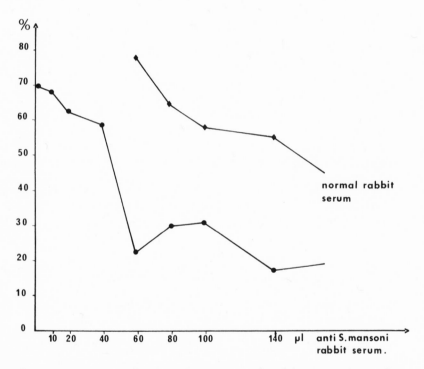

Fig. 5 : Percentage of macrophage-coated schistosomules after
incubation with supernatants of infected rat serum incubated with
increased quantities of anti-S. mansoni rabbit serum.

Table 3 : Inhibition of macrophage adherence after absorption of infected rat serum by anti-S. mansoni.

Solid phase absorption by	Before absorption		After absorption		Eluate
	% coated schistosomules	IgE levels μg/ml	% coated schistosomules	IgE levels μg/ml	IgE levels μg/ml
anti-S. mansoni	71	1.21	7	0.88	0.19
anti-S. mansoni (previously absorbed by host proteins)	91	1.18	0	—	0.20

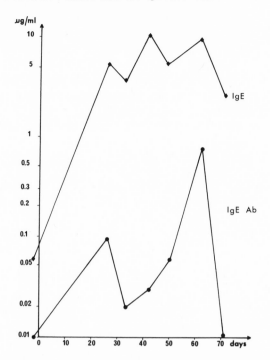

Fig. 6 : Serum IgE level and concentration of anti-schistosome IgE antibody in S. mansoni infected rats, measured by radioimmunoassay. IgE antibody against S. mansoni is isolated by means of S. mansoni saline extract covalently linked to BrCN activated Sepharose 4B.

Using immunization of syngeneic normal Fisher rats by infected Fisher rat serum, it was found that 42 days after initial exposure to cercariae, rat serum contained soluble antigens which were able to elicit precipitating IgG and IgE antibodies in normal rats (up to 2.1 µg/ml). A reaction of identity by gel diffusion with various antigenic extracts of adult schistosomes proved the parasitic origin of this circulating material.

As high levels of IgE were produced in rats immunized by circulating antigens from infected rats, it was attempted to characterize those antigens implicated in IgE production.

Using I^{125} labelled anti-rat IgE (ϵ specific) and radioimmuno-electrophoresis it was possible to demonstrate that at least 2 circulating antigens bind to IgE in 42 days rat serum. One of these antigens was shown to be thermostable and was separated on polyacrylamide gel.

Degranulation of rat mast cells or free basophils by serum from rats infected 42 days was investigated by three techniques.

(i) Passive cutaneous anaphylaxis performed in rats given an intravenous injection of Evans blue followed by separate intradermal injections of 0.05 ml of rat serum (either diluted or undiluted) or saline. After 30 minutes the diameter of dye-infiltrated lesions was measured (18). No difference was observed between lesion diameters obtained with infected rat serum, uninfected serum or saline.

(ii) By the connective tissue air punch technique (19), no degranulation of mast cells was seen with infected rat serum.

(iii) The same negative result was obtained by the rat (peritoneal) basophil degranulation test (20). However, incubation of rat immune serum with S. mansoni antigen (100 µg) led to a significant mast cell degranulation.

Bis diazotized rat myeloma IgE (21) led to mast cell degranulation in the same conditions, but did not induce any macrophage cytotoxicity for schistosomules. Since it has been reported (22) that only IgE complexes formed in moderate antigen excess were able to cause mast cell degranulation, it could be suggested that IgE antibody mediated macrophage cytotoxicity is probably induced by IgE complexes in antibody excess.

MACROPHAGE BINDING

From the experiments described above it appears that the binding of IgE molecules to the macrophage depends upon very strict conditions : optimal binding occurs after 3 to 7 hours incubation at 37°C, no binding occurs at 4°C, and macrophage adherence disappears when the adherent cells are washed after incubation in serum.

The binding of IgE molecules on the macrophage surface was investigated by the techniques of rosette formation and immunofluorescence.

Rosette formation was obtained when normal rat macrophages incubated with rat IgE myeloma protein were put in contact with ε specific anti-rat IgE linked to group O rhesus negative human red cells by glutaraldehyde. Similar results were obtained when macrophages were incubated in serum from rats infected by S. mansoni.

Macrophages incubated with immune rat serum demonstrated a fluorescence surface staining with anti-rat IgE goat serum revealed by fluorescein labelled anti-goat globulins. No staining was obtaine

when the anti-S. mansoni serum was previously heated (56°C for
3 hours) or absorbed by F(ab')$_2$ anti-rat IgE.

ISHIZAKA et al. (23) have reported that rat myeloma IgE
does not bind to rat peritoneal macrophages. However experimental
conditions were different from ours since incubation was carried
out at 0°C during 30 minutes with unaggregated IgE and the cells
were subsequently washed.

It should be noted that unaggregated IgE from human myeloma
does not bind to human monocytes but binding of aggregated IgE was
not explored (24).

The exact mechanism by which unbound or complexed IgE antibodies
induce macrophage adherence and cytotoxicity is still unclear.

However, macrophage activation has been evidenced by both ultrastructural observations and enzyme release measurements as
reported by JOSEPH (25).

Incubation of normal macrophages in infected rat serum led
to a significant increase of the protein content, the lysosomial
β glucuronidase and of the cytoplasmic leucine-aminopeptidase activities.

When the serum was absorbed by anti-IgE no increased activity
was observed (table 4). Phagocytosis of sheep red cells or latex
particles (0.8 μm) was not increased by infected rat serum.

Though experimental conditions leading to macrophage adherence
to schistosomules and their subsequent killing differ from those
used to demonstrate cytophilic antibodies, the characteristics of
macrophage activation by IgE antibodies reported here does not fun-
damentally differ from macrophage activation by IgG cytophilic antibodies (26). The differences may be due to the particular structure
of the IgE molecule.

The in vivo relevance of Ig mediated macrophage cytotoxicity
is presently under investigation.

Preliminary results however suggest that immunization of normal
rats with serum from rats infected 42 days leads to a significant
degree of protection against a challenge infection.

There are some examples in other parasitic infections as well
as in tumor immunity suggesting that IgE antibodies might have a
beneficial function in immune defense mechanisms (27).

Experimental metazoal parasite infections will probably

Table 4 : Compared effects of normal, S. mansoni immune and IgE-depleted rat sera on the protein content, the lysosomial β-glucuronidase and cytoplasmic leucine-aminopeptidase activities of normal Fisher rat peritoneal macrophages after a 16 hours culture. Results with rat myeloma IgE, bis-diazotized benzidine aggregated also included.

	Normal serum	42 days immune serum	Percent increase	Anti-IgE absorbed immune serum	Aggregated rat IgE
Proteins (µg/10^6 cells)	32.92	42.13	+ 28 %	35.84	30.10
β-glucuronidase (10^{-9} M hydrolyzed p. nitrophenyl glucuronidate/10^6 cells/hr)	8.69	16.68	+ 80.4 %	6.56	12.21
Leucine aminopeptidase (10^{-9} M hydrolyzed leucine-β-naphtylamide/10^6 cells/hr)	2.72	3.84	+ 41.2 %	2.19	2.56

represent choice models for studies along this line which might
lead to an important progress in the immunological control of
parasitic infections.

REFERENCES

1 - JOHONSSON, S.G.O., BENNICH, H.H., BERG, T. (1972) Progr. Clin. Immunol., 1, 157.

2 - JARRETT, E.E.E. and BAZIN, H. (1975) Nature, 251, 613.

3 - ISHIZAKA, K. and ISHIZAKA, T. (1967) J. Immunol., 99, 187.

4 - SADUN, E.H. and GORE, R.W. (1970) Exp. Parasitol., 28, 435.

5 - CAPRON, A. et al. (1975) Nature, 253, 474.

6 - SMITHERS, S.R. and TERRY, R.J. (1965) Parasitology, 55, 695.

7 - PEREZ, H., CLEGG, A. and SMITHERS, S.R. (1974) Parasitology, 69, 349.

8 - PEREZ, H. (1974) P.H.D. Thesis, Brunel University, Uxbridge, G.B.

9 - CAPRON-DUPONT, M. (1974) Doctoral Thesis, Lille University (France)

10 - PHILLIPS, S.M. et al. (1975) Cell. Immunol., 19, 99.

11 - SHER, A. et al. (1974) Clin. Exp. Immunol., 18, 357.

12 - DEAN, D.A., WISTAR, R. and MURRELL, K.D. (1974) Amer. J. Trop. Med. Hyg., 23, 420.

13 - BUTTERWORTH, A.E. et al. (1974) Nature, 252, 503.

14 - MADDISON, S.E. et al. (1970) J. Parasit., 56, 1066.

15 - BRUCE, J.I. and SADUN, E.H. (1964) J. Parasit., 50, 23.

16 - CLEGG, J.A. and SMITHERS, S.R. (1970) J. Parasit., 56, 56.

17 - JARRETT, E. and FERGUSON, A. (1974) Nature, 250, 420.

18 - KABAT, E.A. and MAYER, M.M. (1961) Experimental Immunochemistry p. 269 - 271 Charles C. THOMAS Springfield.

19 - HIGGINBOTHAM, R.D. and DOUGHERTY, T.F. (1956) Proc. Soc. Exp. Biol. Med., 92, 493.

20 - KOROTZER, J.L., HADDAD, Z.H. and LOPAPA, A.F. (1971) Immunology, 20, 545.

21 - ISHIZAKA, K., ISHIZAKA, T. and LEE, E.H. (1970) Immunochemistry, 7, 687.

22 - ISHIZAKA, K. and CAMPBELL, D.H. (1959) J. Immunol., 83, 318.

23 - ISHIZAKA, K. et al. (1975) J. Immunol., 115, 1078.

24 - LAWRENCE, D.A., WEIGLE, W.O. and SPIEGELBERG, H.L. (1975) J. Clin. Invest., 55, 368.

25 - JOSEPH, M. (1976) Doctoral Thesis, Lille University, France

26 - BERKEN, A. and BENACERRAF, B. (1966) J. Exp. Med., 123, 119.

27 - CAPRON, A. and DESSAINT, J.P. (1975) I.R.C.S., 3, 477.

DISCUSSION

ISHIZAKA: Does EDTA block the binding of IgE to macrophages and can you wash away the IgE from the macrophages?

In my understanding, IgG is known to combine with macrophages. Why do you think IgG antibody does not work in your experiments?

CAPRON: Macrophage adherence to schistosomules was unaffected if immune serum was previously treated with EDTA (0.002 M).

The important point in our experiments was that adherent cells were not washed after incubation in rat immune serum. When macrophages were washed, no significant adherence to schistosomules was observed.

As shown in Table I cytotoxicity was estimated by ^{51}Cr release. Macrophages incubated with immune serum gave 62% ^{51}Cr release. After absorption of this serum on an anti-IgE (epsilon specific) immunosorbent the ^{51}Cr release decreased to 31%, normal serum controls giving 34%.

Moreover, whereas absorption of rat immune sera by increasing quantities of goat anti-rat IgE antiserum led to a progressive decrease of macrophage adherence to schistosomules, similar experiments with anti-rat IgG (IgG$_1$, IgG$_{2A}$, IgG$_{2B}$) did not give any significant decrease (Capron et al. 1975).

DAVID: If you incubate normal macrophages with serum from immune rats for 4-7 hours at 37°C, do you remove the active IgE - i.e. is the resultant supernatant still active when added to new macrophages?

CAPRON: We have not done this particular experiment but it is an excellent suggestion, and we shall certainly do the experiment very soon.

LICHTENSTEIN: Do you have any evidence whether the IgE on the macrophages was aggregated?

CAPRON: Absorption of rat immune sera by increased quantities of S. mansoni antigens before incubation led to a significant decrease of macrophage adherence to schistosomules. On the other hand absorption of rat immune serum by increased quantities of rabbit anti-S. mansoni IgG also led to a progressive decrease of macrophage adherence. This was confirmed by solid phase adsorption as reported in Table III.

These experiments appeared to us as an indication of the

existence in rat immune serum of IgE immune complexes. From mast cell degranulation experiments it can be suggested that these complexes might be complexes in antibody excess.

AUSTEN: Are there eosinophils in the cells which adhere? Does the removal of IgE from the macrophage by washing occur with buffer alone or is there removal by competing non-specific IgE?

CAPRON: We did not observe in our experiments any eosinophils adhering to schistosomules. Electron microscopy studies showed, from time to time, eosinophils in the cell preparation but they were never seen in close contact with the target.

Concerning your second question, incubation with rat IgE myeloma protein after incubation with rat immune serum led to a decrease of macrophage adherence.

BECKER: Have you carried out the reaction of antigen with IgE antibody on the surface of the macrophage so as to measure lysosomal enzyme secretion into the supernatant?

CAPRON: The enzymatic studies reported here only concern intracellular levels of the lysosomal β-glucuronidase and cytoplasmic leucine aminopeptidase.

We did some experiments to measure β-glucuronidase in the supernatant after addition of S. mansoni antigen. These results were not mentioned here as it appeared that β-glucuronidase present in S. mansoni extracts was interfering with the enzyme released from the macrophage.

BECKER: So that so far there is no evidence as yet that analogous to the reaction of IgE on a mast cell or basophil an IgE on the macrophage in the reaction with antigen leads to exocytosis from the macrophage.

CAPRON: No , we have only indirect evidence, and some studies in progress, will, I hope, allow us to answer this important question.

PERLMANN (Stockholm): Is the Fc-part of the IgE antibody molecule needed for the adherence reaction and can the IgE reaction be inhibited by aggregated IgG?

CAPRON: I am sorry that I am not able to answer these two questions. We have not done these experiments but they are certainly to be done.

DAVID: Those were most beautiful pictures.

Concerning the system Anthony Butterworth has described, cell mediated antibody dependent damage to schistosomula is caused by eosinophils. In this case the antibody is IgG, and the reaction does not require complement. This is found using human or baboon cells.

CAPRON: As I mentioned in my paper, several possible effector mechanisms have been described from the in vitro studies. I do not know if the system of Anthony Butterworth has been observed in rat.

The main problem at the moment is to understand how all

these different immune mechanisms can interact, if they do, and what is their application to the <u>in vivo</u> situation.

MÜLLER-EBERHARD: Can macrophage dependent cytotoxicity be observed using IgG antibody to the parasite instead of IgE antibody?

CAPRON: Yes, in experiments reported by Perez (1974) it was shown that macrophage dependent cytotoxicity could be observed if macrophages were incubated at +4°C with heat inactivated, infected rat serum. The cytophilic antibody involved was identified as IgG_1 if I remember correctly.

IgE-Dependent Activation and
Release of Chemical Mediators

FUNCTION AND STRUCTURE OF IMMUNOGLOBULIN E (IgE)

H. Bennich[*], S.G.O. Johansson, H. von Bahr-Lindström[**] and T. Karlsson

The Biomedical Center, Uppsala University and The Blood Center, University Hospital, Uppsala, Sweden

INTRODUCTION

The function of IgE antibody as mediators in allergic reactions of Type I is explained by their ability to interact both with antigen and with receptor molecules on the membrane of blood basophils and tissue mast cells. However, it is not understood how the interaction of an allergen with cell-bound IgE antibody will induce basophil (mast) cells to release a great number of biologically active substances of which some will be further discussed at this meeting, nor is it known what role the IgE-mast cell system plays in the development and control of a normal immune response.

Our studies on IgE over the past 10 years, initiated by the discovery of the ND myeloma protein (1) and its normal counterpart (2,3), have proceeded along two lines, one aiming at an understanding of the role of IgE antibodies in disease with particular reference to atopic allergy, and the other aiming at the elucidation of the structural features of the IgE molecule and their relation to antigenic and biological activities.

GENERAL PROPERTIES

Immunoglobulin E has the general features common to all

---

[*] Present address: Institute for Molecular Biology
                      Aarhus University, Aarhus, Denmark
[**] Present address: Kemiska Institutionen I,
                      Karolinska Institutet, Stockholm, Sweden.

Table I. Some physico-chemical and immunological properties of IgE compared with the other immunoglobulins

Properties	IgE	IgG	IgA	IgM	IgD
Physicochemical					
Molecular weight	190 000	150 000	150 000	900 000	185 000
Sedimentation constant	8	6.5	6.5	19	6.5
Carbohydrate conc.(%)	12	3	8	12	13
Immunological					
Serum conc.(g/l)	0.0001	12	1.5	0.8	0.03
Placental passage	-	+	-	-	-
Antibody activity	+	+	+	+	+
Complement activation	-	+	-	+	-
Secretory component binding	-	-	+	(+)	-
J-chain binding	-	-	+	+	-
Skin sensitization					
heterologous	-	+	-	-	-
homologous	+	-	-	-	-

Table II. General characteristics of human IgE myelomas. Note
          the high frequency of plasmacell leukemia (Plc. leuk.)

Designation	Light chain type	Peripheral blood	Year	Reference
ND	λ	Plc. leuk.	1965	Johansson & Bennich (1)
PS	λ	Plc. leuk.	1968	Ogawa et al. (44)
DM	κ	Not known	1970	Stoica (45)
Hea	κ	Normal	1971	Fishkin et al. (46)
Yu	κ	Plc. leuk?	1971	Stefani et al. (47)
Be	κ	Not known	1972	Penn (48)
FK	κ	Normal	1975	Mills et al. (49)
KG	κ	Plc. leuk.	1975	Senda et al. (50)
Kam	κ	Normal	1975	Knedel et al. (51)

immunoglobulins. Like IgG, IgA and IgD, the native IgE molecule
consists of a single four-chain unit. The molecular weight is
close to 190,000 and the carbohydrate content is about 12 per
cent. The heavy (epsilon) polypeptide is significantly larger
than the γ polypeptide chain (about 11,000 daltons), but similar in size to the μ chain. The physico-chemical and immunological properties of IgE are summarized in Table I and compared
with those of the other serum immunoglobulins. Noteworthy is the
extremely low concentration of IgE in normal serum, the inability of IgE to activate complement, the lack of affinity for or
binding to a secretory component or a J-chain and the inability
of IgE to pass through the placental membranes. Finally, it
should be noted that IgE can sensitize homologous but not heterologous tissue.

     Elevated levels of IgE are generally found in immediate
hypersensitivity (on the order of 1 mg/l) and in parasitic disorders (on the order of 10 mg/l); some cases of parasitic infestations have been reported having levels as high as 100-500 mg/l
(4). The greatest levels of IgE (on the order of 1-60 g/l) are
found in E myelomatosis. In contrast to its high incidence in
the rat (H. Bazin, this Symposium), the frequency in man is low,
and less than 10 cases of human IgE myeloma proteins are known
today; their characteristics are summarized in Table II.

Table III. The occurrence of circulating IgE antibody as
           measured by RAST to common inhalant allergens
           in children with asthma and/or hay fever. The
           correlation between RAST and provocation test
           (PT) is very good with the exception of "low
           grade allergy" defined as positive PT with un-
           diluted (1/10 w/v) allergen extract. Data from
           Berg and Johansson (10).

| PT | RAST | | |
| Allergen | No. tests | | Correlation |
dilution	Positive	Negative	%
Negative	44	328	88
Positive			
≥1/10	348	112	76
1/10	94	82	53
1/100	118	26	82
1/1000	136	4	97

ANTIGEN BINDING ACTIVITY

The activity of IgE antibodies directed to various kinds
of allergen can be determined in-vitro using radioimmunoassays
(RIA), based on either the precipitation of the complex formed
between IgE antibody and a radiolabelled preparation of allergen
(5,6) or the antiglobulin principle using radiolabelled anti-
IgE antibody (7). The latter test - the radioallergosorbent
test (RAST) - has gained wide application not only in the research laboratory but also in routine allergy diagnostic practice. That RAST indeed measures "reaginic" antibody has been
convincingly demonstrated in several laboratories by comparative studies of RAST, Prausnitz-Küstner reaction, and sensitization of human leucocytes or lung tissue, using a great number
of allergens from pollen, dander and food (4,8).

The clinical importance of a detectable level of IgE antibody in serum has been evaluated by studies of atopic individuals
suffering from asthma and hay fever. A very good correlation was
found between the results of RAST and those obtained by end-point
skin titrations, provocation challenge tests and symptom score
(4,9). In a large study of RAST in routine use for the diagnosis

of allergy (10), the average correlation between RAST and provocation tests was found to be 80 to 90 per cent and, as shown
in Table III the degree of correlation will increase with the
increase in challenge titre. In a study of a selected group of
patients using an isolated allergen, a correlation of 100 per
cent was found (11).

It has been reported that IgE antibody may constitute up
to about 50 per cent of the total IgE present in an atopic

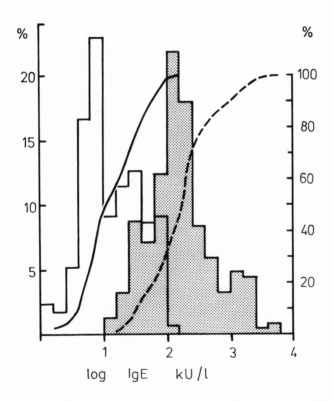

Fig. 1. The distribution and cumulative frequency of serum IgE
levels in healthy adults (solid line) and in adults with asthma
and hay fever (hatched area and broken line). The geometric mean
for the two groups was 13.8 and 140 kU/l respectively. Below
20 kU/l 65 per cent of healthy individuals and 2 per cent of
allergic individuals were found whereas above 100 kU/l the corresponding frequencies are 1 and 63 per cent (From ref. 14).

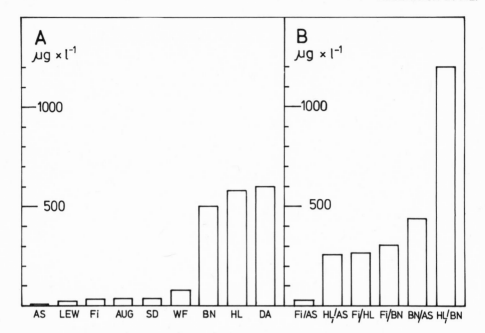

Fig. 2. The IgE level (mean) in different strains of adult rats
(A) and in adult F1 hybrids (B) as determined by a radioimmunoassay. (From T. Karlsson, H. Bazin and H. Bennich, to be published).

serum (6,12). If found to be generally true, these observations
may explain the significant difference in the IgE levels found
in the serum of patients with immediate hypersensitivity and of
healthy individuals, respectively (13). In a study of serum IgE
levels in adults (14) using PRIST - a sandwich-type radioimmunoassay (15) - a geometric mean of 13.8 kU/l was obtained for the
normal sera as compared to 140 kU/l for sera from allergic individuals. As illustrated in Figure 1 an IgE level below 20 kU/l
was found in 65 per cent of normal sera compared to 2 per cent
of allergic sera; above 100 kU/l, the corresponding frequencies
were found to be 1 and 63 per cent, respectively.

Since at this Symposium the IgE response in animal systems
is also subject to discussion, it is of interest to note that
by using PRIST we have found that the IgE level in serum from
apparently healthy rats is strain dependent (T. Karlsson, H.
Bazin and H. Bennich, to be published).

As shown in Fig. 2A the average IgE level in different
strains may differ from less than 10 µg/l to about 500 µg/l. A
potentiating effect is found in F1 hybrids when both parents

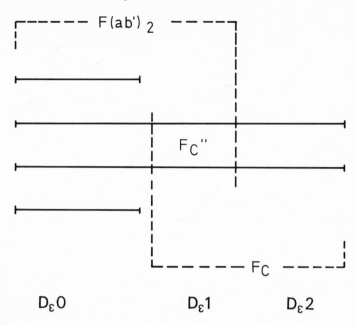

Fig. 3. Schematic structure of IgE, illustrating the molecular
location of the enzymatic fragments Fab'$_2$-ε , Fc"-ε and Fc-ε ,
and the distribution of antigenic determinants (D ε). (Modified
from ref. 16).

come from strains having high IgE, whereas no significant increase in IgE is found in F1 hybrids when only one of the parents
have a high IgE level (Fig. 2B). Strain differences have also
been observed in relation to the effect of potentiation of the
IgE reponse by parasitic infection, which will give IgE levels
on the order of 5 to 200 mg/l (E. Jarrett, this Symposium; T.
Karlsson, H. Bazin, E. Jarrett and H. Bennich, to be published).

IMMUNOCHEMICAL PROPERTIES

Two groups of isotypic antigens - Dε1 and Dε2 - have been
recognized on the epsilon chain (16). By enzymic cleavage of
IgE, the Dε1 activity is recovered with the peptic Fab'$_2$-ε fragment, whereas the Fc- ε fragment will carry both Dε1 and Dε2 activities (17); the disposition of Fab'$_2$-ε and Fc-ε within the IgE
molecule is shown in Fig. 3.

Both fragments are significantly larger (about 40,000 daltons) than the corresponding fragments derived from IgG. The
findings of Dε1 activity both in Fab'$_2$-ε and Fc-ε indicates that

```
                                             10                              20           96
  Glp-Val-Gln-Leu-Val-Gln-Ser-Gly-Ala-Glu-Val-Arg-Lys-Pro-Gly-Ala-Ser-Val-Arg-Val-Ser-Cys-Lys-Ala-Ser-Gly-Tyr-
                          30                              40                      50
  Thr-Phe-Ile-Asp-Ser-Tyr-Val-Gly-Trp-Ile-Arg-Gln-Ala-Pro-Gly-His-Gly-Leu-Glu-Trp-Ile-His-Trp-Ile-Asn-Pro-Asn-
                                  60                              70                  80
V Ser-Gly-Gly-Thr-Asn-Tyr-Ala-Pro-Arg-Phe-Gln-Gly-Arg-Val-Thr-Met-Thr-Arg-Asp-Ala-Ser-Phe-Ser-Thr-Ala-Tyr-Met-   22
                                  90                         100
  Asp-Leu-Arg-Ser-Leu-Arg-Ser-Asp-Asp-Ser-Ala-Val-Phe-Tyr-Cys-Ala-Lys-Ser-Pro-Phe-Trp-Ser-Asx-Tyr-Asx-Phe-
                     110                                     120                          130
  Asx-Tyr/Ser,Ser,Glx,Glx,Gly/Thr-Glu-Val-Thr-Tyr/Thr-Val-Ser-Gly-Ala-Trp/Thr-Leu-Pro-xxx/Val-Phe-Pro-Leu-
                                                      150                 160
  Thr-Arg-Cys-Cys-Lys-Asx-Ile-Pro-Ser-Asx-Ala-Thr-Ser-Val-Thr-Leu-Gly-Cys-Leu-Ala-Thr-Gly-Tyr-Phe-Pro-Glu-Pro-   207
                    L      225                           170                      180
                                         200
  Val-Met-Val-Thr-Trp-Asx-Thr-Gly-Ser-Leu-ASN-Gly-Thr-Thr-Met-Thr-Leu-Pro-Ala-Thr-Thr-Leu-Ser-Gly-His-Tyr-Ala-
C1                              220                           210
  Thr-Ile-Ser-Leu-Leu-Thr-Val-Ser-Gly-Ala-Trp-Ala-Lys-Gln-Met-Phe-Thr-Cys-Arg-Val-Ala-His-Thr-Pro-Ser-Ser-Thr-   153
                              220      139                        230               240  H
  Val-Asx-ASN-Lys-Thr-Phe-Ser-Val-Cys-Ser-Arg-Asp-Phe-Thr-Pro-Pro-Thr-Val-Lys-Ile-Glx-Ser-Ser-Cys-Asx-Gly-
                              250            312                   260                270
  Leu-Gly-His-Phe-Pro-Pro-Thr-Ile-Glx-Leu-Cys-Leu-Val-Ser-Gly-Tyr-Thr-Pro-Gly-Thr-Ile-ASN-Ile-Thr-Trp-Leu-Glx-
                                                      280                         290
                                                310    254                           320
  Asx-Gly-Glx-Val-Met-Asp-Val-Asp-Leu-Ser-Thr-Ala-Ser-Thr-Glu-Ser-Gln-Gly-Glu-Leu-Ala-Ser-Thr-Glu-Ser-Gln-Leu-
                     300
                                                330                      340                350
C2 Thr-Leu-Ser-Gln-Lys-His-Trp-Leu-Ser-Asp-Arg-Thr-Tyr-Thr-Cys-Gln-Val-Thr-Tyr-Gln-Gly-His-Thr-Phe-Gln-Asp-Ser-
                                          360                        370
  Thr-Lys-Lys-Cys-Ala-Asp-Ser-Asn-Pro-Arg-Gly-Val-Ser-Ala-Tyr-Leu-Ser-Arg-Pro-Ser-Pro-Phe-Asp-Leu-Phe-Ile-Arg-
      H                          418
                                          380                         390                         400
  Lys-Ser-Pro-Thr-Ile-Thr-Cys-Leu-Val-Val-Asp-Leu-Ala-Pro-Ser-Lys-Gly-Thr-Val-ASN-Leu-Thr-Trp-Ser-Arg-Ala-Ser-
                                                      410                      420                430
  Gly-Lys-Pro-Val-Asn-His-Ser-Thr-Arg-Lys-Glu-Glu-Lys-Gln-Arg-ASN-Gly-Thr-Leu-Thr-Val-Thr-Ser-Thr-Leu-Pro-Val-
                                                                  358
C3                              440                                    450
  Gly-Thr-Arg-Asp-Trp-Ile-Glu-Gly-Glu-Thr-Tyr-Gln-Cys-Arg-Val-Thr-His-Pro-His-Leu-Pro-Arg-Ala-Leu-Met-Arg-Ser-
                                                         460              470
  Thr-Thr-Lys-Thr-Ser-Gly-Pro-Arg-Ala-Ala-Pro-Glu-Val-Tyr-Ala-Phe-Ala-Thr-Pro-Glu-Trp-Pro-Gly-Ser-Arg-Asp-Lys-
                                 524                              490
                                                   480
  Arg-Thr-Leu-Ala-Cys-Leu-Ile-Gln-Asn-Phe-Met-Pro-Glu-Asp-Ile-Ser-Val-Gln-Trp-Leu-His-Asn-Glu-Val-Gln-Leu-Pro-
                                 490                                   500                     510
  Asp-Ala-Arg-His-Ser-Thr-Thr-Gln-Pro-Arg-Lys-Thr-Lys-Gly-Ser-Gly-Phe-Phe-Val-Phe-Ser-Arg-Leu-Glu-Val-Thr-Arg-
C4                      520           464                           530                         540
  Ala-Glu-Trp-Gln-Glu-Lys-Asp-Glu-Phe-Ile-Cys-Arg-Ala-Val-His-Glu-Ala-Ala-Ser-Pro-Ser-Gln-Thr-Val-Gln-Arg-Ala-
                                 547
  Val-Ser-Val-Asn-Pro-Gly-Lys.
```

Fig. 4

these fragments share an antigenically active portion of the
epsilon chain. By sequence analysis, this overlapping region
has been identified as a disulphide linked dimer of the $C\varepsilon 2$
domain, which is produced as a distinct fragment, Fc"-ε (previously designated Fc-like (18))with retained antigenic properties by peptic digestion of Fab'$_2$-ε or IgE at pH 2.4. The carboxy
terminal portion of the epsilon chain carrying Dε2 activity is
more vulnerable to proteolysis than the Cε2 region. Thus prolonged digestion of IgE with papain will convert initially produced Fc-ε to a smaller papain resistant fragment, which is
antigenically indistinguishable from Fc"-ε. For the same reason,
all efforts to produce enzymic fragments carrying Dε2 activity
have so far been unsuccessful.

CHEMICAL STRUCTURE

The amino acid sequence of epsilon chain ND (19) is shown
in Fig. 4. The epsilon polypeptide is composed of 547 amino
acid residues, and in addition to the Vε region, it contains 4
constant homology regions (Cε1, Cε2, Cε3 and Cε4) (20), thus
confirming our previous hypothesis about the general structure
of the epsilon chain (16). The primary structure of the Vε
region indicates that IgE(ND) represents a VHI subgroup protein
and comparison with "prototype" sequences (21) gives 63, 35
and 47 per cent homology between V ε (ND) and VHI, VHII and VHIII
respectively. These results give further support to the hypothesis that subgroup specificity of a VH region is not restricted to any particular class of heavy chain (22).

Fig. 4.   Tentative amino acid sequence of human ε chain ND,
subgroup VHI.
    Intra-chain disulphide bridges are indicated by an arrow
(the non-linear disulphide bridge in C 1 runs from Cys-139 (or
Cys-138)to Cys-225) and inter-chain disulphide are indicated
by H (inter-heavy) and by L (inter-light-heavy).
    Oligosaccharide side chains are located at Asn-residues
145, 173, 219, 265, 371 and 394; their carbohydrate composition
is shown in Table V.
    Fab'$_2$-ε and Fc"-ε fragments terminate at residues 339
and 338 respectively. The sequence of the peptide 330-334 contains one Asn but its position is not definitely determined.
Note the repetetive sequences 282-287 and 291-296.
    The sequence from residue 110 to residue 132 is not de-
finitely ascertained and the peptides within this region have
been placed by homology. (Extended and modified from ref. 20).

Table IV.   Comparison of the sequence of the 55 amino terminal residues in the variable region of lambda
chain ND with the sequence of two "prototype"
VλII proteins (21) (From H. von Bahr-Lindström
and H. Bennich, to be published).

```
                                                  10
λ(ND)   Glp-Ser-Ala-Leu-Thr-Gln-Pro-Pro-Ser-Ala-Ser-Gly-Ser-Leu-
λ(Nei)                                      Ala       Val           Pro
λ(Vil)His                                   Ala       Val           Leu
```
```
                              20
λ(ND)   Gly-Gln-Ser-Val-Thr-Phe-Ser-Cys-Ser-Gly-Thr-Ser-Ser-Asn-
λ(Nei)              Ile       Ile           Thr           Thr   Asp
λ(Vil)              Ile       Ile           Thr                 Asp
```
```
            30                                          40
λ(ND)   Ile-Gly-Asp-Tyr-Asn-Tyr-Val-Ser-Trp-Tyr-Arg-Glu-His-Pro-
λ(Nei)Val     Ser       Phe                       Gln Gln Asn
λ(Vil)Val     Gly                                 Phe Gln Gln
```
```
                                  50
λ(ND)   Gly-Lys-Ala-Pro-Lys-Leu-Met-Ile-Glx-Val-Thr-Lys-Arg
λ(Nei)                              Glu Gly Asn
λ(Vil)        Thr             Ile       Glu       Arg
```

The structure of light chain ND, which is of Type L, is
still incomplete, but as shown in Table IV the amino acid sequence of the amino terminal 55 residues indicates that VλND
is a representative of the VλII subgroup.

The sequence data of the epsilon chain ND further confirms
that the heavy polypeptide of IgE contains 15 half-cystine residues (17) of which 10 participate in the formation of intra-
chain disulphide bridges, one in each of the 5 homology regions
However, there are only 3 inter-chain bonds present in IgE(ND)
- not 5 as previously suggested (16): one inter-heavy-light cha
bond involving Cys-138 (or Cys-139) and two inter-heavy chain
bonds, which are located at Cys-241 and Cys-328, respectively.
The inter-ε-chain bonds are presumed to be arranged in parallel
in analogy with the inte-γ-chain bridges. The two remaining

Table V. Amino acid sequence and carbohydrate composition of glycopeptide regions in the epsilon chain ND[a]). Monosaccharides[b]) are expressed as number of residues per mole of peptide.

Glycopeptide region[c]	Fucose	Mannose	Galactose	N-acetyl-Glucosamine	Sialic acid
A. -Ile-Pro-Ser-Asn[145]-Ala-Thr-Ser-	1.3	3.3	2.5	3.9	0.5
B. -Gly-Ser-Leu-Asn[173]-Gly-Thr-Thr-	1.5	3.8	2.7	5.0	0.7
C. -Thr-Val-Asx-Asn[219]-Lys-Thr-Phe-	trace	3.3	2.6	3.8	2.3
D. -Gly-Thr-Ile-Asn[265]-Ile-Thr-Trp-	trace	3.0	2.4	3.5	2.1
E. -Gly-Thr-Val-Asn[371]-Leu-Thr-Trp-	0.7	3.4	2.1	3.3	1.3
F. -Lys-Gln-Arg-Asn[394]-Gly-Thr-Leu-	nil	5.7	trace	2.0	nil
Total:	3.5	22.5	12.3	21.5	6.9
Sugar residues per epsilon chain[d])	3.5	22	11	22.5	4.5

a) Modified and corrected from Table 1 in Ref. 20.

b) Determined as TMS-derivatives by GLC as described in Ref. 42.

c) Figures refer to residue position in Fig. 4; Letters refer to position of glycopeptide Fig. 5.

d) Calculated from the carbohydrate composition of IgE(ND) given in Ref. 43.

half-cystines - Cys-139 (or Cys-138) and Cys-225 - are engaged
in the formation of an additional "non-linear" intra-chain bond
located in the Cε1 region. Though not previously found in a
human Ig heavy chain, the presence of two intra-chain brigdes
located in the CH1 domain region has been demonstrated in rabbit γ chain (23).

The attachment of a light chain to a half-cystine residue
located at a position homologous to the Cys-138 in the Vε -
Cε1 inter-domain region has been found in heavy chains of several classes and of different species, with the exception of
human γ1 and γ2 heavy chains (24). The results of chemical
typing of IgE myeloma protein PS (25) confirms the labile nature of the disulphide bonds at Cys-138, Cys-139, Cys-225 and
Cys-328. The finding that the linear intra-chain bond (Cys-153
to Cys-207) in Cε1 is also cleaved by mild reduction, is in
agreement with an earlier observation (16) that 8 of the 20
disulphide bonds in native IgE(ND) can be reduced in the absence of unfolding agents. In this context, it should be mentioned
that the two inter-heavy chain bonds differ with respect to
susceptibility to reduction, and the relative resistance of the
inter-chain bond located at Cys-241 explains the slow production of epsilon chain monomer from IgE when subjected to mild
reduction (26).

By comparison of the sequences for ε, γ, μ and α chains,
their homologous regions can be arranged as shown in Fig. 5.
If it is assumed that the constant portion of an ancestral
heavy chain consisted of 4 homology regions, deletion of a
counterpart to the Cε2 and Cμ2 domains is one possible explanation to the general structure of the bridge (hinge) region
in γ and α chains. The fact that IgG subclass differences (24)
as well as duplications of peptide segments in α (27) and γ3
(28) chains (in the corresponding Cε2 region, see fig. 4) are
restricted to the hinge region, indicates that the gene(s) coding for this segment has (have) been subjected to a unique
evolutionary pressure. Although the inter-domain regions surrounding the CH2 domain of ε and μ chains show little or no
homology with the γ hinge segment, the location of cysteinyl-
residues and Pro/Pro-Pro containing portions, indicates that
the amino terminal portion of the γ hinge is related to an
inter-C1-C2 region, whereas its carboxy terminal half is related to an inter-C2-C3 region in both ε and μ chain.

The high carbohydrate content in IgE is explained by the
presence of 6 oligosaccharide chains attached to the heavy
polypeptide. One side chain is located at Asn-145 in the inter-
V-C region, one in the Cε1 domain at Asn-173, one in the first
bridge region at Asn-219, and one in the Cε2 domain at Asn-265,
whereas two are present in the Cε3 domain located at Asn-371

and Asn-394. The carbohydrate composition and the amino acid
sequence of glycopeptide regions is shown in Table V. The presence of carbohydrate side chains of both complex and simple
structure has also been found in the μ chain (29). Comparison
of the distribution of side chains in ε and μ reveals no obvious homology, with the exception of the side chain in the
CH1 region and the simple carbohydrate chain in the CH3, the
latter being also homologous as regards position with the complex side chain in γ chain. The structure of the carbohydrate
units in IgE(PS) have been determined (30) and the results not
only confirm the presence of one simple type of oligosaccharide unit in the ε chain, but demonstrate that this side chain
includes an α-linked N-acetyl glucosamine residue, unique for
serum glycoproteins.

CYTOTROPIC ACTIVITY

        The skin fixing or cytotropic activity of IgE antibodies
is directed to a specific receptor molecule presumably present

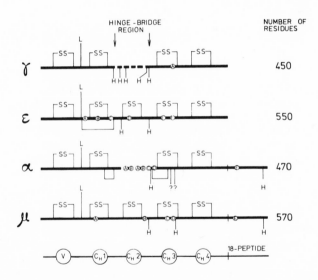

Fig. 5. Diagrammatic representation of homology regions, inter-
chain disulphide bridges (L=light chain; H=heavy chain) and
carbohydrate units (A,B,C etc.) in the chain of IgE ND, IgG Eu
(38), IgM Gal (39), IgA Tro (40), and IgA Bur(41). Deletion of a
counterpart to Cε2 and Cμ2 may explain the presence of only 3
constant domains in α and γ chain, and accordingly gaps have
been inserted in their bridge regions to maximize homology.
Sequence duplications are found in the bridge region of α and
γ3 and in C ε2 (see Fig. 4).

Table VI.   Inhibition of the Prausnitz-Küstner (PK) reaction
by IgE(ND) and its enzymic fragments. Dotted area
represents location of fragment within molecule.
The location of the peptide Asx-Ser-Asx-Pro-Arg,
postulated to have PK inhibitory activity (52) is
indicated by X. (Data taken from ref. 18).

INHIBITOR:	μMOLES x 10^{-5} PER SITE:	INHIBITION OF P-K(%) AFTER: 10´	20´
IgE(ND)	5.25	82	88
Fc-(ND)	5.56	93	95
Fc"-(ND)	12.5	24	18
Fab'$_2$-(ND)	7.14	0	0
Fab-(ND)	10.0	0	7
IgG-monocl.	6.9	60	18
	6.9	64	0

only on the membrane of basophil (mast) cells (31,32). The finding that the E myeloma protein ND will inhibit the Prausnitz-
Küstner reaction (33) and therefore is likely to have retained
the skin fixing activity characteristic for reaginic antibody,
initiated a study of the inhibitory activity of the enzymic
fragments Fab'$_2$-ε , Fc-ε and Fc"-ε (Fig. 3). As shown in Table
VI, the Fc- ε fragment was found to be the only fragment that
gave the same inhibitory activity as intact IgE when compared
on a molar basis (18). Since the 3 fragments have the Cε2 domain in common, the results indicate that the cytotropic activity is likely to be a function of the carboxy terminal domains
(Cε3 and/or Cε4) of the epsilon chain.

The effect of heating on reaginic activity is well known,
and further support for the molecular location of cytotropic
activity has been obtained by comparative studies of the conformational transitions induced by the heating of intact IgE
and its fragments at 56° (34). However, the results of P-K

inhibition studies or heating experiments provide but indirect
evidence, and until isolated Cε3 and Cε4 fragments have been
tested, the additional contribution of neighbouring domains to
cytotropic activity cannot be excluded (26).

   The cytotropic properties of IgE are also affected by reduction. It has long been known that treatment of reaginic serum
with 0.1 M mercaptoethanol will abolish the skin fixing activity.
However, studies of the effect of limited reduction under mild
conditions indicate that cytotropic activity is not affected
when less than 5 of the most labile disulphide bonds are cleaved (35). These results are not neccessarily in conflict with
those of other workers (36), who reported that the cleavage of
only 3 bonds is sufficient to impair the skin fixing properties,
as principally different methods were used. The difficulties
encountered in elucidating the biologic significance of disulphide bonds in IgE are illustrated by the results of a recent
study by Takatsu et al. (37). Cleavage of 4 disulphide bonds -
two between heavy-light chains and two located in the Cε1 region - was found to significantly diminish the affinity of IgE
for basophils, as measured by a reversed-type sensitization
technique. The Fc-ε fragment produced from such partially reduced IgE retained full binding capacity. In contrast, no effect
was found on the capacity of the reduced IgE to block passive
sensitization of target cells with reaginic antibody. By further
reduction, resulting in the cleavage of 5 disulphide bonds, both
sensitization and blocking activities were found to be lost, which
is in agreement with our previous findings (35).

   From our structural work discussed above, it is evident
that the disulphide bonds in IgE differ in susceptibility to reduction. Very mild reduction (i.e., 2 mM DTT or 0.05 M mercaptoethanol), though primarily affecting the heavy-light chain
bridges, will also cleave the neighbouring disulphide bonds between Cys-139 and Cys-225 located in the Cε1 region. Provided
that reduction of these bonds does not affect the binding of
anti-Dε0 antibodies (Fig. 3) used by Takatsu et al. (37) to
evaluate the affinity of reduced IgE for target cells, the results suggest - as these authors point out - that the conformation of Fab regions may interact with or influence the conformation of the binding site (s) located in the Fc region. Though
there is no direct evidence available at present to support this
hypothesis, it might be of interest to mention that the results
of experiments involving ultraviolet difference spectral analyses of IgE and its fragments before and after reduction (Bennich & Dorrington, to be published) seem to be explicable only
in terms of some kind of interaction taking place between the
Fab and Fc regions of intact IgE.

ACKNOWLEDGEMENTS

This work was supported in part by the Swedish Medical
Research Council (grants no. 16X-105 and 13X-3556), Svenska
Livförsäkringsbolags nämnd för medicinsk forskning and the
Wallenberg Foundation.

REFERENCES

1.   Johansson, S.G.O., and H. Bennich, Immunological studies
      of an atypical (myeloma) immunoglobulin, Immunology, 13,
      381, 1967.

2.   Johansson, S.G.O., and H. Bennich, Studies on a new class
      of human immunoglobulins. I. Immunological properties, in
      Nobel Symposium 3, Gamma Globulins, Structure and Control
      of Biosynthesis, Ed. J. Killander, p. 193, published by
      Almqvist and Wiksell, Stockholm, 1967.

3.   Bennich, H., and S.G.O. Johansson, Studies on a new class
      of human immunoglobulins. II. Chemical and physical proper-
      ties, in Nobel Symposium 3, Gamma Globulins, Structure and
      Control of Biosynthesis, Ed. J. Killander, p. 199, pub-
      lished by Almqvist and Wiksell, Stockholm, 1967.

4.   Johansson, S.G.O., H. Bennich, and T. Berg, Clinical sig-
      nificance of IgE, in Progress in Clinical Immunology, Ed.
      R.S. Schwarts, p. 157, published by Grune and Stratton,
      New York, 1972.

5.   Ishizaka, K., and T. Ishizaka, Identification of γ E-anti-
      bodies as a carrier of reaginic activity, J. Immunology,
      99, 1187, 1967.

6.   Zeiss, C.R., J.J. Pruzansky, R. Patterson, and M. Roberts,
      A solid phase radioimmunoassay for the quantitation of
      human reaginic antibody against ragweed antigen E, J.
      Immunol., 110, 414, 1973.

7.   Wide, L., H. Bennich, and S.G.O. Johansson, Diagnosis of
      allergy by an in vitro test for allergen antibodies,
      Lancet, ii, 1105, 1967.

8.   Evans, R., III (editor), Advances in Diagnosis of Allergy:
      RAST, published by Stratton Intercontinental Medical Book
      Corporation, New York, 1975.

9.   Johansson, S.G.O., Comparison of in vivo and in vitro
      tests for diagnosis of immediate hypersensitivity, in
      Laboratory Diagnosis of Immunologic Disorders, Eds. G.N.
      Vyas, and D.P. Stites, p. 225, published by Grune and
      Stratton, New York, 1975.

10.   Berg, T., and S.G.O. Johansson, Allergy diagnosis with the
      radioallergosorbent test. A comparison with the results
      of skin and provocation tests in an unselected group of
      children with asthma and hay fever, J. Allergy Clin.
      Immunol., 54, 209, 1974.

11.   Aas, K., and U. Lundkvist, The radioallergosorbent test
      with a purified allergen from cod-fish, Clin. Allergy,
      3, 255, 1973.

12.   Gleich, G.J., and G.L. Jacob, Immunoglobulin E antibodies
      to pollen allergens account for high percentages of total
      immunoglobulin E protein, Science, 190, 1106, 1975.

13.   Johansson, S.G.O., Raised levels of a new immunoglobulin
      class (IgND) in asthma, Lancet, ii, 951, 1967.

14.   Johansson, S.G.O., Determination of IgE and IgE antibody
      by RAST, in Advances in Diagnosis of Allergy: RAST, Ed.
      R. Evans III, p. 7, published by Stratton Intercontinental
      Medical Book Corporation, New York, 1975.

15.   Ceska, M., and U. Lundkvist, A new and simple radioimmuno-
      assay method for the determination of IgE, Immunochemistry,
      9, 1021, 1972.

16.   Bennich, H., and S.G.O. Johansson, Immunoglobulin E and
      immediate hypersensitivity, Vox Sanguinis, 19, 1, 1970.

17.   Bennich, H., and S.G.O. Johansson, Structure and function
      of human immunoglobulin E, in Advances in Immunology, vol.
      13, Eds. F.J. Dixon and H.G. Kunkel, p.1, published by
      Academic Press, New York, 1971.

18.   Stanworth, D.R., J.H. Humphrey, H. Bennich, and S.G.O.
      Johansson, Inhibition of Prausnitz-Küstner reaction by
      proteolytic cleavage fragments of a human myeloma protein
      of immunoglobulin class E, Lancet, ii, 17, 1968.

19.   Bennich, H., H. von Bahr-Lindström, D. Seecher, and C.
      Milstein, Primary structure of a monoclonal immunoglobulin
      E (IgE,ND).To be published.

20. Bennich, H., H. von Bahr-Lindström, Structure of immuno-
    globulin E (IgE), in Progress in Immunology II, Vol. 1,
    Eds. L. Brent and J. Holborow, p. 49, published by North-
    Holland Publishing Company, 1974.

21. Gally, J.A., and G.M. Edelman, The genetic control of
    immunoglobulin synthesis, Am. Rev. Genetics, 6, 1, 1972.

22. Putnam, F.W., A. Shimizu, C. Paul, and T. Shinoda, Varia-
    tion and homology in immunoglobulin heavy chains, Federa-
    tion Proc. (US), 31, 193, 1972.

23. O'Donnell, I.J., B. Frangione, and R.R. Porter, The disul-
    phide bonds of the heavy chain of rabbit immunoglobulin G.
    Biochem. J., 116, 261, 1970.

24. Milstein, C., and J.R.L. Pink, Structure and evolution of
    immunoglobulins, in Progress in Biophysics and Molecular
    Biology, 21, eds. J.A.V. Butler and D. Noble, p. 211,
    published by Pergamon Press, Oxford and New York, 1970.

25. Mendez, E., B. Frangione, and S. Kochwa, Chemical typing
    of human immunoglobulins E and D, FEBS Letters, 33, 4, 1973

26. Bennich, H., and K.J. Dorrington, Structure and conforma-
    tion of immunoglobulin E (IgE), in The Biological Role of
    the Immunoglobulin E System, Eds. K. Ishizaka and D.H.
    Dayton Jr., p. 19, published by U.S. Government Printing
    Office, Washington DC, 1972.

27. Adlersberg, J.B., E.C. Franklin, and B. Frangione, Repe-
    tetive hinge region sequences in human IgG3: Isolation of
    an 11,000-dalton fragment, Proc. Nat. Acd. Sci. (USA), 72,
    723, 1975.

28. Michaelsen, T.E., and J.B. Natvig, Unusual molecular pro-
    perties of human IgG3 proteins due to an extended hinge
    region, J. Biol. Chem., 249, 2778, 1974.

29. Shimizu, A., F.W. Putnam, C. Paul, J.R. Clamp, and I.
    Johnson, Structure and role of the five glycopeptides of
    human IgM immunoglobulin, Nature New Biol., 231, 73, 1971.

30. Baenziger, J., S. Kornfeld, and S. Kochwa, Structure of the
    carbohydrate units of IgE immunoglobulin, J. Biol. Chem.,
    249, 1889, 1974.

31. Ishizaka, K., H. Tomioka, and T. Ishizaka, Mechanisms of
    passive sensitization, I. Presence of IgE and IgG molecules
    on human leucocytes, J. Immunol., 105, 1459, 1970.

32. Sullivan, A.L., P.M. Grimley, and H. Metzger, Electron microscopic localization of immunoglobulin E on the surface membrane of human basophils, J. Exp. Med., 134, 1403, 1971.

33. Stanworth, D.R., J.H. Humphrey, H. Bennich, and S.G.O. Johansson, Specific inhibition of the Prausnitz-Küstner reaction by an atypical human myeloma protein, Lancet, ii, 330, 1967.

34. Dorrington, K.J., and H. Bennich, Thermally induced structure changes in immunoglobulin E (IgE). J. Biol. Chem., 248, 8378, 1973.

35. Stanworth, P.R., J. Housley, H. Bennich, and S.G.O. Johansson, Effect of reduction upon the PCA-blocking activity of immunoglobulin E. Immunochemistry, 7, 321, 1970.

36. Ishizaka, T., and K. Ishizaka, Biologic function of immunoglobulin E. in The Biological Role of the Immunoglobulin E System, Eds. K. Ishizaka and D.H. Dayton Jr., p. 33, published by U.S. Government Printing Office, Washington, D.C., 1972.

37. Takatsu, K., T. Ishizaka, and K. Ishizaka, Biologic significance of disulphide bonds in human IgE molecules, J. Immunol., 114, 1838, 1975.

38. Edelman, G.M., B.A. Cunningham, W.E. Gall, P.D. Gottlieb, U. Rutishauser, and M.J. Waxdal, The covalent structure of an entire G immunoglobulin molecule, Proc. Natl. Acad. Sci. (USA), 63, 78, 1969.

39. Watanabe, S., H.U. Barnikoe, J. Horn, J. Bertvam, and N. Hilschmann, The primary structure of a monoclonal IgM-immunoglobulin (macroglobulin Gal.). II: The amino acid sequence of the H-chain (μ-type), subgroup H III. Architecture of the complete IgM-molecule, Hoppe-Seyler's Z. Physiol. Chemie, 354, 1505, 1973.

40. Kratzin, H., P. Altevogt, E. Ruban, A. Kortt, K. Staroscik, and N. Hilschmann, The primary structure of a monoclonal IgA-immunoglobulin (IgA TRO). II: The amino acid sequence of the H-chain, α-type, subgroup III: structure of the complete IgA-molecule, Hoppe-Seyler's Z. Physiol. Chemie, 356, 1337, 1975.

41. Low, T.L.K., Y.-S.V. Liu, and F.W. Putnam, Structure,
     function and evolutionary relationship of Fc domains of
     human immunoglobulins A,G,M, and E, Science, 191, 390, 1976

42. Clamp, J.R., T. Bhatti, and R.E. Chambere, The examination
     of carbohydrate in glycoproteins by gas-liquid chromato-
     graphy, in: Glycoproteins, Ed. A Gottschalk, vol. 5: A,
     p. 300, Elsevier Publishing Company, 1972.

43. Clamp, J.R., and I. Johnson, Immunoglobulins, in Glyco-
     proteins, Ed. A. Gottschalk, vol. 5:A, p. 612, Elsevier
     Publishing Company, 1972.

44. Ogawa, M., S. Kochwa, C. Smith, K. Ishizaka, and O.R.
     McIntyre, Clinical aspects of IgE myeloma, N. Engl. J.
     Med., 281, 1217, 1969.

45. Stoica, G.H., personal communication, 1970.

46. Fishkin, B.G., N. Orloff, L.C. Scaduto, D.T. Borucki, and
     H.L. Spiegelberg, IgE multiple myeloma. Report of the third
     case, Blood, 39, 361, 1972.

47. Stefani, D.V., A.I. Gusev, and R.A. Mokeeva, Isolation of
     immunochemically pure IgE from serum of E-myeloma patient
     Yu, Immunochemistry, 10, 559, 1973.

48. Penn, G.M., personal communication, 1972.

49. Mills, R.J., M.N. Fahie-Wilson, P.M. Carter, and J.R. Hobbs
     IgE myelomatosis, Clin. exp. Immunol., 23, 228, 1976.

50. Senda, N., and S.Inai, personal communication, 1975.

51. Knedel, M., A. Fateh-Moghadam, H. Edel, R. Bartl,und D.
     Neumeier, Multiples Myelom mit monoklonaler IgE-Gammopathie,
     Dtsch. med. Wschr., 101, 496, 1976.

52. Hamburger, R.N., Peptide inhibition of the Prausnitz-Küstner
     reaction, Science, 189, 389, 1975.

DISCUSSION

MARSH: I notice that in your figure showing serum IgE levels in allergic and nor-allergic populations there is a substantial overlap between the two populations. The range in which the overlap occurs may be different in different populations, and the time of year when the serum samples are drawn, and may also depend to some extent on the assay system for measuring total IgE (e.g. direct RIST versus double antibody).

However, the main point I wish to make is that one can not really differentiate between allergic and non-allergic people in terms of total IgE level which you seem to be implying. In fact, the highly allergic people with low total IgE turn out to be most interesting from the genetic point of view as I showed yesterday.

BENNICH: I did not imply that it is possible to identify an individual as allergic only on the basis of the serum IgE level. However, the distribution of IgE levels obtained by PRIST shows a very small overlap between normal and allergic individuals. In our study only approximately 2% of allergic patients had an IgE value less than 20 kU/l compared to more than 60% of the normals and for values above 100 kU/l the percentage figures were reversed.

LICHTENSTEIN: As you know both Gleich and Adkinson have been able, by different techniques, to quantitate in absolute terms the IgE antibody levels. We have seen patients with low total IgE levels, 15-20 ng/ml who were anaphylactically sensitive to a honey bee sting. They have only 4-5 ng/ml of bee venom specific IgE and would thus not be considered as allergic by there total IgE, or by present standards for bee venom RAST tests.

BENNICH: The figures for the percentage of specific IgE antibody of the total IgE recently reported by Gleich and Adkinson are generally higher than those reported some years ago by Zeiss et al. The adsorption procedures used by Gleich and Adkinson in our hands are rather inaccurate and tend to give falsely high values.

Rare cases with anaphylactic reactions to less typical allergens, i.e. bee venom and penicilline, have low levels of circulating specific IgE but the concentration can change rapidly in relation to the symptoms. An IgE level below 20 kU/l is very unusual in atopic patients allergic to the common inhalant

allergens. In the RAST commercially available from Pharmacia
the lowest concentration of IgE antibody regarded as positive
is 1 SRU (Specific Reaginic Unit) which would correspond to
approximately 2 ng/ml of IgE. The corresponding figure for
RAST in our laboratory using labeled anti-Dε2 is 0.1-0.2 SRU,
or around 0.2-0.4 ng/ml of IgE.

DIAMANT: Have anybody experienced among allergic patients
a negative RAST, together with a negative skin test but with
a positive histamine release from the patients basophils? We
have found that 2 out of 13 bakers tested in Copenhagen have
this combination of test results. The remaining 11 were positive in all three tests. (Blands er al., to be published).

ISHIZAKA, K.: I am glad to hear that the disagreement between your data and our results was almost solved. I would like
to know your evidence for a possible interaction between the
Fab and Fc portions of the IgE molecule.

BENNICH: There are at present no direct evidence for an
interaction between the Fab(ε) and Fc(ε) regions. However, preliminary results of a study done in collaboration with Dr. K.
Dorrington, University of Toronto, on the conformational changes
that can be observed in IgE and its fragments under various
experimental conditions seem to favour the hypothesis that the
C-terminal portion (Cε3 and Cε4 domains) of the epsilon chain
is non-covalently linked to the Fab portion (CL or Cε1?) and
furthermore that such and interaction may be affected by reduction of presumably the labile disulphide bonds present in the
Cε1 domain region.

ISHIZAKA, K: It is difficult to explain our results simply
by some changes in the Dε O determinants. After mild reduction,
reduced-alkylated protein sensitized skin sites for reversed
P-K reaction for 2 to 3 hr. If one waits for 24 hrs, which is
optimal to get maximal sensitization with native IgE, the reversed P-K was negative. Our explanation was that reduced
alkylated protein did not stay on the mast cells for a long
time.

I would like to ask you another question. I heard from
Dr. Kochwa recently that one of the inter-heavy chain disulphide bond was more susceptible to reduction that the heavy-
light chain bond. This is in conflict with our results. Do
you have such an experience with the IgE(ND) protein?

BENNICH: No.

ISHIZAKA, T: Would you like to make a comment on "the
PK-test inhibiting pentapeptide" reported by Dr. Hamburger?

BENNICH: Yes! Last year Dr. Robert Hamburger reported
(52) his (sensational) findings that a synthetic peptide -
Asp-Ser-Asp-Pro-Arg had the capacity to block a standard Prausnitz-Küstner reaction as well as to inhibit a known positive
skin test reaction, which suggested that the peptide could
compete for IgE binding site on mast (basophil) cells. The
sequence of Dr Hamburger's pentapeptide is found in the tenta-

tive sequence of the epsilon chain ND as reported by us at the
Immunology Congress in Brighton 1974 (see ref. 20).

However, by repeated sequence analysis of the epsilon chain,
we now know that the sequence of a "Hamburger peptide" must contain one asparaginyl (Asn) and one aspartyl (Asp) residue, which
leaves us with the following alternatives for a correct sequence:
Asn-Ser-Asp-Pro-Arg and Asp-Ser-Asn-Pro-Arg. In collaboration
with Dr. U. Ragnarsson (Dept. of Biochemistry, Uppsala University) we have tested the P-K inhibitory activity of a number of
synthetic pentapeptides having both the structure of the "Hamburger peptide" and the "correct" sequences as above, but in
neither of two series of experiments using different batches of
peptides have we been able to varify Dr. Hamburger's findings.
Since the pentapeptide (Asx-Ser-Asx-Pro-Arg) is present in the
Fab'2-ε and Fc"-ε fragments, where it is located vary close
to the carboxyl terminal end, the Fc"-ε fragment was also tested,
but no inhibitory activity could be demonstrated, which is in
agreement with our previous findings (see Table 6).

Furthermore, the fact - as reported by Dr. Hamburger - that
his pentapeptide requires 5 to 24 hours for full inhibitory activity when administered prior to reaginic serum, strongly suggests that the inhibitory activity observed cannot be explained
in terms of an interaction with specific IgE receptor sites on
mast (basophil) cells.

Finally I should mention that Dr. Hamburger was informed
about our failure to verify his findings, some two months, prior
to the publication of his paper in Science.

FUNCTIONS AND DEVELOPMENT OF CELL RECEPTORS FOR IgE[1]

Teruko Ishizaka

The Johns Hopkins University School of Medicine at

The Good Samaritan Hospital, Baltimore, Md. 21239 U.S.A.

It has been established that IgE is present on basophil granu-locytes and mast cells and that the immunoglobulin combines with these cells through the Fc portion of the molecules (1,2). Earlier studies on the cell-bound IgE was carried out in human basophil system using E myeloma protein. The isolation of rat E myeloma protein by Bazin (3) made the rat mast cell system as useful as human basophils for the studies on the mechanisms of sensitization. An advantage of the rat system is that isolation of normal rat mast cells is much easier than purification of human basophils (4). Furthermore, a basophilic leukemia cell line became available for the studies of IgE-binding (5). In this Symposium, I would like to summarize available information on cell-bound IgE and receptors on basophils and mast cells, and present our recent findings on the development of rat mast cells and their receptors by a long-term culture of thymus cells.

I. Cell-bound IgE Molecules and Receptors

The demonstration of IgE on human basophils immediately raised questions of how many IgE molecules are present on basophils and whether the binding of IgE with receptors is reversible. The first question was answered by enumerating IgE molecules per human baso-phil granulocyte by C1 fixation transfer technique. The results of the experiment showed that the average number was 10,000 to 40,000 per cells in most of both normal and atopic individuals (6). The experiment also showed that receptors for IgE on the basophils of normal individuals are not saturated under the physiological condi-tion, but the sites will be saturated by incubation of the cells in 100 μg to 1 mg/ml of E myeloma protein. The total number of

Table I

Binding of Anti-IgE or IgE with basophils exposed to pH 4.0

Pretreat at pH	Incubation with ^{125}I-labeled	Number of grains per basophil			
		<10	11-30	31-50	>50
4.0	Anti-IgE	100	0	0	0
7.6		0	0	9	91
4.0	IgE	0	0	0	100
7.6		0	57	34	9

The numbers in this table indicate percentage of basophils giving a certain number of grains.

receptors per cell was estimated to be 40,000 to 100,000 (6).

It was also found that the binding of IgE molecules with the receptor was a reversible reaction. If normal basophils were sensitized with ^{125}I-labeled IgE and the sensitized cells were incubated with unlabelled IgE, a slow release of cell-bound IgE was demonstrated (6). Subsequent experiments also showed that cell-bound IgE dissociated at acid pH (7). In the experiment shown in Table I, mononuclear cell fraction containing basophils were exposed to pH 4.0 for 5 min at $0^{o}C$, and the cells were treated with ^{125}I-anti-IgE at the neutral pH. Autoradiographs of the cells showed that radioactive anti-IgE combined with untreated basophils but did not combine with the acid-treated cells, and indicated that cell-bound IgE was lost by the acid treatment. Disappearance of IgE from the cell-surface was not due to degradation of receptor sites. If the acid-treated cells were incubated with radio-labeled E myeloma protein, the protein combined with both untreated and acid-treated cells. Indeed, the number of grains on the acid-treated basophils was more than that on the untreated cells. These findings confirmed that the binding of IgE with basophil receptor is reversible and showed that covalent bonding is not involved in the binding reaction.

Based on the proportion of IgE receptors occupied by IgE and the serum IgE concentration of the donors, equilibrium constant of the binding reaction was estimated (Table II). In 9 out of 13 donors studied, equilibrium constant of the reaction was 0.5 to 1.3 x 10^9/mole (6). Subsequently, Kulczycki and Metzger (8) have studied the binding of rat IgE with rat basophilic leukemia cells.

Table II

Receptors for IgE on basophils and mast cells

Target cells	Receptors/cells	Equilibrium const.
	$\times 10^3$	$\times 10^9$
Human basophils	$40 \sim 100$	$0.5 \sim 1.3$
Rat basophilic leukemia cells	$1000^{1)}$ $600^{2)}$	$9.0^{1)}$ $1 \sim 2^{2)}$
Rat peritoneal	$300^{2)}$	$1 \sim 1.5^{2)}$

1) Kulczcki, A., et al   2) Conrad, D.H. et al

As the leukemia cells were cultured in vitro and did not possess IgE on their surface, kinetics of the binding reaction was studied by incubating the cells in various concentrations of radio-labeled E myeloma protein and measuring cell-bound IgE. Dissociation of ^{125}I-IgE from the cells was determined by incubating the labeled cells in a high concentration of unlabelled IgE. Their experiments showed that an average number of receptors per leukemia cell was in the order of 1 million and an average equilibrium constant of the binding reaction was 9×10^9/mole. More recently, Conrad et al (9) carried out a similar experiment using normal rat peritoneal mast cells and compared the binding parameters of the interaction with those of basophilic leukemia cells. As shown in Table II, their results showed that equilibrium constant was in the order of 10^9/mole, comparable for both basophilic leukemia cells and normal mast cells. In their experiment, the average number of receptors on the leukemia cell was 600,000, twice as many as the free receptors on a normal mast cell.

Summarizing the data available for the binding, it appears that equilibrium constants for both human and rat systems are in the order of 10^9/mole. The only significant difference between human basophils and rat mast cells was the number of receptors. If one considers that a diameter of rat mast cell is approximately 2-3 times longer than that of human basophil, it appears that density of receptor sites per unit area of cell surface would be comparable in both cell types. Another factor to be considered is that the number of IgE molecules estimated by the Cl fixation transfer test represents the minimal rather than absolute number. Thus, the results obtained in the human basophil system might be less than the actual number of receptors (6). In any event, all of the findings on the kinetics of IgE binding with human basophils and rat mast

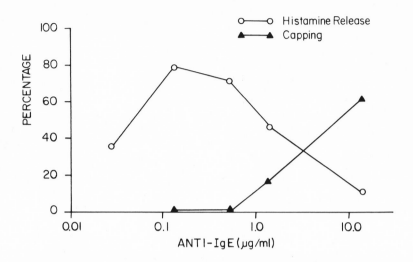

Fig. 1. Optimal concentrations of anti-IgE for histamine release and for cap formation. Percentage of histamine release and the proportion of basophils with capping were plotted against the concentration of fluoresceinated antigen-IgE for incubation.

cells indicate that IgE has high affinity for receptors on the target cell, and this fact will explain why a minute amount of IgE antibody can sensitze target cells and why sensitization with IgE antibody is so persistent.

It is generally accepted that plasma membrane on mammalian cells is in a liquid state. Indeed, IgE molecules on basophil granulocytes are movable at 37°C. When the cell-bound IgE on basophils reacted with divalent anti-IgE, the immunoglobulin form patches and eventually migrate into one pole of the cells (10). The monovalent Fab fragment of the antibody combined with cell-bound IgE but did not induce redistribution of the cell-bound immunoglobulin. This finding is in agreement with the fact that divalent anti-IgE induced histamine release but the Fab fragment of the antibody failed to do so (11). In view of such findings, the relationship between histamine release and cap formation was studied. The leukocyte suspensions were incubated at 37°C with varying concentrations of fluoresceinated anti-IgE. After incubation, the cells were

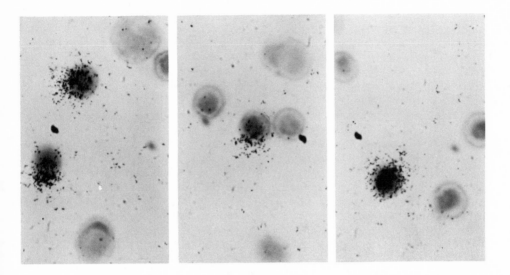

Fig. 2. Autoradiographs of basophils showing redistribution of IgE
        receptors.
a. & b. Cells were treated with fluoresceinated anti-IgE at 37°C
        for cap formation, exposed to pH 3.0 and then treated with
        ^{125}I-E myeloma protein. Radioactive grains are accumulated
        to one-half of the cells (a) or localized on one pole (b).
     c. Basophils were exposed to pH 3.0 to dissociate cell-bound
        IgE and then treated with ^{125}I-E myeloma protein at
        neutral pH.

examined by fluorescent microscope for cap formation, and histamine
released into the supernatant fluid was measured. As shown in Fig.
1, the dose-dependence of cap formation was entirely different from
the dose-response curve of histamine release. Maximum histamine release was obtained with a low concentration of anti-IgE where redistribution of IgE was not observed. More or less complete inhibition of histamine release was observed with higher dose of anti-
IgE which redistributed IgE molecules most effectively. We have
also studied the distribution of IgE upon antigen-induced histamine
release. After incubation of cells from ragweed-sensitive patients
with varying concentration of antigen E, the cells were incubated
with fluoresceinated Fab fragment of anti-IgE to demonstrate cell-
bound IgE. In all instances, the cells showed a uniform diffuse
staining and neither cap nor patch formation was observed. These
results clearly showed that cap formation is not involved in the
process of histamine release. It should be noted, however, that
both histamine release and patch or cap formation required divalent
anti-IgE and indicated that bridging of cell-bound IgE molecules
initiated both processes.

As the IgE molecules are firmly bound with cell receptors, one can expect that the receptors will migrate together with IgE upon capping. Experiments were carried out to confirm the movement (12). The mononuclear cells were first incubated with fluoresceinated anti-IgE. After evaluation of cap formation by fluorescence microscopy, the cells were washed and exposed to pH 3.0 to dissociate cell-bound IgE-anti IgE complexes. The cells were then incubated with ^{125}I-E myeloma protein at neutral pH and their autoradiographs were examined. If the receptors moved to one pole of the cells upon capping, one can expect that radioactive IgE would be localized to one side of the cells. Indeed, distribution of grains on the cell was not homogeneous after capping. In one-third to one-half of the basophils, grains were accumulated on one half of the cell and the other cell circumference was free of grains (Fig. 2a). On some basophils, grains were localized on one pole of the cells (Fig. 2b). Such a cell was not detected on the cell preparation which was not treated with anti-IgE prior to the exposure to pH 3.0 (Fig. 2c).

A question arose as to whether the free receptors may migrate together with IgE-bound receptors. In order to answer this question, we have selected donors of basophils in which less than 50% of receptors are occupied by IgE. A portion of mononuclear cells from such donors was incubated in 100 µg/ml of E myeloma protein to saturate receptors. Both sensitized and unsensitized cells from the same donor were then incubated in fluoresceinated anti-IgE. After cap formation, both cell suspension were exposed to pH 3.0 to dissociate cell-bound IgE and then treated with ^{125}I-E myeloma protein at neutral pH. Autoradiographs of each cell suspension were taken

Table III

Effect of Sensitization with IgE
on the Redistribution of IgE Receptors

Donor	Sensitization with IgE	IgE molecules per basophils			
K.I.	−	5,000*	15	42	43
	+	36,000	16	32	52
J.H.	−	25,000	8	46	46
	+	62,000	9	43	48

*As the number of cell-bound IgE was low, 250 µg/ml of anti-IgE were employed for maximal cap formation.

to examine the distribution of ^{125}I-IgE on the cells. Representative results of the experiments are shown in Table III. After maximal cap formation, the proportion of basophils showing polar distribution of ^{125}I-IgE was comparable, whether the IgE receptors are saturated or not. It should be noted that 85% of total receptors on KI cells and 60% of receptors on JH cells were free of IgE before sensitization. If these free receptors did not migrate together with IgE-bound receptors upon capping, they should have remained all over the cell surface. As the free receptors should combine with radioactive IgE, most of the unsensitized cells would have given uniform distribution of grains. Actual results of autoradiography, however, showed that grains were localized to one side of the cells in more than 50% of unsensitized basophils. These findings strongly suggested that not only IgE-bound receptors but also free receptors migrated to the same pole upon capping with anti-IgE. The results seem to indicate that a group of receptor sites are associated with each other at the cell membrane or that receptor molecules on basophil membrane are multivalent with respect to the combining sites for IgE.

Attempts were made to obtain subcellular components of rat mast cells which have the ability to combine IgE. Bach and Brashler (13) disrupted rat peritoneal mast cells by exposure to distilled water and found that cell ghost had the ability to absorb rat reaginic antibodies. König and Ishizaka (14) have destructed normal rat mast cells by sonication and demonstrated the PCA blocking activity in the 200,000g supernatant. Gel filtration of the supernatant fraction through a sepharose 6B column gave active components in the void volume fraction. The same fraction combined ^{125}I-rat IgE. Incubation of the protein with the membrane fraction followed by gel filtration showed that a significant proportion of ^{125}I-IgE was bound with the components. The binding was inhibited by preincubation of the membrane component with a serum of rat infected with Nippostrongylus brasiliensis which contained a high concentration of IgE, but normal rat serum failed to block the binding (15).

More recently, Conrad et al (16) obtained IgE receptor complexes. Purified rat mast cells and basophilic leukemia cells were surface-labeled with ^{125}I and incubated with E myeloma protein to saturate their receptors. The cells were treated with Nonidet P-40 to solubilize plasma membrane and IgE in the supernatant was precipitated with anti-IgE. Analysis of the precipitate by SDS-polyacrylamide gel electrophoresis showed a radioactive component with the molecular weight of approximately 60,000. As the radioactive components should be derived from plasma membrane and were bound with IgE, they proposed that the component represents IgE-receptor. The nature of the receptor is unknown, however, one can expect that further studies on this line will characterize the receptor.

II. Development of Rat Mast Cells and Their Receptors

Basophilic leukemia cells would be the best source for the studies of receptors, however, these cells sensitized with IgE failed to release histamine upon challenge with either antigen or anti-IgE (17). Attempts were therefore made to develop rat mast cells which bear no IgE but have the ability to be sensitized by IgE antibody. Many years ago, Ginsburg and Sachs (18) described that mouse thymus cells seeded on mouse embryonic fibroblast mono-layer differentiated to mast cells. In view of these observations, experiments were undertaken to obtain rat mast cells by a long term culture of rat thymus cells on rat embryonic monolayer (19).

The monolayer was prepared from the embryos of 15 to 16th day of gestation. Thymus cell suspension was obtained from young Sprague-Dawley rats and 20 to 50 million cells were seeded on the tertiary or quaternary embryonic monolayer. Approximately 95 to 97% of the thymus cells for seeding were small and medium lympho-cytes. Mast cells were detected in some thymus cell suspension but the number of the cells was less than 0.05%. Thymus cells were cultured on Eagle's minimum essential medium enriched with 10% fetal calf serum and 3 mM L-glutamine. The passages were performed every 7 to 8 days.

Within a few days after seeding, the majority of lymphocytes rapidly degenerated. Remaining lymphocytes and other cells, such as epithelial cells and macrophages, gradually settled in the mono-layer. On the 6th or 7th day, just before the first passage, blast cells in various sizes and shapes appeared on the monolayers (Fig. 3). Some of the blast cells contained unique foamy regions in their cytoplasm but no metachromatic materials. The number of blast cells increased in the monolayers during the 10th to 14th day. At the same time, the foamy region in the cells increased intensively (Fig. 4a). At this stage, metachromatic materials appeared in the foamy regions indicating that these blast cells were mastoblasts. These cells in the monolayer were recovered by digesting the mono-layer with trypsin, incubated with ^{125}I-labeled IgE or IgG and their autoradiographs were examined. As shown in Fig. 4b, the mastoblast gave a small but significant number of grains, whereas the other cells, such as lymphocytes, macrophages and fibroblasts did not give a significant number of grains. The results clearly showed that the mastoblast obtained as early as the 14th day of culture was capable of binding IgE. It was also found that none of the cells, including mastoblast, bound IgG.

Metachromatic granules in the mastoblasts continued to in-crease and the cells developed to young mast cells. As shown in Fig. 5, their cytoplasm were filled with granules. After about 20 days culture, mature mast cells in the monolayer began to be-come free in the culture medium. The number of free mast cells

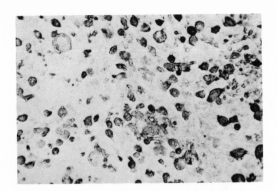

Fig. 3. Blast cells in various sizes and shapes on the feeder layer,
7 days after seeding thymus cells. Wright staining, x 160.

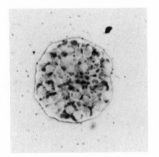
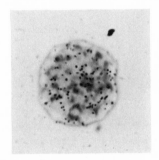

Fig. 4. Autoradiograph of a mastoblast (14 days culture). Cells
were treated with ^{125}I-IgE, Wright staining, x 960. Microscope was focused to the cell (a) or to radioactive grains
on the cell (b). Cytoplasm is filled with foamy regions.
Sparse, but definite, metachromatic granules are seen.

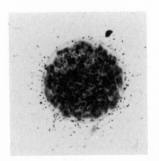
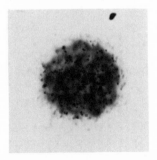

Fig. 5. Autoradiograph of a mature mast cell (35 days culture).
Mast cells were treated with ^{125}I-IgE, Wright staining,
x 960. Microscope was focused to the cell (a) or to the
grains on the cell (b). Cytoplasm was loaded with metachromatic granules.

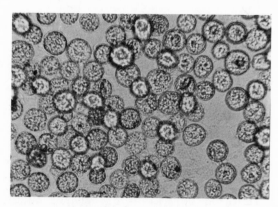

Fig. 6. Living culture of mature mast cells (35 days culture),
X 400. Most of them are floating freely in the culture
medium.

gradually increased by 35 to 40 days. After 40 days culture with
5 to 6 passages, most of the free cells in the medium were mast
cells (Fig. 6). Mature mast cells obtained from the culture were
heterogeneous with respect to their size and density of metachromatic
granules, but morphologically identical to tissue mast cells. The
yield of mast cells from the original culture of 2 to 5 x 10^7 thymus
cells was 5 x 10^5 to 10^7.

As shown in Fig. 7, IgE receptors on the mature mast cells was
demonstrated by autoradiography. The increase in the number of
grains on the mature cells suggested that the number of receptors
for IgE increased along with maturation of the cells. No IgG was
bound by mature mast cells.

In the course of the experiment, however, we have observed a
substantial differentiation of mast cells from embryonic monolayer
without seeding thymus cells. Therefore, attempts were made to
culture thymus cells without feeder layer. Thymus cells were obtained from 3 to 5 day old rats and seeded on tissue culture petri
dish without embryonic monolayer. By the 7th to 9th day, mastoblasts in various shapes and sizes appeared on the surface of the
petri dish (Fig. 8). These mastoblasts formed colonies and then
their cytoplasms were gradually filled with metachromatic granules
and developed to mast cells. A representative mast cell colony at
the 26th day of culture is shown in Fig. 9. The results clearly
show that the thymus cells actually contained precursors of mast
cells.

Since pure mast cells were obtained by culture, we have studied
the biological function of culture mast cells. First of all, the

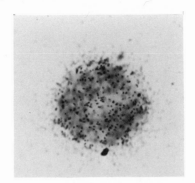

Fig. 7. Autoradiograph of a mature mast cell (56 days culture).
Mast cells were treated with ^{125}I-IgE. Toluidine blue
staining, x 960. The number of grains on the cell is
much more than that shown in Fig. 5b.

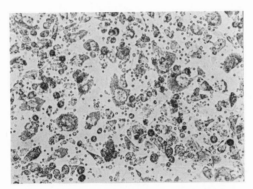

Fig. 8. Blast cells appeared 7 days after seeding thymus cells in
petri dish, (no feeder layer), living culture, no staining,
x 160.

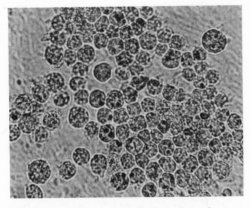

Fig. 9. Mast cell colonies developed in the thymus cell culture
without feeder layer (26 days culture), living culture,
no staining, x 400.

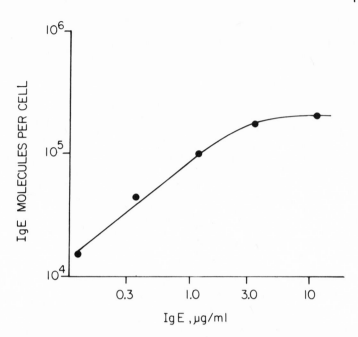

Fig. 10. Binding of ^{125}I-IgE with cultured mast cells. Aliquots of
cultured mast cells were incubated with different concentrations of ^{125}I-IgE at 37°C for 60 min, and the number
of IgE molecules bound per mast cell was calculated. Variation among triplicate tubes was within 5 percent.

Table IV

Histamine content in cultured mast cells

Source of thymus cells	Period of culture days	Histamine content $\mu g/10^6$ cells
Young adult	40	3.1
	45	2.8
	52	1.5
	56	4.5
3 to 5 day old rats	20	0.1, 0.3
	26	0.8
	28	0.8
	30	0.5
	32	1.6
	34	0.8, 2.7
	36	2.0
	40	1.1, 2.1

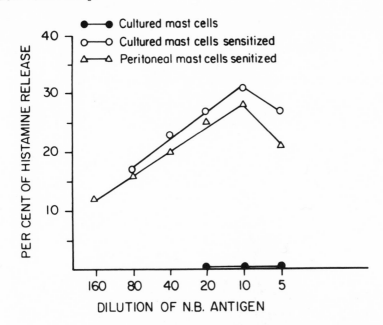

Fig. 11. Dose response curves of antigen-induced histamine release
from mast cells. Both cultured mast cells and peritoneal
mast cells were sensitized in vitro with an IgE-rich fraction of the serum of rats infected with NB. Sensitized
cells (o---o) and unsensitized cultured mast cells (●---●)
were incubated in serial dilutions of NB antigen.

number of IgE-receptors on the cultured mast cells was determined
by the method described by Kulczycki and Metzger (8). Cultured
mast cells were incubated in different concentrations of ^{125}I-IgE
at 37°C for 60 min, and the number of IgE molecules bound per mast
cell was calculated. A representative binding curve is shown in
Fig. 10. The number of IgE molecules bound per cultured mast cell
reached to maximum at approximately 5 μg/ml of IgE. Maximum number
of IgE molecules bound per mast cell was 100,000 to 400,000. From
this binding curve, the equilibrium constant between IgE and receptor was estimated to be in the order of 10^8 per mole.

Histamine content in the cultured mast cells was measured by
spectrofluorometric technique. As shown in Table IV, histamine
content in the cultured mast cells was varied depending on the
culture, but mast cells recovered after a long culture period generally had higher histamine content than those obtained before 30
days culture. It seems that histamine content increases with
maturation. Even after 50 days culture, however, histamine content
in the cultured mast cells was much less than that in peritoneal

mast cells.

As the cultured mast cells possess IgE receptors and contain histamine, attempts were made to sensitize these cells with IgE antibody for antigen-induced histamine release. The IgE-rich fraction was obtained from the serum of rats infected with Nippostrongylus brasilienis. Both cultured mast cells and puri-fied peritoneal mast cells were incubated with a 1:8 dilution of the IgE-rich fraction in culture medium at 37°C for 60 min for passive sensitization. After washing, cells were suspended in Tyrode solution containing 25 µg/ml of phosphatidyl serine and aliquots of the cells were incubated in serial dilutions of Nippostrongylus antigen (Fig. 11). Both the culture mast cells and peritoneal mast cells released histamine. Since unsensitized mast cells did not release histamine upon exposure to the antigen, it is clear that cultured mast cells were sensitized with IgE anti-body for antigen-induced histamine release.

The cultured mast cells released histamine upon exposure to compound 48/80. Both cultured mast cells and purified peritoneal mast cells released histamine in dose-response fashion. It seems that mast cells which are developed from thymus cells in vitro culture are not only morphologically identical to normal mast cells but also have biological functions similar to those of normal mast cells.

SUMMARY

Both basophil granulocytes and mast cells bear specific recep-tors for IgE. The number of receptors per human basophil granu-locyte is 40,000 to 100,000 and the number of receptors per rat mast cell is 300,000 to 400,000. The binding of IgE molecules with the receptors is reversible and does not involve covalent bonding. The equilibrium constant of the binding reaction was estimated to be in the order of 10^9 mole $^{-1}$ in both human basophil and rat mast cell systems. Evidence was obtained that cap-forma-tion of cell-bound IgE by anti-IgE was accompanied by migration of free receptors into the same pole. The results indicated that a group of receptor sites are associated with each other at the cell membrane.

Rat mast cells were developed successfully by a long-term culture of rat thymus cell suspension. Receptors for IgE became detectable at the early or young stage of differentiation. Mature mast cells obtained in the culture could be passively sensitized with rat IgE antibody for antigen-induced histamine release. Since histamine content of cultured mast cells was much less than that present in peritoneal mast cells, cultured mast cells are not suitable for the analysis of biochemical mechanisms of histamine release. Differentiation of mast cells in the culture, however, will provide a useful system to follow the development of IgE receptors during maturation.

REFERENCES

1. Ishizaka, K., Tomioka, H. and Ishizaka, T., J. Immunol., 105: 1459, 1970.
2. Ishizaka, I., Ishizaka, K. and Tomioka, H., J. Immunol., 108: 513, 1972.
3. Bazin, H., Beckers, A. and Querinjean, P., Eur. J. Immunol., 4: 44, 1974.
4. Bach, M.K., Bloch, K.J. and Austen, K.F., J. Exp. Med., 133: 752, 1971.
5. Kulczycki, A., Jr., Isersky, C. and Metzger, H., J. Exp. Med., 139: 600, 1974.
6. Ishizaka, T., Soto, C.S., and Ishizaka, K., J. Immunol., 111: 500, 1973.
7. Ishizaka, T. and Ishizaka, K., J. Immunol., 112: 1078, 1974.
8. Kulczycki, A.,Jr. and Metzger, H., J. Exp. Med., 140: 1676, 1974.
9. Conrad, D.H., Bazin, H., Sehon, A.H. and Froese, A., J. Immunol., 114: 1688, 1975.
10. Becker, K.E., Ishizaka, T., Metzger, H., Ishizaka, K. and Grimley, P.M., J. Exp. Med., 138: 394, 1973.
11. Ishizaka, K. and Ishizaka, T., J. Immunol., 103: 588, 1969.
12. Ishizaka, T. and Ishizaka, K., Annals of the New York Academy of Sciences, 254: 462.
13. Bach, M.K. and Brashler, J.R., J. Immunol., 111: 324.
14. König, W. and Ishizaka, K., J. Immunol., 113: 1237, 1974.
15. König, W. and Ishizaka, K., Immunochemistry - in press.
16. Conrad, D.H. and Froese, A., J. Immunol., 116: 319, 1976.
17. Kulczycki, A.,Jr., Siraganian, R., Mendoza, G. and Metzger, H., Fed. Proc. 34: 985, 1975.
18. Ginsburg, H. and Sachs, L., J. Nat. Cancer Institute, 31: 1, 1962.
19. Ishizaka, T., Okudaira, H., Mauser, L.E. and Ishizaka, K., J. Immunol. - in press, 1976.

[1] This work was supported by Research Grant AI-10060 from the U.S. Public Health Service and a grant from Lillia Babbitt Hyde Foundation. This is publication #215 from The O'Neill Laboratories at The Good Samaritan Hospital.

DISCUSSION

BENNICH: My question is related to your studies of the membrane receptor. When you solubilize with NP 40, how much of the bound (radiolabeled) IgE is recovered in the supernatant?

ISHIZAKA, T.: The mast cells were first surface labelled with ^{125}I and then saturated with cold IgE before they were solubilized by NP-40. The proportion of radiolabelled subcellular components co-precipitated with the IgE anti-IgE precipitate was only a small fraction.

In Dr. König's experiment, mast cells were coated with ^{125}I-labelled IgE and disrupted by sonication. In this case, most of the cell bound ^{125}I-labelled IgE was recovered in the void volume fractions from a Sepharose 6B column.

AUSTEN: Has any one attempted to isolate "receptors" from membranes of mast cells beginning with membrane obtained by subcellular fractionation before study?

ISHIZAKA, T.: As far as I know, no one has isolated the membranes from the mast cells before the preparation of the "receptors".

When mast cells were disrupted by sonication and the 20,000 g supernatant was filtered through a Sepharose column, most of the membrane associated enzymes were recovered in the void volume fractions. Purification of receptors from this fraction was not successful.

BENNICH: Isolation of membrane receptors from intact cells is for sure a different business than isolation of the receptors from the plasma cell fraction.

BAZIN: Have you studied the homing properties of cultured pure mast cells by injecting them in normal or infected rats.

ISHIZAKA, T.: We have not done such an experiment yet.

AUSTEN: Do mast cells derive in culture from T cells or connective tissue elements? Do you found T cell markers on these mast cells?

ISHIZAKA, T.: We tried to demonstrate the presence of θ

antigen on the mast cells, using anti-rat thymocyte antiserum, but the results were not convincing. We can not exclude the possibility that a small amount of anti-mast cells was present in the antiserum. As anti-mouse θ antiserum was more reliable, we have treated mouse peritoneal mast cells with rabbit anti-brain θ antiserum, followed by ^{125}I-labelled anti-rabbit IgG. The results of the autoradiography was also not convincing.

Burnet has proposed that basophils and mast cells are postmitotic derivatives of thymus derived cells. At the moment, however, we do not have any evidence which indicates that the precursors of the mast cells are T cells. Further studies are required to answer your question.

DAVID: In reference to your studies in which mast cells were cultured from the thymus - do you know if nude (or thymectomized) mice have a normal component of mast cells.

ISHIZAKA, T.: One of our co-workers, Dr. Okudaria examined the number of peritoneal mast cells in nude mice and found a number comparable to that in normal control mice.

BECKER: Have you incubated your cultured mast cells with histidine and found any increase in their histamine content?

ISHIZAKA, T.: I have increased the concentration of histidine in the regular medium or cultured the cells in α-medium which contains much higher concentration of histidine. However, the results were inconsistant and the histamine content never reached the level of normal peritoneal mast cells.

COCHRANE: Have you attempted to release histamine from the cultured mast cells using peptide activators such as the anaphylatoxins?

ISHIZAKA, T.: I have not tried anaphylatoxins, but as I mentioned, compound 48/80 released histamine from the cultured mast cells.

UVNÄS: When your mast cell degranulate, do the expelled granules dissolve in your incubation medium?

ISHIZAKA, T.: After histamine release the cultured mast cells were degranulated. However, the condition of granules expelled into the supernatant was not examined.

MODES OF ACTION OF ANTIGEN-ANTIBODY REACTION AND COMPOUND 48/80 IN HISTAMINE RELEASE

Börje Uvnäs

Department of Pharmacology, Karolinska institutet

S-104 01 Stockholm 60, Sweden

There is general agreement today about the mast cell being a secretory cell. It reacts to a multitude of agents with the release not only of histamine and heparin but of a whole battery of biologically active materials, either preformed and stored in the basophil granules or formed during the secretory process. The mast cells are the specific target cells for allergens because of the very high affinity of their cell membrane for IgE globulins. These IgE molecules, are assumed to act as specific receptors for circulating allergens. The mast cell response to other "releasing" or "degranulating" agents is also supposed to require an attachment of these agents to specific receptors on the mast cell surface. These receptors are so far not identified. The attachment to the receptor is assumed to be the crucial step in the activation of the mast cell response, initiating a series of biochemical events ending with exocytosis, partial degranulation and the release of biologically active materials.

Biochemistry of the mast cell response

Current theories on the mechanism of the mast cell response are rather speculative and to a great extent based on pharmacological evidence. Certain facts are generally agreed upon. Calcium ions are essential in the stimulus-secretion coupling and energy yielding metabolism - either aerobic or anaerobic - is indispensable. However, the opinions apart as soon as we come to a closer definition of the biochemical events behind the mast cell response. There are those who believe the primary and essential step to be an opening of "calcium gates" in the mast cell membrane. The entry of calcium ions should activate the exocytotic process and thereby the release process. Those Ca^{++} enthusiasts emphasize the degranulating effects of ionophores (1) and intracellular application of

217

Ca^{++} (2). However, in my mind these people may oversimplify the
role of calcium. The fact that an experimentally induced intracellular calcium flood will cause a mast cell response with exocytosis and release merely shows that Ca^{++} ions are able to elicit
a response. But, they might do this by activating either simultaneously several calcium requiring processes, or only the final
exocytotic step thereby circumventing the normally occurring prior
chain of events. One might compare the action of intracellularly applied calcium with the effect of gasoline injected directly into the
carburator. The motor starts if the ignition is on, but the activity
is beyond the normal control system.

Others have presented more sophisticated schemes to fit available experimental observations. Högberg and Uvnäs (3) observed that
compound 48/80-induced degranulation of rat mesentary mast cells
was inhibited by the phosphorylating agent phosphoimidazol. They
ascribed this inhibition to the inactivation of a phospholipase,
assumed to be located to the mast cell membrane and instrumental
in the initiation of the mast cell response. Since DFP (di-isopro-
pyl-fluoro-phosphate) and various phosphonates inhibit antigen-
-induced histamine release the activation of a serine dependent esterase has been suggested as an initial calcium dependent step
(4,5). c-AMP is assumed to be of importance for the modulation of
subsequent biochemical processes required for the exocytosis and
degranulation (6,7,8). Accordingly, an increase in c-AMP levels
have been seen on inhibition of histamine release with various
drugs which stimulate adenyl cyclase activity (prostaglandin E_1,
adrenaline, isoproterenol, cholera toxin etc) or reduce the breakdown of c-AMP (inhibitors of phosphodiesterase like theofylline and
other xanthines). The addition of c-AMP itself is reported to inhibit anaphylactic histamine release. Sullivan et al. reported
that carbamylcholine, adenine and diazoxide reduced the mast cell
c-AMP levels and potentiated the histamine release induced by compound 48/80. α-adrenergic stimuli (noradrenaline, phenylephrine)
enhanced antigen-induced histamine release. Concomitantly, the
c-AMP levels decreased. Similar effects were seen after treatment
with the phosphodiesterase-stimulating drug imidazol. However, the
reports are conflicting about changes in c-AMP levels in association with histamine release induced from mast cells by compound
48/80. Sullivan et al. report a correlation between changes in
c-AMP levels in mast cells and the ability of compound 48/80 to
release histamine. On the other hand, we have not observed any
correlation between the effects of drugs (9) on the c-AMP level
and their inhibitory effects on 48/80 induced histamine release.
A 4-6 fold increase in the c-AMP level produced by cyclase activation (PG E_1) or even a 15-fold increase produced by the phosphodiesterase inhibitor IBM X had no effect on the histamine release.
Only papaverine produced an almost total inhibition of histamine
release in doses assumed to inhibit phosphodiesterase activity.
However, a closer analysis of this inhibitory phenomenon showed it
to be due to metabolic inhibition and not to inhibition of a phos-

phodiesterase. Accordingly, the inhibition of papaverine on histamine release was completely abolished by the addition of glucose
to the incubation medium and the resulting restoration of cellular
ATP.

There are other pecularities characteristic for the action of
compound 48/80 (see also Table I). External calcium is not necessary for the mast cell response. It cannot be blocked by DFP - assumed
to block a serine esterase essential for the antigen induced mast
cell response (4,5). The inhibitory or excitatory effects of drugs
activating β or α -receptors are weak or absent. If the biochemical
mechanism depicted in fig. 1 is valid, at least in principle, for
the mast cell response to allergens, then one has to assume a different point of attack for compound 48/80. Either one might think
- as a calcium enthusiast will probably do - that this amine due
to its strong charge is able to mobilize intramembraneous or intracellular Ca^{++} stores essential for the exocytotic process or that
the amine circumvents some of the initial steps. One possibility
is depicted in fig. 1 where compound 48/80 is proposed to surpass
the esterase activation step and the c-AMP system by activating
directly the c-AMP modulated protein kinase essential for the
phosphorylations required for the metabolic and exocytotic processes. Other polymer amines like histone, protamine and poly-L-lysine
have been shown to activate protein kinase in vitro by removing
- by virtue of their strong electric charges - the acid inhibitory
protein assumed to modulate the activity of the protein kinase
systems.

I have dealt with the differences in the effects of drugs on
the mast cell responses to allergens and to compound 48/80 for two
reasons. Firstly, one should be careful in interpreting data obtained from a pharmacological analysis. The drugs used for such
analysis usually lack the necessary specificity and we usually
know too little about their mechanisms of action to justify the
far reacting conclusions frequently drawn. Secondly, biochemical
evidence should be required - identification of the enzymes postulated or the products of their activation. Evidently, much remains
to be done in this respect before a clear picture can be drawn of
the biochemical processes behind the secretory response of the
mast cell to allergens and other "releasing agents".

The exocytosis and the final release step
     The morphological changes triggered by allergens and other
"degranulating" agents can be characterized as a sequential exocytosis (10,11). Beginning at the cell periphery, normal, electron-
-dense, membrane-limited granules swell and lose their electron
density. At the same time fusions of the granule membrane occur,
both with the plasma membrane and with membranes of adjacent granules. The process continues with the formation of more or less
complicated cavities seen to contain numerous swollen, less electron

Table I:

Factors influencing the mast cell respone <u>to antigen</u> <u>to compound 48/8</u>

	Ca^{2+}	to antigen	to compound 48/8
		essential	not essential
serine esterase blockade	{ DFP	inhibition	no inhibition
cyclase stimulation	{ PGE$_1$ β-receptor stimulants	inhibition	no inhibition
phosphodiesterase inhibition	{ methylxanthines	inhibition	no inhibition
metabolic block	{ lack of oxygen, glucose Enzyme inhibitors	inhibition	inhibition

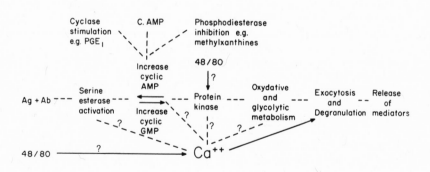

Fig. 1: Schematic picture of the mast cell response to allergens and to compound 48/80.

dense and membrane-free granules. Some of the altered granules are expelled from the cell but many appear to remain inside them. However, by the use of marker substances all the cavities have been shown to be in direct communication with the extracellular space. Consequently, all the changed granules - whether they are expelled from the cell or remain inside it - become exposed to the extracellular fluid (fig. 2). Since all these granules are devoid of a surrounding membrane there will be no barrier to prevent an exchange of ions between the granules and the fluid. A series of studies in Stockholm has shown that the mast cell granules are composed mainly of a complex between heparin and a basic low moleuclar weight peptide. The complex has the properties of a weak cationic exchanger with the free carboxyls of the peptide acting as the cation-binding sites. The cation binding capacity of the granules in vitro is sufficient to explain the binding of all the endogenous mast cell histamine on the basis of binding to such carboxyl groups. Mast cell granules charged in vitro with histamine to the level normally occuring in the mast cell release all their histamine on exposure to cation-containing media, such as physiological saline or serum. The release of histamine is paralleled by the uptake of an equivalent amount of sodium. The cation exchanger properties of the granules are further corroborated by the fact that the uptake and release satisfy the Rothmund-Kornfeld equation for cation exchangers (fig.3) - a modification of the Law of Mass Action valid for cation exchangers (12). Accordingly, when the ratio between the concentrations of cationic and hydrogen ions in the granules is plotted against the corresponding ratio in the suspension fluid the values obtained lie on a straight line (13). Fig. 4 shows such a plot for sodium and histamine uptake in mast cell granules in vitro.

The consequences of the cation exchanger properties of the mast cell granules are clear. Regardless of the agent initiating exocytosis all altered granules, both those expelled from the cell and those remaining in the formed cavities will be exposed to the extracellular fluid. Since all the altered granules are devoid of a surrounding membrane there will be an exchange of cations between the granules and the extracellular fluid. The affinity of histamine and sodium for the granule sites is the same and furthermore, the extracellular sodium concentrations are about 10 times higher than those required for saturation of the granule sites. Consequently, the granule histamine will be immediately exchanged for sodium and released from the altered granules.

The mechanism of storage of the other granule components and therefore their mode of release is less well documented. 5-HT is probably ionically stored (14) as is also claimed for the ECF-A (eosinophil chemotactic factor of anaphylaxis) (15). The other components (chymotrypsin, neutrophil chemotactic factor etc) remain to be studied in these respects.

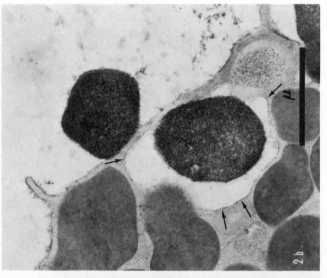

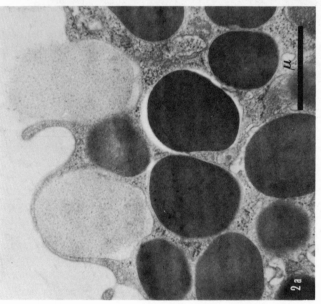

Fig. 2: Electron micrographs of isolated rat mast cells treated with compound 48/80 (0.4 µg/ml, 20 sec, 17°C). 2a. Two of the peripherally located granules show a swollen, reticular, net-like, less electron dense appearance compared to the normal, homogeneous, electron dense granules, which all are surrounded by a perigranular membrane. Magnification 25.000 X. 2b. After glutaral- dehyde fixation an extracellular tracer substance (lanthanum) was added to the cells to show the extent of the extracellular space. The precipitate formed is localized to the cell periphery and is also seen lining the cavity containing a swollen granule (arrows). Changed granules, both outside and inside the cell, have taken up the precipitate and are even more electron-dense than the normal ones.

$$\left[\frac{B_r}{A_r}\right] \times \left[\frac{A_W}{B_W}\right]^{\beta} = K$$

A_r and B_r = ions in resin

A_W and B_W = ions in solution

β and K = empirical parameters

Fig. 3: The Rothmund-Kornfeld equation for cation exchangers

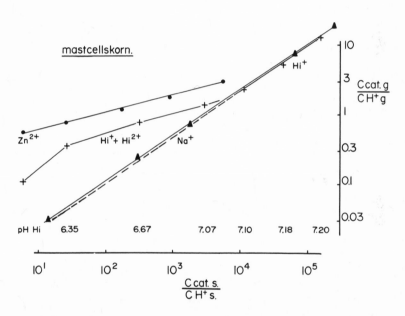

Fig. 4 : Plots illustrating the cation exchange properties of isola-ted mast cell granules exposed to various cations and amines in vitro. Ordinates: ratio between cation conc. and hydrogen ion conc. in granules. Abscissae: ratio between cation conc. and hydrogen conc. in suspension medium. The deviation of the Hi-line below pH 7 is due to protonization of the ring -N whereby histamine is becoming divalent.
Histamine (Hi), sodium (Na) and zinc (Zn).

REFERENCES

1. Foreman, J.C., Mongar, J.L., Gomperts, B.D., Calcium ionophores and movement of calcium ions following the physiological stimulus to a secretory process. Nature, 245, 249-251, 1973.

2. Kanoe, T., Cochrane, D.E., Douglas, W.W., Exocytosis (secretory granule extension) induced by injection of calcium into mast cells. Can. J. Physiol. Pharmacol. 51, 1001-1004, 1973.

3. Högberg, B. and Uvnäs, B., The mechanism of the disruption of mast cells produced by compound 48/80. Acta physiol. scand. 41, 345-369, 1957.

4. Becker, E.L. and Austen, K.F., Mechanism of immunologic injury of rat peritoneal mast cells. I. The effect of phosphonate inhibitors on the homocytotrophic antibody-mediated histamine release and the first component of the rat complement. J. Exp. Med. 124, 379-396, 1966.

5. Ranadive, N.S., Cochrane, C.G., Mechanism of histamine release from mast cells by cationic protein (band 2) from neutrophil lysosomes. J. Immunol. 100, 506-516, 1971.

6. Kaliner, M. and Austen, K.F., Cyclic nucleotides and modulation of effector systems of inflammation. Biochem. Pharmacol. 23, 763-771, 1974.

7. Sullivan, T.J., Parker, K.L., Stenson, W., Parker, C.W., Modulation of cyclic AMP in purified rat mast cells. I. Responses to pharmacologic, metabolic and physical stimuli. J. Immunol. 114, 1473-1479, 1975.

8. Sullivan, T.J., Parker, K.L., Eisen, S.A., Parker, C.W., Modulation of cyclic AMP in purified mast cells. II. Studies on the relationship between intracellular cyclic AMP concentrations and histamine release. J. Immunol. 114, 1480-1485, 1975.

9, Fredholm, B.B., Gushin, I., Elwin, K., Schwab, G. and Uvnäs, B., Cyclic AMP independent inhibition by papaverine of histamine release induced by compound 48/80. Biochem. Pharmacol. 25, 1976 (in press).

10. Röhlich, P., Anderson, P., Uvnäs, B., Electron microscope observations on compound 48/80-induced degranulation in rat mast cells. Evidence for sequential exocytosis of storage granules. J. Cell Biol. 51, 465-483, 1971.

11. Anderson, P., Slorach, S.A., Uvnäs, B., Sequential exocytosis of storage granules during antigen-induced histamine release from sensitized rat mast cells in vitro. An electron microscopic study. Acta physiol. scand. 96, 512-525, 1976.

12. Samuelsson, O., Ion exchangers in analytical chemistry. Almqvist & Wiksell, Stockholm 1972.

13. Uvnäs, B. and Åborg, C.-H., An in vitro-formed protamine-heparin complex as a model for a two-compartment store for biogenic amines. Acta physiol. scand. 96, 512-525, 1976.

14. Bergendorff, A., Uvnäs, B., Storage properties of rat mast cell granules in vitro. Acta physiol. scand. 87, 213-222, 1973.

15. Austen, K.F., Biochemical characteristics and pharmacological modulation of the antigen-induced release of the chemical mediators of immediate hypersensitivity. In: Allergology. Proceedings of the VIII International Congress of Allergology. Tokyo, October 14-20, 1973. Eds. Y. Yamamura et al. Excerpta Medica. 1974. American Elsevier Publishing Co. Inc., New York, pp. 306--315.

DISCUSSION

BENNICH: Does the "histamine-free" granulae contain protein.

UVNÄS: The main constituent of the granulae matrix is a water insoluble complex between a basic low molecular weight polypeptide and heparin. This matrix complex dissociates first at high salt concentrations (e.g. 1-2 M NaCl).

BENNICH: What is the function of this low molecular weight protein?

UVNÄS: The complex functions as a weak cation exchanger with carboxyl groups in the polypeptide as ion binding sites for histamine. Since the granulae matrix is insoluble in the tissue fluid the protein remains in the complex after histamine is released.

COCHRANE: Regarding the question of DFP susceptible esterases in mast cells, Dr. Ranadive working in our laboratory several years ago employed DFP to inhibit the release of histamine from rat peritoneal mast cells. The release of histamine in these studies was induced by certain cationic peptides (band 2 protein of rabbit neutrophils). The evidences that DFP was acting in one sensitive step in the release process, and therefore not by non-specific general injury to the cells, were the following.

Firstly, treatment with DFP together with peptide activation led to inhibition of release, while pretreatment of the cells and DFP, followed by washing, and exposure of the cells to peptide activator allowed full release to occur.

Secondly, by exposing cells to peptide activator in non-releasing conditions, i.e. in the absence of an energy system, or at 10°C, followed by re-establishment of normal releasing conditions, DFP was no longer able to inhibit. These data were published several years ago in the J. of Immunology.

Aside from showing that the DFP inhibition did not result from general toxic injury to the cells, the data also allowed one to separate the process of release of histamine into two stages, an early, DFP inhibitable stage that precedes need for energy, and a second stage in which energy systems are needed.

UVNÄS: I am well aware of your observations on the inhibitory effect of DFP but these are still only indirect evidence for the activation of an esterase.

AUSTEN: Studies with human lung tissue have shown that antigen challenge with DFP present and no extra cellular calcium ions does not activate the proesterase. This suggests that activation is extra cellular calcium ion dependent and autocatalytic. Sequence studies have further shown that proesterase activation precedes the energy dependent step (Kaliner & Austen, J. Exp. Med. 1973).

Further studies in collaboration with Dr. Becker using phosphonate inhibitors have developed particular profiles from the immunologically activatable mast cell proesterase.

DIAMANT: Since I will discuss this in my presentation later today I have better declare already now, that in my hands, DFP as well as theophylline block histamine release also when induced by 48/80.

I have two questions. Do you know the localization of the protein kinase and when you exposed the rat mast cells to ^{32}P ATP, what concentration did you use?

FREDHOLM (Stockholm): During experiments with cells $\gamma - ^{32}P$ ATP was added 5 seconds before the addition of compound 48/80 and to a final concentration of approximately $10^{-7}M$.

BECKER: The general basis for the use of DFP and other similar organphosphorus inhibitors is that the given reaction is blocked when the inhibitor is present when the cell is stimulated but no inhibition occurs when the cell or stimulus is treated alone. In addition there is the very large assumption that these organophosphorus inhibitors act only in the reaction as an irreversible inhibitor.

Dr. Cochrane has mentioned one situation when this assumption has been partially met. Dr. Austen has mentioned another situation where again this assumption has been partially but only partially met. Drs. Pruzansky and Patterson has presented other evidence which even more stronlgy but still not completely has met this assumption in the antigen induced release of histamine from sensitized basophils.

GOMPERTS: I think it would be helpful to see the mast cell in the wider context of secretory and other excitable tissues.

It might therefore be useful to ask what polycations do to Ca^{2+} fluxes in other systems, because I think we can agree that it is internal Ca^{2+} which initiates exocytosis. Certainly polycations have effects on Ca^{2+} flux in isolated mitochondria, and turning to model systems, it is known that polycations can reverse the ion charge specificity of model membranes treated with excitability inducing antibodies such as alamethicin (Mueller and Rudin).

If we seek an enzyme mediated step to occur before Ca^{2+} entry, it could be helpful to look at the phosphatidylinositol (PI)-phosphatidic acid cycle. This is an invariable accompaniment of every cellular activation system in which it has been measured. It is an early event and it is not dependent on the presence of Ca^{2+}. R.H. Michell (BBA Biomembrane Reviews) argues most persuasively that activation of the PI cycle could be a regulator of Ca^{2+} flux.

DISCUSSION REMARK:

PROTEIN KINASES IN RAT MAST CELLS

B.B. Fredholm and B. Uvnäs

Department of Pharmacology, Karolinska institutet

104 01 Stockholm 60, Sweden

Most if not all the known actions of cyclic nucleotides are mediated over protein kinases (1). In view of the recent data implicating cyclic AMP and cyclic GMP as modulators or even mediators of
histamine release from mast cells (2) it was of interest to examine the mast cell protein kinases. The following is a brief report of our preliminary findings.

The first point to be made is that rat mast cells contain protein
kinase activity. This is illustrated in Fig. 1, which illustrates
a Sephadex chromatography of a crude mast cell extract. The fractions containing cyclic GMP-stimulated protein kinase activity also
contained material that inhibited basal and cyclic AMP stimulated
kinase activity of purified skeletal muscle protein kinase. The inhibition may have been caused in part by heparin from the mast cell
granules since heparin is a potent inhibitor of protein kinase.
However, mast cells also contained material that could be purified
by the same procedure as that described for the protein kinase modulator in skeletal muscle (3). This is of interest since this protein has been found to enhance cyclic GMP dependent protein kinase
activity at the same time as it inhibits cyclic AMP dependent protein kinase activity (4). Indeed after removal of the protein kinase
inhibitor by DEAE-cellulose chromatography the mast cell protein kinase was no longer stimulatable by cyclic GMP. Furthermore, a cell
membrane fraction of mast cells essentially devoid of mast cell
granular material and protein kinase inhibitor had protein kinase
activity that was uninfluenced by cyclic GMP. In contrast, auto-
phosphorylation of the membranes as well as phosphorylation of exogenous substrate (kaseine or histone) was stimulated by cyclic AMP
(20 μM).

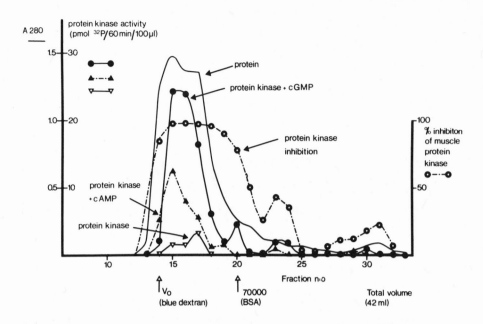

Fig. 1. Mast cells were isolated from 30 rats (24 x 10⁶ cells)
which were lysed in distilled water. Protein was precipitated with
70% saturated (NH₄)₂SO₄ and resuspended in assay buffer (5 mM
Tris-C 1, 1 mM EDTA pH 7,0, pH 6,0), dialysed against the same
buffer and put on a Sephadex G-100 column (0.9-60 cm) equilibtated
with the same buffer. The effluents were collected in 0.9 ml fractions. Protein kinase was assayed in a total volume of 250µl containing 30 mM Na-acetate, 5 mM Mg-acetate, 0.6 mM ³²P-ATP (appr.
0.3µCi) and 350 µg/ml histone.

The present data therefore show that mast cell membranes contain
protein kinase activity capable of phosphorylating components of
the membranes. In the purified membranes this activity is stimulated by cyclic AMP. However, mast cells also contain substantial
amounts of protein kinase modulator, which inhibits cyclic AMP -
dependent and enhances cyclic GMP - dependent protein kinase. Thus,
the degree of activation of the different protein kinases may be
a complex function of the cyclic nucleotide concentrations as well
as the local concentration of the protein kinase modulator. Further
studies are obviously needed to clarify the physiological significance of these findings. In particular, it is necessary to determine the substrate(s) for the membrane-associated protein kinase.

One further point is worthy of mention. Purified protein kinase is
stimulated by compound 48/80 (as well as by other polybasic compounds). Purified skeletal muscle protein kinase is stimulated
2-3 fold by 10 μg/ml 48/80, lower concentration being ineffective.
No activation was seen when the assay was conducted in the presence of 20 μM cyclic AMP, suggesting that compound 48/80 activates
the protein kinase by removing the somewhat acidic regulatory subunit from the catalytic subunit.

We have some preliminary evidence that ^{32}P incorporation into mast
cell proteins from ^{32}P-ATP (7×10^{-7} M) present in the incubation
medium is also stimulated by compound 48/80. This may represent
an activation of protein kinase activity in intact mast cells by
the histamine releasing agent. Incorporation at 22°C was maximal
30 sec. after the addition of compound 48/80 at which time histamine release was still submaximal (maximal histamine release was
seen after 45-60 sec. At 0°C there was no incorporation of ^{32}P
into protein and no histamine release by compound 48/80.

These studies were supported in a part by a grant from Svenska
Livförsäkringsbolagens Nämnd för Medicinsk Forskning and by the
Swedish Medical Research Council (No. 2553).

REFERENCES

1. Langan, T.A.: Protein kinases and protein kinase substrates.
    Adv. Cyclic Nucleotide Res. 3: 99-153, 1973.

2. Parker, C.W., T.J. Sullivan and H.J. Wedner: Cyclic AMP and
    the immunic response. Adv. Cyclic Nucleotides Res. 4: 1-79,
    1974.

3. Walsh, D.A., C.D. Ashby, C. Gonzales, D. Calkius, E.H. Fischer
    and E.G. Krebs: Purification and characterization of a protein
    inhibitor of adenosine 3',5'-monophosphate-dependent protein
    kinases. J. Biol. Chem. 246: 1977-1985, 1971.

4. Kuo, J.F.: Divergent actions of protein kinase modulator in
    regulating mammalian cyclic GMP-dependent and cyclic AMP-
    -dependent protein kinases. Metabolism. 24: 321-329, 1975.

THE INTERDEPENDENCE OF ALLERGIC AND INFLAMMATORY PROCESSES*

Lawrence M. Lichtenstein

The Johns Hopkins University School of Medicine at

The Good Samaritan Hospital, Baltimore, Maryland 21239

In a widely accepted system of classification, allergic reactions have been divided by Gell and Coombs into four different categories (1). Their definition of allergy is the classical one, rather than the limited modern or clinical definition, and, therefore, purports to encompass the totality of reactions which involve the immune system. While this classification has served a useful role, it will be the purpose of this discussion to review recent data which suggests that allergic reactions are an integral part of the whole range of inflammatory responses, and, perhaps, should no longer be divided in this fashion. It will be suggested, instead, that these responses, which are of major importance in both defense mechanisms and in disease processes, have a pathogenesis in which each of the traditional types of allergic response are so inextricably intermingled that they are best considered as constituting a continuum.

This thesis has been generated as a result of three lines of evidence which have emerged from our research efforts and those of others:

(1) The mediators which are involved in the inflammatory response, whether we consider histamine release from mast cells or basophils, lysosomal enzyme release from polymorphonuclear cells or lymphokine release from T lymphocytes, are generated as

* Supported by U. S. Public Health Service Grants Nos. AI 07290 and AI 11334.
This work was carried out in collaboration with several of my colleagues: Drs. M. C. Conroy, H. H. Newball, R. C. Talamo, W. König, B. M. Czarnetzki, and M. Plaut.

the result of secretory processes which are in no way different from the secretory response of endocrine cells. Moreover, the release of these mediators is controlled in an intimate fashion by membrane bound hormone receptors linked with adenylate cyclase. In each cell type cited above, endogenous hormones such as epinephrine, the prostaglandins, or histamine cause an increase in adenylate cyclase activity, an increase in cyclic AMP, and a diminution of the release response. This characteristic control mechanism, which seems to involve all inflammatory cell types, is quite different from that found for most other secretory cells, in which a stimulus which increases intracellular cyclic AMP appears to facilitate release. It seems logical, therefore, in view of these stereotyped secretory control mechanisms, that there must be marked similarities in the patterns of response of inflammatory cells.

(2) The second major line of evidence suggesting the indivisible nature of inflammation is the experiments showing that mediators released from one or another of the cell types control the function of other cell types. Perhaps the best example, considered here as a prototype, is histamine release from mast cells or basophils: It has been shown that histamine, when released, can "feedback" to inhibit the release of both histamine and the other mediators of immediate hypersensitivity. More importantly, released histamine, operating through a histamine-2 receptor, has been shown to have dramatic effects on the secretory processes of the human polymorphonuclear cells and lymphocytes, in each case causing inhibition of the response. There is now evidence, which will be cited below, indicating that histamine has in vivo activity on such diverse inflammatory functions as the evolution of the delayed skin response, antibody production, and the development of the lesions in immune glomerulonephritis. As noted, histamine is only a prototype; there is evidence that prostaglandins are released from the same cell types on appropriate stimulation, and it is clear that these ubiquitous hormones can also modulate the release of mediators from other cells.

Not only do the mediators themselves regulate the inflammatory process, but they also serve to bring new cell types to the site of inflammation and to involve the serum cascade systems in these responses. We refer, first, to the antigen-IgE generated release of a mediator with kallikrein activity. This allows the generation of bradykinin from serum kininogen, thereby bringing into play the complex kinin-complement cascade. Similarly, IgE mediated reactions can involve the clotting system. Further to this point is the release from basophils and mast cells of an eosinophil chemotactic factor, which brings this cell type to the inflammatory response, and the release of lymphokines which are chemotactic for granulocytes or basophils. There are, of course, many other chemotactic molecules which could be cited.

(3)   The final line of evidence bearing on our thesis is the recent observation that mediators which have been considered to be relevant only in immediate hypersensitivity, i.e., to be released from basophils and mast cells by an IgE-mediated reaction, are also released from other cell types. Specifically, we will present evidence that a molecule which appears to be identical to SRS-A can be released from human polymorphonuclear cells by a general secretory stimulus. Additionally, a molecule which is similar to the ECF-A released by basophils and mast cells can be shown to be generated by human polymorphonuclear cells during the process of phagocytosis. When two such apparently different release processes, IgE-mediated and phagocytic, lead to the generation of the same mediator, the lines of classification become vanishingly faint.

The studies which I will review involve primarily human peripheral blood leukocytes (2). This system has many advantages for studying immediate hypersensitivity reactions, but is particularly useful for addressing questions relating to the interrelationship between the activities of the different cell types. It is possible, since the basophils are the only cell type with IgE on their cell membrane, to selectively release mediators from these cells by challenging whole leukocyte preparations with anti-IgE (3). The other cell types, eosinophils, polymorphonuclear cells, and lymphocytes, can be obtained in good yield with a degree of homogeneity ranging from 80 to 99+% by standard and relatively simple techniques.

With respect to immediate hypersensitivity reactions, the basophil and the mast cell seem to have marked functional similarities, although in control mechanisms some differences have been noted. In particular, the whole range of mediators which were first described in mast cells are also released from basophils by antigen or anti-IgE stimulation. While the leukocyte system has been used to study histamine release for many years, in the recent past it has been possible to demonstrate, as well, the release of SRS-A, ECF-A, and the platelet-activated factor (PAF) from the same cell types (4-6). Moreover, as we will consider below, the kallikrein-like esterase activity which is obtained from basophils appears, as well, to be released from human lung mast cells (7).

The control of mediator release by hormone-induced changes in cyclic nucleotide concentrations was described in the leukocyte system (8). It was demonstrated that antigen or anti-IgE induced histamine release was markedly diminished by β-adrenergic

agonists, theophylline or by dibutyryl cyclic AMP itself. Extensive studies with these and other agonists, both with respect to
dose response relationships and kinetics, have established that
changes in the leukocyte cyclic AMP level parallel quite exactly
the degree of inhibition of histamine release (9). In this, as
in all primate systems, the parallelism provides only circumstantial evidence of control, since the histamine or other mediator
release is being measured from a distinct minority of the cells
present, while the cyclic AMP measurements reflect the entire cell
population. Only in the rat system, in which it is possible to
obtain purified peritoneal mast cells, has it been shown that the
antigen-IgE antibody interaction leads to a fall in cyclic AMP
level and that the agonists in question prevent release because
they cause an increase in the cyclic AMP concentration (10, 11).

This work was confirmed and extended by Austen, Ishizaka and
others who demonstrated that similar control mechanisms were
operative in the mast cells when mediator release was initiated
from chopped monkey or human lung (12, 13). Austen and his colleagues made the novel observation that changes in cyclic GMP
levels, presumably as a result of cholinergic stimulation,
potentiate release processes (see Austen's manuscript, this book)
(14). Weissmann, Henson and others showed the generality of
these observations by studying the release of lysosomal enzymes
from human polymorphonuclear cells on phagocytosis and the release of serotonin during platelet stimulation (15, 16). Our own
experiments, with Chris Henney, demonstrated that the control of
T cell killing, which appears to be a secretory response, is
modulated in an entirely analogous fashion (17, 18). In the
latter system, cyclic nucleotide measurements have been carried
out in considerably more homogeneous cell populations and, in
each case, correlate with the agonist inhibition of the inflammatory response. It is, perhaps, unnecessary to further consider
this stereotyped release and control mechanism in inflammatory
cells, since it is relatively well known. Table I will suffice
to summarize both the in vivo and in vitro aspects of these control mechanisms in the inflammatory response and to point out
effects on diverse phenomena ranging from the response to chemotactic agents to lymphocyte motility. It should be pointed out
that this table is by no means comprehensive.
The second line of evidence bearing on our thesis regarding
the inflammatory response concerns the release from one cell type
of mediators which control or involve other systems. This is a
broad area to which many have contributed, but I will consider it
primarily with respect to our own research efforts.

Table I.   Effects of cyclic AMP on Inflammatory Responses

INCREASED cAMP LEVELS DEPRESS:

Basophil/mast cell IgE mediated release reaction in vitro
     and in vivo

PMN chemotaxis; phagocytosis; release of lysosomal enzymes, and
     intracellular killing

Platelet random motility, agglutination, and release reaction

Lymphocyte motility; proliferative response to mitogens;
     induction and expression of cytotoxicity; delayed skin
     reactivity; graft rejection; granulomatous response to
     parasites; antibody induction, production and secretion
     in vitro and in vivo*

Macrophage response to MIF

* Under certain conditions, cAMP increases B cell responses to
  antigen and T cell helper functions.

The complex mechanism of the cascade which leads to the
generation of bradykinin has been laboriously elucidated by many
investigators over the last two decades (19, 20). This potent
mediator has many of the biologic effects of histamine and, in
addition, the ability to cause pain; it has, therefore, been
thought to be intimately involved in the inflammatory response.
The puzzle in assessing the pathogenetic importance of bradykinin
has concerned the conditions under which it is generated from
serum kininogen in order to contribute to inflammation.   It
seemed likely from previous work that a kallikrein-like activity
might be released during an IgE-mediated reaction and, since most
molecules with kallikrein activity hydrolyze TAMe, Dr. Newball
used this exquisitely sensitive assay to explore the potential
release of such a mediator from the basophils (21). Figure 1
demonstrates that leukocyte preparations from virtually all individuals challenged with antigen or anti-IgE release a material
which has TAMe esterase activity. The kinetics of release,
temperature dependence, and the antigen (or anti-IgE) dose
response relationships are identical for the release of histamine
and the esterase. It is possible to compare the quantity of each
mediator released since the kallikrein is a preformed mediator,

as is histamine. A very considerable number of experiments indicate that there is no fixed relationship between the percent of
total release of histamine and the esterase. This is similar to
the lack of a quantitative relationship between histamine and
SRS-A or ECF-A release and suggests different sites of storage or
mechanisms of generation (22).

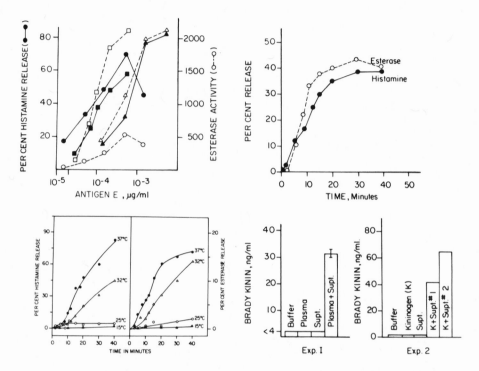

Fig. 1. A comparison of the dose response and kinetic
relationships and the temperature dependence of histamine and
TAMe esterase release from antigenically challenged preparations
of human leukocytes. The lower right panel shows that the
esterase containing supernate can generate a molecule which
reacts with antibodies to bradykinin from either plasma or
purified kininogen.

It is true that not all TAMe esterases are kallikreins.
The supernates containing the esterase activity were, therefore,
incubated with appropriately treated plasma or purified kininogen
and the product of this reaction was analyzed by an immunoassay

for bradykinin (23). Dr. Talamo has, on ten separate occasions,
demonstrated the generation from plasma of highly significant
amounts of bradykinin, or a molecule which contains the same non-
apeptide as bradykinin. Furthermore, as may be noted in Fig. 1,
the esterase has the ability to convert purified kininogen to
bradykinin. This activity is, incidentally, not due to prekallikrein activator activity in the basophil supernate. Isolation and characterization of the kallikrein activity is in progress; this work has gone slowly, but on simple procedures, such
as Sephadex G200 chromatography, the esterase and kallikrein
activities co-elute. It would, thus, appear that one pathway
leading to the involvement of the kallikrein-kinin system in inflammation is through an IgE-mediated immediate hypersensitivity
reaction. While this is the first immune pathway to be described,
it seems likely that the kallikrein system can be activated
through other immune mechanisms. Another example of IgE-mediated
responses which lead to involvement of serum cascade systems may
be found in Pinckard's work: He has described marked alterations
in the coagulation system which occur when rabbits containing
only IgE antibody are challenged with the appropriate antigens
(24).

In addition to the release of agents which can involve the
kinin and clotting systems, and mediators which are chemotactic
and thereby bring in other inflammatory cells (see below), another important means of cell-cell interaction concerns the
modulation of inflammatory cell function by released mediators.
In the narrow context of the present discussion, an early description of this phenomenon was the observation that histamine
could "feedback" to inhibit histamine release (25). This series
of experiments was initiated on the basis of reports delineating
histamine's ability to stimulate adenylate cyclase in other tissue types. It was readily observed that the exogenous administration of histamine in concentrations ranging from 10^{-7} to
10^{-5} M caused a dramatic inhibition of IgE-mediated histamine
release; these concentrations of histamine also caused a clear-
cut increase in the cyclic AMP level of the leukocyte preparations (Fig. 2).

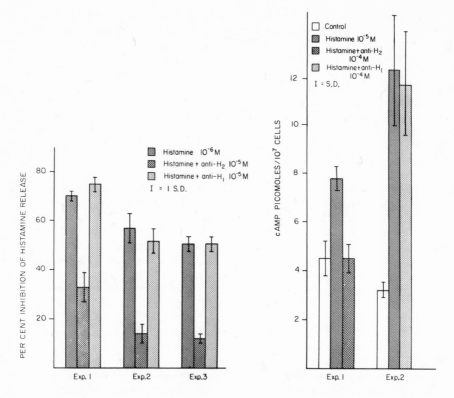

Fig. 2. <u>Left</u>. The inhibition of antigen-induced histamine release from human basophils by histamine: There is reversal of this effect by the anti-H_2 antagonist (burimamide) while the anti-H_1 antagonist (pyrilamine) has no effect. <u>Right</u>. The increase in leukocyte cAMP levels by histamine. The histamine antagonists are the same as above and have similar effects.

Our attempts to define the receptor responsible for histamine's activity in this respect were entirely dependent upon Black's brilliant synthesis of a series of compounds which specifically antagonized histamine's activity on histamine type 2 receptors (26). These agents, burimamide and metiamide, were found to block histamine's inhibitory activity and its ability to raise leukocyte cyclic AMP levels. Using these antagonists, it was possible to define the K_B which describes the affinity of the basophil receptor for histamine: it was found to be similar to that described for histamine-2 receptors in other tissue types (27).

This observation was first generalized by virtue of our collaboration with Dr. Henney's laboratory in which Dr. Plaut

carried out the work which began to describe histamine's effects
on cell-mediated immunity. In addition to the expected observation that histamine blocked the T lymphocyte killing of target
mastocytoma cells through stimulation of adenylate cyclase, this
work led to the interesting observation that the density of
histamine receptors on T lymphocytes changed with the time after
immunization (28). That is, early in immunization, when T lymphocyte killing is maximal, histamine inhibits only modestly,
whereas later in the course, when the killing activity of the
lymphocytes decreases, their responsiveness to histamine, in
terms of inhibition, increases dramatically. Other studies by
Dr. Plaut demonstrated that lymphocytes obtained from several
sites were differentially sensitive to histamine inhibition (29).
For example, peritoneal T lymphocytes are, at any given time,
more potent "killers" than splenic lymphocytes and, at the same
time, are clearly less inhibitable by histamine. Work by
Roszkowski and Plaut in our laboratory has confirmed the findings
that thymic lymphocytes are completely unresponsive to histamine
(30). Additional studies on histamine receptors have been carried out in a number of laboratories, using cells which are
putatively separated by virtue of their histamine receptors.
This work suggests that cells with histamine receptors have quite
different functional abilities when compared to cells which do
not (31). It, thus, seems evident that histamine can have a
striking modulatory role on lymphocyte function in immune and inflammatory conditions and that a means of diversity is provided
by different densities of histamine receptors on the lymphocytes.

Table II.   Effects of Histamine on Inflammatory Processes

HISTAMINE INHIBITS:	H2 Receptor
Mediator Release from basophils (human)	+
Mediator Release, lung and skin (monkey)	+
PCA reaction (rabbit)	+
Neutrophil Phagocytosis (human)	+
Neutrophil Chemotaxis (human)	+
Neutrophil Lysosomal Enzyme Release (human)	?
Eosinophil Chemotaxis (high dose) (human)	+
T cell Cytotoxicity (murine)	+
MIF Production (G. pig)	+
Delayed Skin Reactivity (G. Pig)	+
Ab Production or Secretion (murine)	?

HISTAMINE PERMITS:	
Immune Glomerulonephritis (rabbit)	H1
Foot Pad Swelling (murine)	?

As summarized in Table II, histamine has other activities which are quite widespread: It has been shown to inhibit lyso-somal enzyme release from human polymorphonuclear cells, to stop the platelet release reaction, and to inhibit chemotaxis (15, 32). Moreover, Rocklin has shown that MIF production is blocked by histamine operating through the H2 receptor (33). Finally, these observations have been extended in vivo to show that hista-mine modulates cell-mediated immunity, i.e., it can inhibit the delayed skin test (33). Further evidence for the operation of a histamine feedback control mechanism in vivo is the observation made in chopped tissues that immediate hypersensitivity reactions carried out in the presence of H2 antagonists are clearly poten-tiated, while histamine itself inhibits the PCA reaction (34, 35).

The role of histamine in controlling inflammatory responses is just beginning to be appreciated. It is obvious, however, that it has profound effects which are permissive in some in-stances and inhibitory in others. In the context of inflamma-tion, it is clear that the early response of an animal to a foreign agent, i.e., that which is characterized by IgE-induced mediator release, controls the subsequent development of both the inflammatory response and the mounting of an immune response to the inciting agent. It should be appreciated that histamine is merely a prototype for the interactions of primarily released mediators on the function of other inflammatory cell types. The prostaglandin system is rapidly emerging as a second such system. It has been shown, for example, by Zurier, that PGE1, which has potent inhibitory effects on most inflammatory cell responses, is released by human polymorphonuclear cells during phagocytosis (36). Other workers have shown that one result of an IgE-mediated challenge of chopped lung tissues is the release of prostaglandins which cause an increase in the cyclic AMP level of the lung fragments (37). Whether the prostaglandin release is primary or secondary in this situation remains to be established. Furthermore, because it has been previously shown that E prosta-glandins are potent inhibitors while, in some instances, the F prostaglandins enhance, the balance between the prostaglandins which are released needs to be adequately understood (38). This whole area has been further complicated by the observations of Samuelson's group who provided evidence that what are now known as the classical prostaglandins are probably metabolic end products, while thomboxanes and endoperoxides with short half-lives are playing a more active role (39). This area, obviously, is one that deserves considerable attention in the immediate future (see manuscript by Strandberg, this book).

The final line of experimentation which supports the thesis of this discussion is also the most recent and, in fact, repre-sents the data which forced this reexamination of the classifi-cation of allergic reactions. As is not uncommon, the relevant

observations were made not because they were anticipated, but
rather as the serendipitous result of the use of the calcium
ionophore A23187. We had been engaged in studying the mechanism
of histamine release with the ionophore and had found that in
this system, as in others, the ionophore provided a general
secretory stimulus (40).   The nature of this stimulus was interesting in that it short-circuited the cyclic nucleotide-
associated, early events of the release process, but this observation is not central to the main thread of the present argument.
When we used the ionophore to study the release of mediators
other than histamine, a surprising result was obtained.   As
described in Figure 3, Dr. Conroy repeatedly obtained more SRS-A,
for example, from identical leukocyte preparations which were
challenged with the ionophore as compared to anti-IgE or antigen;
the amount of histamine released was, however, the same.   One
possible explanation for this phenomenon was that other cell
types, in addition to the basophils, could produce this mediator.
Cell fractionation studies were carried out, and the results
clearly indicated that the human polymorphonuclear cell was
capable of generating and/or releasing SRS-A (Fig. 3) (41).

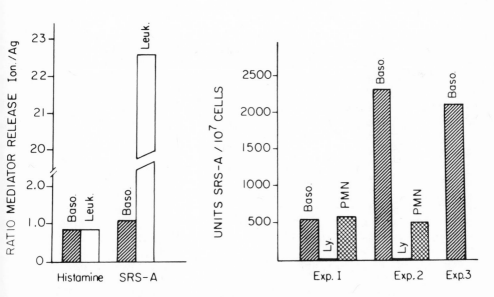

Fig. 3. Left. The ratio of the amount of histamine and
SRS-A released from human leukocytes by antigen and the calcium
ionophore A23187. Right. Ionophore induced SRS-A release from
purified cell fractions. The lymphocytes were >99% and the polymorphonuclear cells were >90% homogeneous. The basophils represented 3-6% of the total cells and were contaminated by lymphocytes. The 3rd experiment shows only a basophil preparation.

This mediator, which has not as yet been structurally defined, has been characterized by Orange, Austen and their colleagues as being purified, with increased specific activity, through a series of extractions and chromatographic steps (42). The SRS-A derived by ionophore stimulation of 98% pure human polymorphonuclear cells appeared identical with the antigen-induced SRS-A released from human lungs, in the experiments which were carried out by Dr. Orange. Furthermore, within the rather broad limits of our ability to quantitate SRS-A, the number of units obtained per neutrophil were similar to quantities obtained from the basophils.

There is a precedent for this observation in its description some years ago that there was a non-mast cell source for SRS-A utilizing rat peritoneal cells (43). With respect to primate systems, however, the observations cited above were a rather surprising demonstration of the release of a mediator associated with immediate hypersensitivity from a cell type which is clearly not associated with this type of response. We have not pursued a more physiologic mechanism for the release of granulocyte SRS-A because of our difficulties in quantitating this mediator. Once this precedent was established, however, the question arose as to whether similar findings could be obtained with respect to other mediators; this has been pursued by a study of the release of an eosinophil chemotactic factor.

The eosinophils themselves represent one of the more interesting "interface" cells in considering the continuity of the inflammatory response. They are present in a number of different types of pathological lesions, although mainly associated with parasitic or IgE-mediated responses. Until recently, however, neither the stimulus that elicited their accumulation nor their function was known. Work by Kay and Austen has, however, delineated an eosinophil chemotactic factor (ECF-A) which is released from mast cells and we have confirmed their work in describing its release from basophils; in both instances the release is IgE-mediated (6, 44). Furthermore, some hints as to eosinophil function are beginning to appear, in that the eosinophil has been reported to contain an arylsulfatase which can destroy SRS-A as well as an enzyme which leads to the destruction of histamine (45, 46). It may be speculated, therefore, that the eosinophils function to "mop up" the first phase of inflammation.

Our original experiments in this area followed those just described: Drs. Czarnetzki and König studied the release of ECF-A with an immunologic stimulus and with ionophore from identical aliquots of leukocyte preparations (47). It was apparent that ionophore stimulation led to a more massive release of ECF (since this does not represent anaphylactic release, we have dropped the suffix, A). Cell fractionation studies (Fig. 4) again

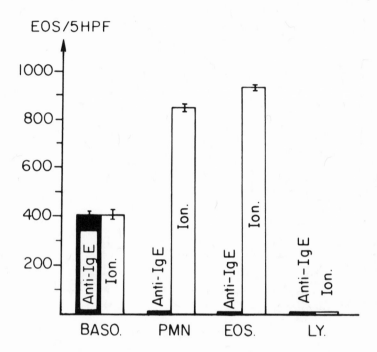

Fig. 4.   The release of ECF from purified cell preparations
by anti-IgE and the calcium ionophore. The polymorphonuclears
and eosinophils were >90 and the lymphocytes >99% homogeneous
while the basophils represented 3-6% of the total cells and were
contaminated by lymphocytes.

demonstrated that the polymorphonuclear cell was the cell of
origin; in this instance, further studies with eosinophils produced data which suggested that this cell as well contains and
can release ECF.

The experiments with the ionophore were of interest in that
they demonstrated in neutrophils the presence or capability of
synthesizing these mediators, but they revealed little in terms of
the nature of the possible in vivo stimulus which might lead to
the release of these products. We therefore carried out further
experiments with human polymorphonuclear cells, posing the question of whether phagocytosis was an appropriate stimulus for the
release (48). As a phagocytic stimulus, zymosan was chosen and
used either in its native state (Z) or coated with serum (complement) components and washed (Z$_{(x)}$), or in the presence of

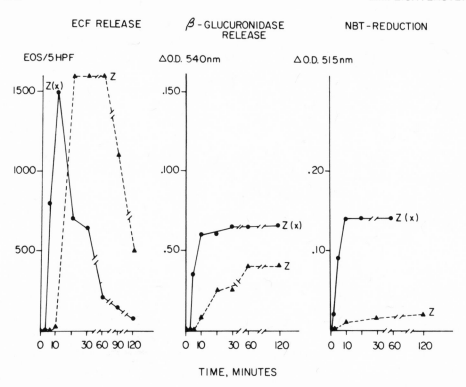

Fig. 5.   The kinetics of ECF and β-glucuronidase release and NBT reduction on treatment of identical aliquots of purified human polymorphonuclear cells with Z or $Z_{(x)}$.

serum ($Z_{(s)}$). The results of some of these experiments are shown in Figure 5. When homogeneous populations of human polymorpho-nuclear cells were provided with $Z_{(x)}$, there was rapid NBT reduction indicating that phagocytosis was occurring and, as has been described by others, a concomitant release of the lysosomal enzyme, β-glucuronidase. Not shown is the fact that there was no release of the cytoplasmic marker, lactic dehydrogenase. What is of interest is that as a parallel to the release of the lyso-somal enzyme, ECF appears in the supernatant fluid. The original kinetics of ECF release are quite similar to that of β-glucuroni-dase release. However, while the enzyme is released and remains at a stable level in the supernatant fluid, it is apparent that with time the amount of ECF which is assayable in the supernatant fluid decreases. The reason for this decrease in ECF is current-ly under investigation, but preliminary evidence suggests that

late in the phagocytic cycle the granulocytes release a substance
which destroys the activity of ECF: whether this is by binding or
enzymatic action is not yet clear. Of further interest is the
different pattern obtained when zymosan alone (Z) is the stimulus
for phagocytosis. In this instance, there is little in the way
of NBT reduction and a significantly lower amount of β-glucuroni-
dase is released. Although the release of ECF is delayed, the
total amount released is as great or greater than when the cells
are stimulated with $Z_{(x)}$. A still different pattern of release
is obtained with $Z(s)$. Thus, different stimuli lead to a dis-
parity in the release of lysosomal enzymes as compared to the
eosinophil chemotactic factor, suggesting either different mechanisms of release or storage in two distinct types of granules.
This latter question has not been addressed.

In contrast to what has been described for mast cell ECF-A,
the lysis of human polymorphonuclear cells leads to no recovery of
ECF. Within seconds, however, after the cells have been exposed
to either the ionophore or the zymosan particles, ECF is readily
obtainable on sonication of the cells. Thus, in this instance
ECF is not preformed. Preliminary studies suggest that the modulation of ECF release by the agonists described above is entirely
similar to what has been described for the release of lysosomal
enzymes from polymorphonuclear cells or histamine from the
basophils.

We have pursued, as well, the question of whether the ECF
produced by the neutrophils is similar to that released by basophils with an anti-IgE stimulus. The materials released from
basophils and that from granulocytes challenged with either
ionophore or zymosan chromatographs on Sephadex G25 with identical elution patterns and an apparent molecular weight of
approximately 500 daltons. Of the several eosinophil chemotactic
factors which have been described, only ECF-A has this molecular
size. While the identity of PMN ECF with the ECF-A which has
been characterized by Kay and Austen cannot be assumed, it seems
likely.

In summary, then, we have adduced data from three independent lines of experimentation, all of which bear on the marked
interrelationship between inflammatory cells as they participate
in inflammatory processes. With rare exceptions as, for example,
acute anaphylactic shock, it would appear that there is virtually no human disease process which can be characterized as
being even primarily caused by one or another of the pathogenetic
categories defined by Gell and Coombs. There are, in fact, many
other lines of experimentation which lead to the same conclusion.
One fascinating example is the recently described basophil
cutaneous hypersensitivity in which basophils and lymphocytes
participate in what was earlier described as the Jones-Mote

phenomenon (49). Another such instance derives from work by
Gleich and Dolovich and their colleagues who showed that purely
IgE-mediated reactions, the pathogenesis of which is not clear,
can have a temporal sequence which extends over many hours (50,
51). The marked efficacy of steroids for treatment of allergic
rhinitis, as contrasted to their very minor effect, if any, on
IgE-mediated release processes, is a clinical example which bears
on this question. In conclusion, it seems not unreasonable to
suggest that we concentrate less on attempting to define the
various types of allergic responses but rather accept the inter-
relatedness which is so abundantly clear and attempt to begin to
understand the pathogenesis of allergic and inflammatory
responses in these terms.

1. Gell, P.G.H. and Coombs, R.R.A. Clinical aspects of immuno-
    logy. 2nd Edit. F.A. Davis, Phil., Pa. 1968 (p. 575).

2. Lichtenstein, L.M. and Osler, A.G. Studies on the mechanisms
    of hypersensitivity phenomena. IX. Histamine release from
    human leukocytes by ragweed pollen antigen. J. Exp. Med.,
    120: 507, 1964.

3. Ishizaka, T., DeBernardo, R., Tomioka, Hisao, Lichtenstein,
    L.M. and Ishizaka, K. Identification of basophil granulo-
    cytes as a site of allergic histamine release. J. Immun.,
    108: 1000, 1972.

4. Grant, J.A. and Lichtenstein, L.M. Release of slow reacting
    substance of anaphylaxis from human leukocytes. J. Immun.,
    112: 897, 1974.

5. Lewis, R.A., Goetzl, E.J., Wasserman, S.I., Valone, F.H.,
    Rubin, R.H. and Austen, K.F. The release of four mediators
    of immediate hypersensitivity from human leukemic basophils.
    J. Immunol. 114: 87, 1975.

6. Czarnetzki, B.M., Konig, W. and Lichtenstein, L.M. Antigen-
    induced eosinophil chemotactic factor (ECF) release by human
    leukocytes. Inflammation, In Press.

7. Newball, H.H., Talamo, R.C., and Lichtenstein, L.M. Release
    of leukocyte kallikrein mediated by IgE. Nature 254: 635,
    1975.

8. Lichtenstein, L.M. and Margolis, S. Histamine release in
    vitro: Inhibition by catecholamines and methylxanthines.
    Science, 161: 902, 1968.

9. Bourne, H.R., Lichtenstein, L.M. and Melmon, K.L. Pharmaco-
    logic control of allergic histamine release in vitro: Evi-
    dence for an inhibitory role of 3',5'-adenosine monophosphate
    in human leukocytes. J. Immun., 108: 695, 1972.

10. Kaliner, M. and Austen, K.F. Cyclic AMP, ATP and reversed
    anaphylactic histamine release from rat mast cells. J.
    Immunol. 112: 664, 1974.

11. Gillespie, E. Compound 48/80 decreases adenosine 3',5'-mono-
    phosphate formation in rat peritoneal mast cells. Experien-
    tia 29: 447, 1973.

12. Ishizaka, T., Ishizaka, K., Orange, R.P. and Austen, K.F.
    Pharmacologic inhibition of the antigen-induced release of
    histamine and slow-reacting substance of anaphylaxis (SRS-A)

from monkey lung tissues mediated by human IgE. J. Immunol.
106: 1267, 1971.

13. Orange, R.P., Austen, W.G. and Austen, K.F. Immunologic re-
     lease of histamine and slow-reacting substance of anaphylaxis
     from human lung. I. Modulation by agents influencing cellu-
     lar levels of cyclic 3',5'-adenosine monophosphate. J. Exp.
     Med. **134**: 1365, 1971.

14. Kaliner, M., Orange, R.P. and Austen, K.F. Immunological
     release of histamine and slow reacting substance of anaphyl-
     axis from human lung. IV. Enhancement by cholinergic and
     alpha adrenergic stimulation. J. Exp. Med. **136**: 556,
     1972.

15. Zurier, R.B., Weissmann, G., Hoffstein, S., Kammerman, S. and
     Tai, H.H. Mechanisms of lysosomal enzyme release from human
     leukocytes. II. Effects of cAMP and cGMP, autonomic agon-
     ists, and agents which affect microtubule function. J. Clin.
     Invest. **53**: 297, 1974.

16. Henson, P.M. Mechanisms of activation and secretion by pla-
     telets and neutrophils. Prog. Immunol. II. **2**: 95, 1974.

17. Henney, C.S., Bourne, H.R. and Lichtenstein, L.M. The role
     of cyclic 3',5'-adenosine monophosphate in the specific cy-
     tolytic activity of lymphocytes. J. Immun., **108**: 1526,
     1972.

18. Lichtenstein, L.M., Henney, C.S., Bourne, H.R. and Greenough,
     W.B. Effects of cholera toxin on in vitro models of immedi-
     ate and delayed hypersensitivity: Further evidence for the
     role of cAMP. J. Clin. Invest. **52**: 691, 1973.

19. Colman, R.W. Formation of human plasma kinin. N. Engl. J.
     Med. **291**: 509, 1974.

20. Cochrane, C.G., Revak, S.D., Aikin, B.S. and Wuepper, K.D.
     The structural characteristics and activation of Hageman fac-
     tor. In Inflammation: Mechanisms and Control. I.H. Lepow
     and P.A. Ward, editors. Academic Press, New York. 1972.
     pp. 119-138.

21. Prado, J.L. Proteolytic enzymes as kininogenases. In Hand-
     book of Exper. Pharmacol. E.G. Erdos, editor. Springer-
     Verlag, New York. **25**: 156, 1970.

22. Orange, R.P. The formation and release of slow reacting sub-
     stance of anaphylaxis in human lung tissues. Prog. Immunol.
     II. **4**: 29, 1974.

23. Talamo, R.C., Haber, E. and Austen, K.F. A radioimmunoassay
     for bradykinin in plasma and synovial fluid. J. Lab. Clin.
     Med. 74: 816, 1969.

24. Halonen, M. and Pinckard, R.N. Intravascular effects of IgE
     antibody upon basophils, neutrophils, platelets and blood
     coagulation in the rabbit. J. Immunol. 115: 519, 1975.

25. Bourne, H.R., Melmon, K.L. and Lichtenstein, L.M. Histamine
     augments leukocyte cyclic AMP and blocks antigenic histamine
     release. Science, 173: 743, 1971.

26. Black, J.W., Duncan, W.A.M., Durant, C.J., Ganellin, C.R. and
     Parsons, E.M. Definition and antagonism of histamine H2-
     receptors. Nature 236: 385, 1972.

27. Lichtenstein, L.M. and Gillespie, E. The effects of the H1
     and H2 antihistamines on "allergic" histamine release and its
     inhibition by histamine. J. Pharm. Exp. Therap. 192:
     441, 1975.

28. Plaut, M., Lichtenstein, L.M. and Henney, C. Increase in
     histamine receptors on thymus-derived effector lymphocytes
     during the primary immune response to alloantigens. Nature
     244: 284, 1973.

29. Plaut, M., Lichtenstein, L.M. and Henney, C.S. Properties of
     a subpopulation of T cells bearing histamine receptors. J.
     Clin. Invest. 55: 856, 1975.

30. Makman, M.H. Properties of adenyl cyclase of lymphoid cells.
     Proc. Nat. Acad. Sci. USA 68: 885, 1971.

31. Weinstein, Y., Melmon, K.L., Bourne, H.R. and Sela, M.
     Specific leukocyte receptors for small exogenous hormones.
     Detection by cell binding to insolubilized hormone prepara-
     tions. J. Clin. Invest. 52: 1349, 1973.

32. Hill, H.R., Estenson, R.D., Quie, P.G., Hogan, N.A. and
     Goldberg, N.D. Modulation of human neutrophil chemotactic
     responses by cyclic 3',5'-guanosine monophosphate and cyclic
     3',5'-adenosine monophosphate. Metabolism 24: 447, 1975.

33. Rocklin, R.E. Modulation of cellular immune response in
     vitro and in vivo by histamine. J. Clin. Invest., in press.

34. Chakrin, L.W., Krell, R.D., Mengel, J. et al. Effect of a
     histamine H-2 receptor antagonist in immunologically induced
     mediator release in vitro. Agents and Actions 4: 297,
     1974.

35. Kravis, T.C. and Zvaifler, N.J.   Alteration of rabbit PCA
    reaction by drugs known to influence intracellular cyclic
    AMP. J. Immunol. 113: 244, 1974.

36. Zurier, R.B. and Sayadoff, D.M.   Release of prostaglandins
    from human polymorphonuclear leukocytes. Inflammation.
    1: 93, 1975.

37. Barrett-Bee, K.J. and Green, L.R.   The relationship between
    prostaglandin release and lung c-AMP levels during anaphyl-
    axis in the guinea pig. Prostaglandins 10: 589, 1975.

38. Lichtenstein, L.M., Gillespie, E., Bourne, H.R. and Henney,
    C.S. The effects of a series of prostaglandins on in vitro
    models of the allergic response and cellular immunity.
    Prostaglandins 2: 519, 1972.

39. Hamberg, M., Svensson, J. and Samuelsson, B.   Thromboxanes:
    A new group of biologically active compounds derived from
    prostaglandin endoperoxides. Proc. Natl. Acad. Sci. 72:
    2994, 1975.

40. Lichtenstein, L.M. The mechanism of basophil histamine re-
    lease induced by antigen and by the calcium ionophore
    A23187. J. Immunol. 114: 1692, 1975.

41. Conroy, M.C., Orange, R.P. and Lichtenstein, L.M. Slow re-
    acting substance (SRS-A) release from human granulocytes by
    the calcium ionophore A23187. J. Immunol., in press.

42. Orange, R.P., Murphy, R.C., Karnovsky, M.L. and Austen, K.F.
    The physicochemical characteristics and purification of slow
    reacting substance of anaphylaxis. J. Immunol. 110: 760,
    1973.

43. Orange, R.P., Valentine, M.D. and Austen, K.F.   Antigen in-
    duced release of slow reacting substance of anaphylaxis
    (SRS-A^{rat}) in rats prepared with homologous antibody. J.
    Exp. Med. 127: 767, 1968.

44. Kay, A.B. and Austen, K.F.   The IgE-mediated release of an
    eosinophil leukocyte chemotactic factor from human lung. J.
    Immunol. 107: 899, 1971.

45. Wasserman, S.I., Goetzl, G.J. and Austen, K.F.   Inactivation
    of slow reacting substance of anaphylaxis by human eosinophil
    arylsulfatase. J. Immunol. 114: 645, 1975.

46. Zeiger, R.S., Yurdin, B.A. and Colten, H.R.   Histamine cata-
    bolism: Localization of histaminase and histamine methyl

transferase in human leukocytes. J. Allergy Clin. Immunol., in press.

47. Czarnetzki, B.M., Konig, W. and Lichtenstein, L.M. Eosino-phil chemotactic factor (ECF) I: Release from polymorpho-nuclear leukocytes by the calcium ionophore A23187. J. Immunol., in press.

48. Konig, W., Czarnetzki, B.M. and Lichtenstein, L.M. Eosino-phil chemotactic factor (ECF) II: Release during phagocy-tosis of human polymorphonuclear leukocytes. J. Immunol., in press.

49. Richerson, H.B., Dvorak, H.B. and Leskowitz, S. Cutaneous basophil hypersensitivity I. A new look at The Jones Mote Reaction, general characteristics. J. Exp. Med. 132: 546, 1970.

50. Dolovitch, J., Hargreave, F.E., Chalmers, R., Shier, K.J., Gouldie, J. and Bienenstock, J. Late cutaneous allergic responses in isolated IgE dependent reactions. J. Allergy Clin. Immunol. 52: 38, 1973.

51. Solley, G.O., Larson, J.B., Jordon, R.E. and Gleich, G.J. Late cutaneous reactions due to IgE. J. Allergy Clin. Immunol. 55: 112, 1975.

DISCUSSION

BENNICH: I was pleased by your attempt to integrate the IgE induced mast cell reactions and to relate the release of mediators to other cell systems.

LICHTENSTEIN: I realize that I somewhat overstate the case - but I hope that my speculations are valuable in suggesting new approaches to inflammation.

BECKER: You carefully qualified your remarks so that you cannot be accused of being a "histaminiac". Nevertheless, do you believe that it is possible to obtain concentrations in vivo of histamine which reach the levels required to affect the response in vitro.

LICHTENSTEIN: It is quite possible to get concentrations of histamine in vivo of 10^{-5} to perhaps 10^{-4} M. We have experi-ments in which we biopsied human skin which had been tested with injection of an allergen. The measured decrease in histamine con-tent presumably was a result of histamine release. It is then possible to calculate the concentration of histamine per gram of tissue and it closely corresponds to the concentrations I have mentioned.

DIAMANT: Do you believe that a decrease in cAMP is among

the first biochemical events that triggers off histamine release? If so what are the exact biochemical proof for this triggering?

LICHTENSTEIN: That is my belief, based on the inhibition of histamine release obtained by agents which increase cAMP and the actual measurements of cAMP decrease in the rat mast cell system after stimulation by 48/80 (Gillespie) or antigen (Kaliner et al.).

DIAMANT: If there really occurs a decrease of cAMP in mast cells and basophils upon stimulation it could be either secondary to an increased ATP utilization or to the uptake of Ca^{2+} which would activate phosphodiesterase and inhibit adenylcyclase. Would you consider these possibilities?

LICHTENSTEIN: I would certainly consider these as real possibilities. My own view, substantiated by evidence, is that the membrane crosslinking caused by anti-IgE or allergen decrease the activity of the membrane bound adenylcyclase.

COCHRANE: There is no doubt that in many if not most immunopathologic reactions the various aspects of inflammatory processes take place, from acute release of vasoactive amines to accumulation of neutrophils and mononuclear cells.

However, it is worth emphasizing that in certain reactions, one phase of the process may be dominant. For example, in acute nephrotoxic nephritis, complement and neutrophils can dominate the mediator systems so that removal of neutrophils alone will prevent the injury. Antihistamines that can block completely a PCA reaction in such rabbits have no effect on the glomerular injury. And of course there are other examples of this.

LICHTENSTEIN: I do, of course, agree and I have mentioned acute anaphylaxis or intravascular hemolysis as examples of in vivo reactions of one "type". I only stress that most in vivo immunopathogenic mechanisms involve multiple cell types and serum systems.

INFLUENCE OF CALCIUM IONS AND METABOLIC ENERGY (ATP) ON HISTAMINE RELEASE

Bertil Diamant

Department of Pharmacology, Univ. of Copenhagen

20, Juliane Maries Vej, DK-2100 Copenhagen

Rat mast cells can be stimulated by a number of different agents to secrete histamine (Paton 1956). Some of these, including antigen, the polymer amine compound 48/80, ATP, and the ionophore A23187, act selectively on the cells in the sense that stimulation is coupled to secretion through the influence of certain coupling factors. These factors are, in agreement with so many other secretory systems, calcium and endogenous ATP (Fig. 1). Both factors are equally important for secretion to occur. Omit calcium (Krüger et al. 1974, Krüger & Bloom 1974, Cochrane & Douglas 1974) or inhibit ATP production (Yamasaki et al. 1970) in the cells, and none of the typical morphological changes occur upon stimulation, and consequently no histamine is released. On the other hand, decylamine, the ionophore X537A, and chlorpromazine stimulate histamine secretion completely independent of calcium or metabolic energy (Högberg & Uvnäs 1960, Frisk-Holmberg 1971, Foreman et al. 1973). The molecular nature of the coupling reactions which depend on calcium and ATP is far from solved. From a theoretical point of view it should be considered if calcium and ATP might act directly on the perigranular membrane. Grosman & Diamant (1976) have recently concluded from studies on isolated membrane-containing mast cell granules which retain their histamine in a balanced salt solution that ATP and calcium do not interfere directly with the permeability of the perigranular membrane, since ATP and calcium did not induce release of histamine from this preparation. Experimental data

point to that stimulation of the cell membrane by selective releasing agents is followed by an increased association of calcium with the cells. This has been shown
to precede histamine secretion when induced by extracellular ATP (Dahlquist & Diamant 1972, Dahlquist 1974).
An enhanced association of calcium has also been demonstrated after stimulation of mast cells with antigen as
well as the ionophore A23187 (Foreman et al. 1973).
Furthermore, Kanno et al. (1973) found that microinjec-
tions of calcium directly into the mast cell induced
morphological changes consistent with the expulsion of
granular material. It could be argued that metabolic
energy is needed somehow in the uptake mechanism of calcium following stimulation. However, Foreman et al.
(1975) have recently demonstrated an increased association of 45-calcium with the cells after stimulation with
antigen, even in the presence of a metabolic inhibitor
(antimycin A), which depletes the cell of metabolic energy
and consequently does not allow histamine secretion to
occur.

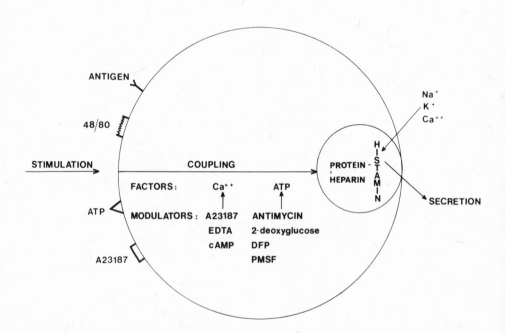

Fig. 1. Schematic representation of stimulus-secretion
coupling in rat mast cells.

The information presently available suggest that from a mechanical point of view stimulation of rat mast cells with selective releasing agents makes calcium available at critical sites within the cell. Provided cellular energy is available simultaneously (Diamant & Patkar 1975), conditions are established which allow histamine bound to the cellular matrix to exchange for cations according to the model given by Uvnäs (1971). Röhlich (1975) has recently demonstrated actin filaments in rat mast cells attaching the perigranular membrane to the plasma membrane. In glycerinated mast cells these filaments bind heavy meromyosin. It seems therefore likely that a contractile mechanism is the underlying cause for the fusion of the perigranular membrane with the plasma membrane. At the junction the permeability properties would change (Satir 1974) and as a consequence the granular matrix be exposed to extracellular cations. The possible involvement of calcium and ATP as coupling factors in this fusion process is obvious and might correlate well to what is known concerning other contractile mechanisms.

The access of these coupling factors can be influenced by various modulating agents which consequently indirectly modulate the secretory response. In case of metabolic energy, the secretory response of mast cells stimulated by selective agents is directly dependent on the concentration of intracellular ATP (Peterson & Diamant 1972, Peterson 1974a, Johansen & Chakravarty 1972, 1975). When glucose is supplied to rat mast cells, ATP can be furnished by anaerobic glycolytic reactions to an extent sufficient to allow secretion to occur upon stimulation. The generation of ATP through anaerobic glycolysis,when glucose is not limiting, has about the same efficiency as aerobic glycolysis, when the cells rely on their endogenous substrate alone (Diamant 1975). It has further been established that during secretion, ATP is utilized by the cells (Kaliner & Austen, 1974, Peterson & Diamant 1974, Johansen & Chakravarty 1975), which in itself supports the possibility of the activation of an intracellular contractile process.

Although histamine release is generally inhibited by agents interfering with oxidative phosphorylation in various species and cellular preparations, provided the incubation medium is not fortified with glucose (Diamant 1962), the influence of 2-deoxyglucose varies. Under aerobic conditions, 2-deoxyglucose inhibits anaphylactic histamine release from guinea pig lung tissue (Chakravarty 1962, Yamasaki & Endo 1965), from human leukocytes

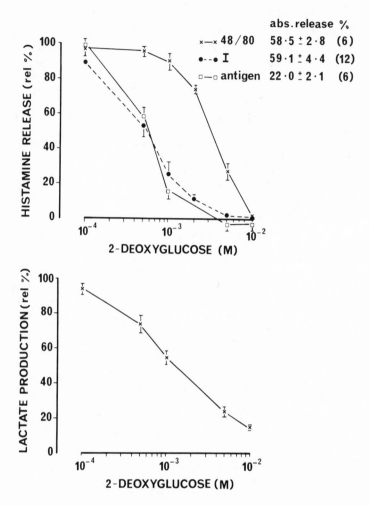

Fig. 2. The influence of 2-deoxyglucose on histamine release induced by compound 48/80 (0.6 μg/ml), ionophore
A23187 (10⁻⁶ M), and antigen (horse serum) (0.75% v/v).
Mast cells were incubated for 10 min in a medium containing antimycin (10⁻⁶ M), glucose (2 mM), calcium
(1 mM), and 2-deoxyglucose before addition of histamine
releasing agents. All values related to histamine release and lactate production in control samples incubated in the absence of 2-deoxyglucose. These values are
presented in the figure.

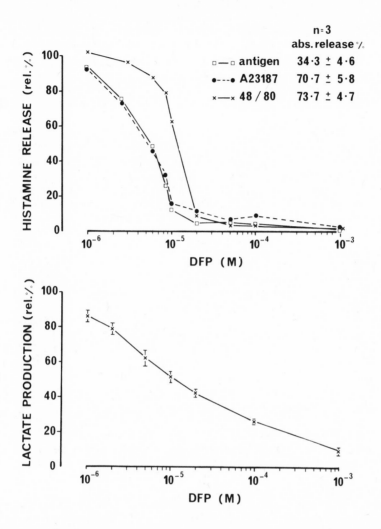

Fig. 3. The influence of DFP on histamine release induced
by compound 48/80 (0.6 µg/ml), ionophore A23187 (10^{-6} M),
and antigen (horse serum) (0.75% v/v). Mast cells were
incubated for 10 min in a medium containing antimycin
(10^{-6} M), glucose (2 mM), calcium (1 mM), and DFP before
addition of histamine releasing agents. All values related to histamine release and lactate production in
control samples incubated in the absence of DFP. These
values are presented in the figure.

(Lichtenstein 1975), and from human lung tissue (Orange
et al. 1971). Under similar conditions Chakravarty (1968)
found, however, that 2-deoxyglucose was ineffective to
inhibit histamine release induced by compound 48/80 or
antigen from isolated rat mast cells. However, when oxidative phosphorylation in mast cells was blocked by cyanide and the energy production relied on the utilization
of glucose present in the incubation medium, 2-deoxyglu-
cose became a pronounced inhibitor of the histamine release. Diamant & Patkar (to be published) have recently
reinvestigated the inhibitory action of 2-deoxyglucose
on histamine release from isolated rat mast cells induced
by 48/80, antigen, as well as the ionophore A23187 under
conditions where oxidative phosphorylation was blocked by
antimycin and where the energy production relied on the
utilization of glucose present in the incubation medium.
The inhibitory action of 2-deoxyglucose on histamine release (Fig. 2) and on lactate production of the cells
correlated well. The lactate production reflected the ATP
generation under the experimental conditions used (Peterson 1974a). It is notable that the secretion induced by
compound 48/80 was less sensitive to this metabolic effect as compared to antigen and A23187. This agrees well
with earlier observations by Johansen & Chakravarty (1972)
and Peterson (1974b), who demonstrated that it is possible
to depress the steady state level of ATP in mast cells by
25-30% without inhibiting compound 48/80-induced histamine
release. On the other hand, antigen-induced release was
shown by Johansen & Chakravarty (1975) to be much more
sensitive to changes in the ATP concentration of the cells.
The same experimental design was used in order to study
the effect of various agents considered to depress histamine release through an esterase inhibiting action (Orange
et al. 1971). DFP in concentrations between $10^{-6} - 10^{-3}$ M
gradually depressed the lactate production as did 2-deoxy-
glucose and parallel to this effect the histamine release
decreased (Fig. 3). In agreement with observations for 2-
deoxyglucose, secretion caused by compound 48/80 was again
less sensitive to this action as compared to the ionophore
and antigen. The same results have been obtained with
another "esterase inhibitor" phenyl-methyl-sulphonyl-flu-
ride (PMSF) (Fahrney & Gold 1963).

        In agreement with the observations by Chakravarty
(1968) 10 mM of 2-deoxyglucose was completely ineffective to inhibit histamine release induced by either antigen, compound 48/80, ATP, or A23187 from rat mast cells
incubated under aerobic conditions in the absence of extracellular glucose (Table 1). Under the same conditions,

Table 1. The effect of 10 mM 2-deoxyglucose on histamine release from mast cells. (Glucose absent; calcium (1 mM) present except for ATP (0.25 mM)). Preincubation time 10 min with 2-deoxyglucose.

Releasing agent	Histamine rel. (%) Mean $\pm$ S.E.M.	
( ) = No. of exp.	2-deoxyglucose (10 mM)	
	−	+
Antigen (13)	29.0 $\pm$ 3.1	31.3 $\pm$ 2.8
48/80 (0.6 µg/ml) (5)	62.8 $\pm$ 7.5	60.8 $\pm$ 5.5
ATP (6×10^{-5} M) (4)	68.9 $\pm$ 6.4	70.4 $\pm$ 4.2
A23187 (10^{-6} M) (5)	46.2 $\pm$ 9.2	48.0 $\pm$ 8.2

Table 2. Mast cells incubated 15 min with or without DFP before addition of glucose (2 mM). 15 min later they were challenged with 48/80 (0.6 µg/ml); calcium (1 mM) present at all stages.

	Lactate prod. (rel. %)	Histamine rel. (rel. %)
Cells − DFP	100	100
Cells + 2.5 mM DFP	44.2 $\pm$ 6.2	67.7 $\pm$ 6.0
Cells + 5 mM DFP	17.3 $\pm$ 5.3	41.3 $\pm$ 3.9
Cells + 10 mM DFP	$<5.6 \pm 1.3$	9.0 $\pm$ 0.5

n = 3; mean $\pm$ S.E.M.

however, DFP inhibited histamine release induced by all four agents, but markedly higher concentrations (5-10 mM) were needed for efficient inhibition (Table 2). The most obvious explanation to these results is that when oxidative phosphorylation in the cells is blocked by antimycin A, 2-deoxyglucose as well as low concentrations of DFP inhibit the utilization of extracellular glucose by the cells. Under anaerobic conditions in the absence of extracellular glucose, the utilization of endogenous

substrates is not sufficient to maintain the ATP production in the cells to a degree sufficient for secretion
to occur (Diamant 1975). The inhibitory action of DFP
under aerobic conditions might then be ascribed to that
DFP at higher concentrations (5-10 mM) would affect the
aerobic glycolysis at some additional critical enzymatic
step. The inhibitory action noted for DFP on histamine
release, which has been ascribed to inhibition of an
esterase activated early in the release process (Kaliner
& Austen 1973, 1974),could therefore, according to the
present results, just as well be explained on the basis
that DFP inhibits metabolic energy production. To further
test this possibility, direct measurements of cellular
ATP in the cells under the influence of DFP are now in
progress.

Turning to the second coupling factor to be discussed, namely calcium, it has been known for some time
that even if mast cells are isolated in the absence of
calcium and challenged with selective releasing agents

Table 3

Histamine release (% of total histamine content)

	-	Ca^{++}	n
I $\longrightarrow$ 48/80	2.9 ± 2.1	66.1 ± 3.8	5
I $\longrightarrow$ ATP	1.4 ± 1.8	44.8 ± 7.0	5
I $\longrightarrow$ I	1.3 ± 0.4	75.2 ± 1.7	6
I $\longrightarrow$ Antigen	2.6 ± 1.1	30.6 ± 12.3	3
Controls			
48/80	47.7 ± 8.3	66.0 ± 5.3	5
ATP	6.8 ± 2.1	52.7 ± 6.0	5
I	9.4 ± 2.3	76.6 ± 2.9	6
Antigen	15.3 ± 6.2	26.1 ± 1.0	3

48/80: 0.6 µg/ml, ATP: 6×10^{-5} M, ionophore A23187 (I):
10^{-6} M, antigen (horse serum): 0.75% v/v, calcium: 1 mM,
for ATP 0.25 mM.

like antigen, 48/80, ATP, and the ionophore A23187 in
the absence of extracellular calcium, there always occurs
a slight, but significant release. In case of compound
48/80, this release is comparatively high. In all instances this release is suboptimal as compared to that
occurring in the presence of extracellular calcium (Table
3). The question to answer now is, if the suboptimal release, which occurs in the absence of extracellular calcium, is caused by a non-selective mechanism or if it is
due to utilization of cellular calcium present for example
in the plasma membrane of the cells. This was recently
resolved partly by Douglas & Ueda (1973), who used EDTA
as an experimental tool, and partly by us (Patkar & Diamant 1974, Diamant & Patkar 1975). Insteady of EDTA we
have used the ionophore A23187 as a tool to deplete the
mast cells of cell-bound calcium. When mast cells were
preincubated with micromolar concentrations of the ionophore in the absence of calcium for a few minutes, and
the ionophore was then washed out or diluted out to ineffective concentrations, the suboptimal release which
occurred in non-treated cells completely disappeared
(Table 3). This effect of the ionophore was fast with a
half time of about 20 seconds (Diamant & Patkar 1975).

The response of the cells, however, was unaffected
by ionophore treatment, provided the cells were exposed
to the releasing agents in the presence of optimal concentrations of calcium (Table 3). This indicates that
the main action of the ionophore on the cell is to quick-
ly transport cell-bound calcium out from the cell, thereby limiting one of the coupling factors needed in the
release process.

In continuation of these experiments it became apparent that the insensitive state which occurred after ionophore treatment could be spontaneously reversed even in
the absence of extracellular calcium. When ionophore-pre-
treated cells were incubated at 37°C for various lengths
of time before challenge with 48/80, the secretory response gradually returned close to the levels seen in
control cells not exposed to the ionophore (Fig. 4).

The return of this response was found to be markedly
sensitive to the presence of chelating agents (EDTA or
EGTA) (Table 4). When control cells, e.g. cells not
treated with the ionophore, were incubated in the absence
of calcium for 30 minutes before challenge with 48/80,
they released 47% of their total histamine content and

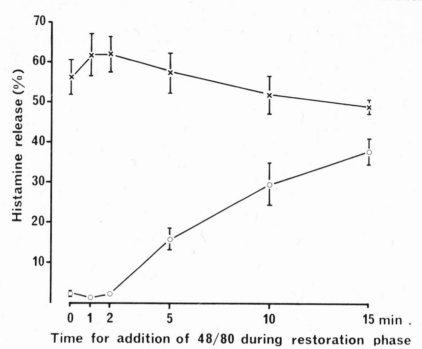

Fig. 4. Ionophore-treated cells incubated for increasing lengths of time at 37°C before challenge with compound 48/80 (0.6 µg/ml): o———o. Histamine release from control cells not exposed to the ionophore incubated identically: x———x. Mean and S.E.M. of 3 experiments.

the presence of EDTA during these 30 minutes did not influence the release at all, neither at 10^{-3} nor at 5 x 10^{-5} M concentrations (Table 4, samples 5, 6, 7). Ionophore-treated cells responded poorly to compound 48/80 when challenged directly after treatment with the ionophore (sample 8), but the sensitivity of these cells was markedly restored by preincubation of the cells for 30 minutes before stimulation with 48/80 (sample 9). If EDTA was included in the incubation medium from the beginning of the restoration period, the cells remained insensitive to 48/80 even at 5 x 10^{-5} M of EDTA (sample 11) Interesting enough, if ionophore-treated cells were incubated for 15 minutes before the addition of EDTA, 1 mM did not any longer inhibit the secretory response induced by compound 48/80 15 minutes later (sample 12).

Table 4

No.	Pretreatment	Incubation time			Histamine rel. (%) (n = 3) Mean ± S.E.M.
		15 min	15 min	10 min	
1	I	-	-	-	2.3 ± 0.5
2	-	-	-	-	2.7 ± 0.1
3	I	EDTA 10^{-3} M	-	-	2.6 ± 0.5
4	-	EDTA 10^{-3} M	-	-	2.7 ± 0.1
5	-	-	-	48/80	47.3 ± 4.3
6	-	EDTA 10^{-3} M	-	48/80	54.2 ± 2.6
7	-	EDTA 5×10^{-5} M	-	48/80	51.2 ± 3.4
8	I	48/80	-	-	9.8 ± 0.4
9	I	-	-	48/80	39.4 ± 6.7
10	I	EDTA 10^{-3} M	-	48/80	9.7 ± 1.3
11	I	EDTA 5×10^{-5} M	-	48/80	8.9 ± 1.3
12	I	-	EDTA 10^{-3} M	48/80	35.7 ± 6.4
13	I	-	EDTA 5×10^{-5} M	48/80	35.7 ± 6.9

Pretreatment with ionophore (I): 2.5 x 10^{-7} M 3 min + 7.5 x 10^{-7} M 3 min in small tubes. Incubation: 20 μl cells diluted to 2 ml.

In order to interpret these results it is useful
to construct a working model. From such a model certain
predictions can be made and tested experimentally in
order to test its validity. Such a model is presented
in Figs. 5 and 6 and constitutes a schematic picture of
a mast cell divided into various experimental situations.
The model is based on the assumption that calcium bound
to the plasma membrane can be utilized for suboptimal
release of histamine. When mast cells are challenged
with 48/80 in the absence of extracellular calcium, the
calcium in the membrane is assumed to be mobilized into
the cytosol, and if metabolic energy is available, the
conditions for secretion of histamine are established
(Fig. 5, 1). After exposure of the cells to the ionophore for a few minutes, this membrane-bound calcium
disappears (Fig. 5, 3a). Therefore, when these cells are

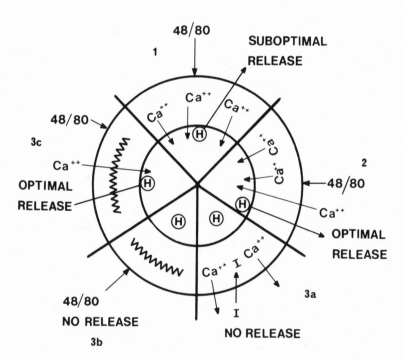

Fig. 5. Schematic representation of the interaction of
the ionophore A23187 with calcium and secretory response
induced by compound 48/80.

challenged with 48/80 immediately after pretreatment with
the ionophore, histamine release will occur (Fig. 5, 3b)
unless extracellular calcium is available (Fig. 5, 3c).
However, if ionophore-treated cells are incubated for
increasing lengths of time, they gradually begin to respond again, indicating that during the restoration phase
calcium is transferred to the plasma membrane from some,
so far, non-defined intracellular pool, which retains its
calcium during exposure of the cells to the ionophore
(Fig. 6, 1c). Thereby calcium will be available again at
the time the cell membrane is stimulated with 48/80.

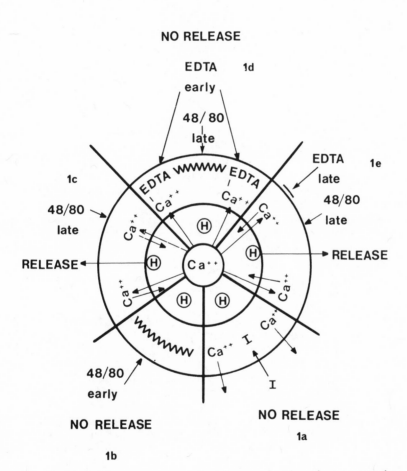

Fig. 6. Schematic representation of the interaction of
the ionophore A23187 and EDTA with intracellular calcium
and secretory response induced by compound 48/80.

Evidently, in cells not pretreated with the ionophore,
EDTA penetrates poorly into the cell membrane. Mast cells
exposed to 1 mM of EDTA for 30 minutes before challenge
with 48/80 responded completely unaffected by EDTA (Table
4). In contrast, when ionophore-treated cells were incubated with EDTA at a concentration as low as 5×10^{-5} M,
the spontaneous restoration of the secretory response
was abolished. This indicates that when the plasma membrane is depleted of its calcium (Fig. 6, 1a and b), the
permeability properties are changed so that EDTA can pene
trate into the membrane and thereby chelate all the calcium that is transferred to the membrane during the
restoration period (Fig. 6, 1d). However, if EDTA is
added to the cells at a late stage in the restoration
phase, EDTA no longer inhibits the secretory response.
This indicates that before the addition of EDTA, calcium
has already returned to the plasma membrane, where it
has restored the original permeability properties of the
membrane, i.e. EDTA is no longer able to reach the calcium pool in the membrane which functions for suboptimal
release (Fig. 6, 1e).

From this model it can be predicted that agents
which cause redistribution of intracellular calcium
should effect the secretory response. The most obvious
agent to investigate in this system is cyclic AMP, which
has been shown to release calcium from mitochondria
(Borle 1974, Matlib & O'Brien 1974) and which has for a
long time been known to cause association of calcium
with various membranes (for ref. see Calcium Transport
in Contraction and Secretion 1975). In fact, Rasmussen
(1970) has proposed that the role of cyclic AMP as a
second messenger might actually be due to its action to
change the local concentrations of calcium within cells.

Before going into the effect of dibutyrylic cyclic
AMP on histamine release from ionophore-treated cells
it is of interest to note (Table 5) that control cells
incubated in a calcium-free medium responded with increased histamine secretion when challenged with 48/80
after they had been preincubated with 1 mM of cyclic
AMP for 20 minutes. The simultaneous presence of 5×10^{-5} M of EDTA neither influenced the release observed
in the presence nor in the absence of cyclic AMP. These
results conform well to what to expect from the model.

Table 5. The influence of EDTA (5×10^{-5} M) and dib. cAMP (1 mM) on histamine release from isolated rat mast cells incubated in the absence of calcium. The cells were not pretreated with the ionophore.

Incubation time		Histamine rel. (%)
20 min	10 min	Mean $\pm$ S.E.M., n = 6
1 -	48/80	36.6 $\pm$ 3.9
2 EDTA	48/80	38.4 $\pm$ 2.7
3 dib. cAMP	48/80	54.0 $\pm$ 3.3
4 EDTA + dib. cAMP	48/80	51.2 $\pm$ 2.7

P_{diff} 1 - 3 <0.01; 3 - 4 > 0.05   48/80: 0.6 µg/ml.

When 1 mM dibutyrylic cyclic AMP was included in the incubation medium during the restoration phase of ionophore-treated cells (Fig. 7), not only did cyclic AMP shorten the restoration phase, but it also caused a significant increase of the secretory response to compound 48/80 as compared to ionophore-treated cells incubated in the absence of cyclic AMP.

From the model it could now be predicted that if the action of cyclic AMP was to enhance the binding of calcium to critical sites in the cell membrane, the effect of cyclic AMP should be completely abolished by a renewed, short-lasting exposure of the cells to the ionophore prior to stimulation with 48/80. It could further be predicted that the presence of a chelating agent (5×10^{-5} M) from the beginning of the restoration phase should also abolish the action of cyclic AMP. Both these effects are shown in Table 6. Furthermore, it has been established that more EDTA was needed to counteract the restoration of the secretory response of ionophore-treated cells in the presence of cyclic AMP than in its absence (Fig. 8). This could also be predicted from the model, since restoration of the secretory response induced by cyclic AMP on these cells should, according to the model, reflect an increased amount of calcium bound to the plasma membrane.

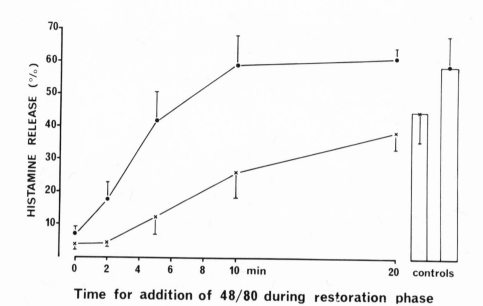

Time for addition of 48/80 during restoration phase

Fig. 7. Histamine release from ionophore-treated cells incubated for increasing lengths of time in the absence x——x or the presence ●——● of 1 mM dib. cAMP before stimulation with compound 48/80 (0.6 µg/ml). Controls represent histamine release from mast cells identically incubated for 20 min before challenge with compound 48/80 but not pretreated with the ionophore. Mean ± S.E.M. of 3 experiments.

Table 6. The influence of A23187 (I) (10^{-6} M) and EGTA (5 x 10^{-5} M) on the action of dib. cAMP (1 mM) to restore the sensitivity of ionophore-treated isolated rat mast cells incubated in the absence of calcium to the secretory action of compound 48/80 (0.6 µg/ml).

Incubation time after ionophore treatment		Histamine release (%) (n = 3; mean $\pm$ S.E.M.)
10 min	10 min	
-	48/80	12.9 $\pm$ 1.7
EGTA	48/80	2.2 $\pm$ 0.5
cAMP	48/80	55.1 $\pm$ 0.8
cAMP + EGTA	48/80	3.2 $\pm$ 1.7
cAMP + I[x]	48/80	- 1.2 $\pm$ 0.6

[x] present during last 2 min.

Finally, if cyclic AMP increased the redistribution of intracellular calcium to the cell membrane, cyclic AMP should also be able to enhance the release induced by other selective agents like antigen, ATP, and the ionophore A23187. According to the model this effect should again be overcome by the presence of EDTA (5 x 10^{-5} M) during the restoration phase (Table 7). As in earlier experiments the cells were pretreated with the ionophore for a few minutes. The ionophore was washed out and the cells were then incubated for 20 minutes either in the presence of EDTA (5 x 10^{-5} M) or dibutyrylic cyclic AMP (1 mM) or a combinations of both agents before challenge with the releasing agents. The secretory response was poor after the restoration period for 20 minutes in the absence of cyclic AMP, especially regarding the response induced by A23187. A slight restoration towards stimulation by ATP or antigen was observed which, in both cases, was depressed by the simultaneous presence of 5 x 10^{-5} M of EDTA. However, when dibutyrylic cyclic AMP (1 mM) was included in the incubation medium during the restoration phase, the cells showed an enhanced

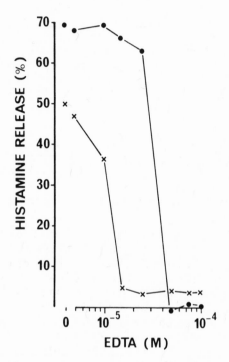

Fig. 8. Histamine release from isolated rat mast cells which, after ionophore treatment, were incubated with-out x———x, or with ●———● 1 mM dib. cAMP for 20 min before stimulation with compound 48/80 (0.6 μg/ml). The influence of increasing concentrations of EDTA during the restoration phase (20 min) is shown.

Table 7

Incubation time after ionophore treatment

20 min	+	10 min

	% Histamine release (mean $\pm$ S.E.M.)		
	A23187	ATP	Antigen
-	3.8 ± 1.1	7.8 ± 2.1	12.0 ± 2.7
EGTA (5×10^{-5} M)	not determ.	3.2 ± 1.1	2.0 ± 1.1
cAMP (10^{-3} M)	24.4 ± 3.3	17.1 ± 2.4	19.3 ± 3.7
EGTA + cAMP	4.4 ± 3.3	3.8 ± 0.7	1.9 ± 0.7
n	7	3	5

After ionophore treatment the cells were washed before incubation. Calcium absent at all stages. A23187: 10^{-6} M, ATP: 6×10^{-6} M, antigen (horse serum): 0.75% v/v.

responsiveness towards all three stimulating agents, which in each instance was depressed by the simultaneous presence of EGTA during the restoration phase.

In summary, the present results obtained with rat mast cells incubated in a calcium-free medium concern the utilization of endogenous calcium for the secretion of histamine. For each selective releasing agent studied cell-bound calcium could function for suboptimal release and seemed to be more effectively utilized after pre-treatment of the cells with cyclic AMP. This suboptimal release was enhanced in all cases by the presence of extracellular calcium, consistent with the view that more calcium would then become available at critical sites within the cells at the time of stimulation. So far, all predictions have favoured the experimental model presented. However, much remains to be established. One important point concerns the specificity of cyclic AMP to restore the secretory response of ionophore-treated cells, another whether the spontaneous restoration studied is due to endogenous cyclic AMP production.

Note added in proof

The suggestion that the spontaneous restoration
of the secretory response of ionophore-treated cells
towards 48/80 (Fig. 4) as well as the activating action
of cyclic AMP (Fig. 7) might be attributed to a transfer of calcium to the plasma membrane from some, so
far non-defined, intracellular pool during the restoration phase might have to be changed. Recent evalua-
tions of the model presented in Fig. 6, assuming contaminating calcium in the "calcium-free" incubation
medium to be the source from which calcium became
associated with the membrane during the restoration
phase, have shown that this could well be true. When
ionophore-treated cells (following washing) were exposed to 48/80 together with 10^{-5} M of calcium no
release occurred. However, allowing the cells to be in
contact with 10^{-5} M of calcium for 10 minutes prior to
challenge with 48/80 resulted in a pronounced release
of histamine. It cannot be excluded that the "calcium-
free" incubation medium as well as the preparation of
dibutyrylic cyclic AMP used (Boehringer & Söhne, Mann-
heim) were contaminated with at least 10^{-5} M of calcium. In fact, calcium determinations (atomic absorption spectophotometry) of the dibutyrylic cyclic AMP
preparation used have revealed a 2% contamination of
calcium, which at a concentration of 1 mM of dibutyrylic cyclic AMP in the experimental situation would add
2×10^{-5} M of calcium to the incubation medium. If this
is the ultimate explanation to the observed spontaneous
restoration of the secretory response of ionophore-
treated cells as well as to the activation induced by
dibutyrylic cyclic AMP remains to be finally established.
If so, the inhibition exerted by chelating agents (EDTA)
demonstrated in Fig. 8 might well be looked upon as a
titration curve of contaminating calcium in the incubation medium.

The financial support of the Danish Medical Research
Council (Grant No. 512-5044) and Hesselman's Foundation,
Sweden is gratefully acknowledged.

References

Borle, A.B., 1974, J. Membrane Biol. 16, 221.

Calcium Transport in Contraction and Secretion, Eds. E. Carafoli, F. Clementi, W. Drabikowski & A. Margreth, North-Holland Publishing Co. Amsterdam 1975.

Chakravarty, N., 1962, Nature (Lond.) 194, 1182.

Chakravarty, N., 1968, Acta physiol. scand. 72, 425.

Cochrane, D.E. & Douglas, W.W., 1974, Proc. Nat. Acad. Sci. 71, 408.

Dahlquist, R., 1974, Acta pharmacol. toxicol. 35, 11.

Dahlquist, R. & Diamant, B., 1972, Proc. 5th Int. Congr. Pharmacology, San Fransisco, p. 50.

Diamant, B., 1962, Acta physiol. scand. 56, 103.

Diamant, B., 1975, Int. Arch. Allergy 49, 155.

Diamant, B. & Patkar, S.A., 1975, Int. Arch. Allergy 49, 183.

Diamant, B. & Patkar, S.A. to be published.

Douglas, W.W. & Ueda, Y., 1973, J. Physiol. Lond. 234, 98.

Fahrney & Gold, 1963, J. Am. Chem. Soc. 85, 997.

Foreman, J.C., Gomperts, B.D. & Mongar, J.L., 1973, Nature 245, 249.

Frisk-Holmberg, M., 1971, Acta physiol. scand. 83, 412.

Grosman, N. & Diamant, B., 1976, Agents & Actions in press.

Högberg, B. & Uvnäs, B., 1960, Acta physiol. scand. 48, 133.

Johansen, T. & Chakravarty, N., 1972, Naunyn-Schmiede-berg's Arch. Pharmacol. 275, 457.

Johansen, T. & Chakravarty, N., 1975, Naunyn-Schmiede-berg's Arch. Pharmacol. 288, 243.

Kaliner, M. & Austen, K.F., 1973, J. Exp. Med. 138, 1077.

Kaliner, M. & Austen, K.F., 1974, J. Immunol. 112, 664.

Kanno, T., Cochrane, D.E. & Douglas, W.W., 1973, Canad. J. Physiol. Pharmacol. 51, 1001.

Krüger, P.G. & Bloom, G.D., 1974, Int. Arch. Allergy 46, 740.

Krüger, P.G., Bloom, G.D. & Diamant, B., 1974, Int. Arch. Allergy 47, 1.

Matlib, A. & O'Brien, P., 1974, Biochem. Soc. Trans. 2, 997.

Lichtenstein, L.M., 1975, J. Immunol. 114, 1692.

Orange, R.P., Kaliner, M. & Austen, K.F., 1971, Biochemistry of the Acute Allergic Reactions, Second International Symposium, Eds. K.F. Austen & E.L. Becker, p. 189, Blackwell, Oxford.

Patkar, S.A. & Diamant, B., 1974, Agents & Actions 4, 200

Paton, W.D.M., 1956, Ciba Foundation Symposium on Histamine, p. 59, Churchill, London.

Peterson, C., 1974a, Acta pharmacol. toxicol. 34, 356.

Peterson, C., 1974b, Acta physiol. scand. Suppl. 413.

Peterson, C. & Diamant, B., 1972, Acta pharmacol. toxicol. 31, Suppl. 1, 80.

Peterson, C. & Diamant, B., 1974, Acta pharmacol. toxicol. 34, 337.

Rasmussen, H., 1970, Science 170, 404.

Röhlich, P., 1975, Exp. Cell Res. 93, 293.

Satir, B., 1974, J. Supramol. Structure 2, 529.

Uvnäs, B., 1971, Biochemistry of the Acute Allergic Reactions, Second International Symposium, Eds. K.F. Austen & E.L. Becker, p. 175, Blackwell, Oxford.

Yamasaki, H. & Endo, K., 1965, Jap. J. Pharmacol. 15, 48.

Yamasaki, H., Fujita, T., Ohara, Y. & Komoto, S., 1970, Arch. Histol. Jap. 31, 393.

DISCUSSION

GOMPERTS: Do you really believe that EDTA penetrates through the phospholipid bilayer of the cell membrane? I suspect that you will have to search for an alternative explanation of this particular phenomenon.

DIAMANT: In normal cells EDTA seems to penetrate the plasma membrane of rat mast cells very slowly.

Douglas and Ueda (1973) have shown that mast cells lost their responsiveness to 48/80 after prolonged (3 hr) exposure to EDTA (2 mM) in the absence of calcium. After washing the addition of calcium to such cells caused the secretory responsiveness to return, when the cells were challenged with 48/80. We have confirmed their results. I would appreciate if you could suggest an alternative explanation to this phenomenon.

The point I wanted to make concerning the ionophore is that the ionophore depletes the cell of membrane bound calcium. After that the cells do not respond when stimulated, unless beforehand the calcium in the membrane has been restored either from intracellular stores, which it has been assumed that dibutyrylic cyclic AMP facilitates, or from the outside of the cell, provided the incubation medium is fortified with calcium.

UVNÄS: Do you believe that your results with cAMP in 10^{-3}M concentration reflect a biological function of this substance?

DIAMANT: The future will show if the observed effects are a physiological function of cAMP.

It is becoming more and more acccepted that cAMP might act by modulating calcium concentrations in the cytosol and membranes and that calcium in fact should be considered as the second messenger in many secretory processes as already proposed by Rasmussen several years ago.

AUSTEN: It will be extremely useful to have data on the effects of raising endogenous cyclic AMP.

DIAMANT: I completely agree. Unfortunately we have not yet investigated the influence of "cAMP-active" drugs in our system, but it is on the program.

LICHTENSTEIN: I wanted to be sure your cAMP experiments were all with Ca^{2+} depleted cells (ionophore)and no extra cellular Ca^{2+}.

DIAMANT: Yes.

LICHTENSTEIN: If so, Gilliespie can confirm that, as we have shown cAMP to enhance histamine release under certain conditions. The Ca^{2+} extracellular was 0.1 mM and not the usual 0.6 mM.

DIAMANT: Your experience agrees in that respect very well with my results.

UVNÄS: Which is the mechanism of action of cAMP on the calcium passage through membranes?

DIAMANT: I would consider a similar mechanism as that working when calcium is taken up and bound to the sercoplasmic reticulum in muscle cells.

FREDHOLM (Stockholm): Do you think that butyrate formed from db cAMP as part of the activation sequence to db cAMP will have any influence on your results?

DIAMANT: cAMP has a similar effect although less prominent than its dibutyrylic form.

BECKER: Have you made any direct measurements of the content of the mast cell Ca^{2+}, especially after various ionophore treatment?

DIAMANT: No because we do not have methods available which are sensitive enough. The 45-calcium binding methods are open to criticism since they do not distinguish non-specifically bound calcium from specific and because it is not possible to separate uptake from exchange.

However, we are presently loading rat mast cells with 45-calcium before stimulation and thus hope to follow the efflux instead of uptake. By this we hope to get some information until we can measure the calcium changes with direct methods.

AUSTEN: Do you have any data on cyclic GMP?

DIAMANT: We have made one experiment only as yet and dib. cGMP gave similar effects as dib. cAMP. We are however continuing to look into the question of specificity for the nucleotides.

MOLECULAR EVENTS IN MEMBRANE FUSION OCCURRING DURING MAST CELL DEGRANULATION

Durward Lawson, Martin C. Raff* Bastien Gomperts**
Clare Fewtrell*** and Norton B. Gilula****

*Medical Research Council Neuroimmunology Project,
Department of Zoology, University College London,
***and the Pharmacology Dept. University College,
** The Department of Experimental Pathology,
University College Hospital, Medical School, London
WC1E 6JJ. and **** the Rockefeller University New York
NY 10021, U.S.A.

Mast cells provide an unusually attractive system for considering the molecular events involved in membrane fusion. When either antigen, (1) anti-immunoglobulin (Ig) antibody (2) or concanavalin A (con A) (3,11) bind to and cross link cytophilic IgE (9,11, 13) on the surface of sensitized mast cells in the presence of extracellular Ca^{2+}(7), they induce exocytotic histamine release (degranulation) within seconds (16). Degranulation involves the fusion of granule membranes with plasma membrane (and subsequently with other granules) followed by the opening of the granule contents to the extracellular space (3,12). Histamine contained in the granules is released by a process of cation exchange; histamine bound to granule matrix exchanges mainly with extra-cellular Na^{+} (16). Histamine release leads to easily recognisable ultra-structural changes in the granules, including loss of electron density and homogeneity, and an increase in size (3,4,12). Since the cells degranulate all over their surface there is always an extensive amount of membrane interaction and fusion taking place. They are, therefore, an excellent system in which to study the molecular events that occur during membrane fusion.

Histamine secretion is Ca^{2+} dependent (7). There is indirect evidence that, following the binding of a stimulating ligand, an influx of Ca^{2+} initiates exocytosis. Introducing Ca^{2+} into mast

279

cells by micro-injection (10), for example, or by using the divalent
cation carrier A23187 induces energy dependent degranulation
mimicking ligand induced secretion (8).

We have studied the behaviour of membrane lipids and proteins
during the degranulation process, using rat peritoneal mast cells
stimulated by A23187, Ferritin (FT) - coupled anti Ig, or ConA.
Our studies suggest that (i) fusion takes place between protein
depleted lipid bilayers and (ii) that these fused bilayers subsequently bleb from the cell surface and pinch off.   This process
exposes the granules to the extracellular space and allows the cell
to dispose of excess lipid while retaining membrane proteins.

There is always a risk in attempting to define the sequence of
events in a dynamic process by studying static pictures.   Therefore
the sequence we propose is necessarily tentative.

MEMBRANE FUSION, BLEBBING, AND THE EXPOSURE OF GRANULES TO THE EXTRACELLULAR SPACE

The earliest membrane changes that can be detected in a stimulated mast cell are a ruffling of the granule membrane and the development of a halo between it and the granule.   These are followed by
fusion of the granule and plasma membranes to form a pentilaminar
structure 125-135 Å in width(Fig 1). The dense central line is
formed by the merged cytoplasmic leaflets of the two membranes.
The fused areas of membrane then bulge outwards from the cell to
form a bleb.   While the majority of blebs are found over altered
granules(Fig. 2),some are seen over granules which show no apparent
morphological changes (Fig 3). This observation suggests that
blebbing may precede histamine release.   The blebs then pinch off
by a process that Farquhar and Palade refer to as 'fission', so that
plasma and granule membranes are now in continuity.   The granules
are now exposed to the extracellular space and histamine is released.
The granule matrix usually remains within the cell circumference but
may be discharged.

The blebs formed from these membrane interactions are of varying
sizes.   They are invariably multivesiculate, with an outer limiting
membrane formed by a continuation of the plasma membrane.   The
vesicles contained within this membrane appear to be derived from
granule membrane which has pinched off along its own length.
Following the fusion of plasma and granule membrane, granule
membranes fuse with each other as peripheral degranulation spreads
inwards.   Blebbing which follows granule membranes fusing with
each other leads to the formation of multilamellor myelin like
whorls (Fig 4)which are discharged from the cell and appear to be
phagocytosed by macrophages.

MEMBRANE PROTEIN DISPLACEMENT AND CONSERVATION

We have observed that mast cells stimulated to release histamine by FT-coupled ligands such as anti-rat Ig or conA show a consistant absence of binding of these ligands to areas where plasma and granule membranes have fused, or where granule membranes have fused with each other.   We have also found that, in regions where these membranes are in close apposition but still separated by a layer of cytoplasm, there is a reduction and sometimes an absence of ligand binding (Fig 5) This observation suggests that protein loss precedes fusion.   Furthermore, we have never detected any conA·FT or anti rat Ig-FT label on developing or fully mature blebs (Fig 6). We have excluded the possibility that the absence of ligand binding in these areas is secondary to ligand induced redistribution of IgE or conA receptors by two types of experiments: (a) FT-coupled monovalent Fab fragments of anti-rat Ig, which we have previously shown binds in a random manner to the surface of mast cells   (13), does not bind to blebs (Fig 7) and (b) cells released with A23187, fixed with glutaraldehyde and then labelled with conA-FT show   no label on blebs (Fig 8). The tendency for anti-Ig-FT and conA-FT to be clustered at the edges of fused membranes suggests that these proteins are displaced laterally during fusion and, as a result, are conserved during exocytosis.

In order to look at other membrane proteins, we have studied degranulating mast cells by freeze fracture electron microscopy. These studies show that plasma and granule membranes are devoid of intramembrane particles (IMPs) on both external (E) and protoplasmic (P) fracture faces in regions where these membranes are interacting and/or are fused (Fig. 9).   Thus, the plasma and granule membrane proteins which show up as particles in freeze-fracture electron microscopy, and which presumably represent a heterogenous group of transmembrane proteins, are also excluded during the fusion process.

CONCLUSIONS

The most striking finding of our studies is that large scale displacement of membrane proteins takes place during membrane fusion occuring in the course of mast cell degranulation.   We cannot be certain that all membrane proteins are excluded.   However, since we have shown that IgE, the heterogeneous population of glycoproteins to which conA binds, and IMPs on both P and E fracture faces are displaced, it seems likely that the majority of proteins are excluded.

Although it seems likely that an influx of Ca^{2+} normally initiates the exocytosis process, it is unclear how Ca^{2+} acts inside the cell to trigger membrane fusion.   Our studies give no indication as to the nature of the recognition system which must be involved to allow fusion between plasma and granule membranes, and the fusion of granule membranes with each other, but with no other membranes in the cell.   However, immediately prior to fusion, when membranes are in close apposition but still separated by an intervening layer of cytoplasm, there is a dramatic reduction, or absence, of both ConA and anti-Ig binding sites.   This suggests the possibility that protein displacement preceeds fusion and can provide the necessary signal for lipid - lipid fusion.   The mechanism(s) involved in such protein displacement is unknown.

Prior to our observations, blebs were generally dismissed as artifacts and were thought to play no central role in mast cell degranulation (12).   We have shown that regions of fused membranes bulge out and bleb from the cell membrane.   They then appear to pinch off by 'fission'.   This same process occuring between granule membranes leaves large, released granule-containing cavities within the cell.   Since blebbing may preceed histamine release, it seems possible that it is the mechanism whereby granule contents come into contact with the extracellular mileu.   Previously it was suggested that the fusion of plasma and granule membranes results in the formation of an ion transmitting diaphragm which allows histamine-Na^+ exchange to take place. (15)   Since one might expect ion conducting channels to be visualised as IMPs in freeze fracture preparations, it seems unlikely that ion exchange could occur through the particle free pentilaminar structures that result from membrane fusion in mast cells.

Blebbing also offers a route for the loss of excess lipid during degranulation; if lipids were not lost during this process the cell would greatly enlarge.   This, clearly, does not happen.   The large amount of lipid seen in the vesicles contained by a bleb comes presumably from several granule membranes which flow into continuity when plasma membranes fuse.   Excess lipid is also lost in the form of multilamellar membrane whorls which develop from the fusion of several granule membranes.   These are probably the intracellular equivalent of surface blebs.

The mechanism of bleb formation is unknown.   It may be that displacement of protein 'weakens' the areas of fused membranes which are then blown out by intra-granule pressure.   Alternatively, the blebs could grow by the accretion   of lipid in a manner similar to that described for certain solvent-free black lipid membranes which expand continuously at the expense of adjacent pools of bulk phase lipid (6).

Besides providing some insight into the process of mast cell degranulation these studies serve to point up the usefulness of mast cells as models for studying the molecular events in membrane fusion.

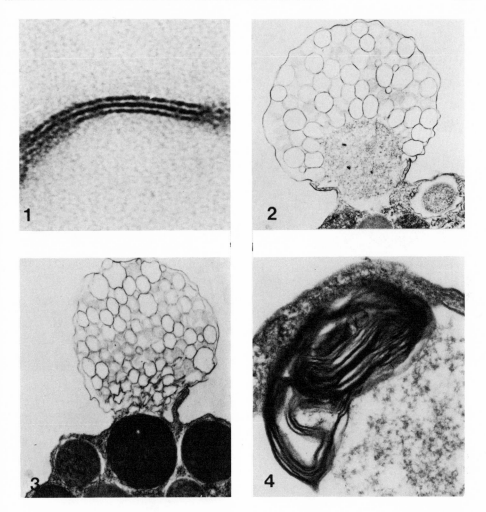

Fig. 1. High magnification view showing the fusion of plasma and
        granule membranes to form a structure 125 - 135 Å in width.
        The intermediate dense line represents the merged cyto-
        plasmic leaflets of the two membranes. x 423,000.

Fig. 2. Multivesiculated bleb overlying an apparently altered
        granule x 28,000.

Fig. 3. Multivesiculated bleb overlying an apparently unaltered
        granule. x 42,000.

Fig. 4. Multilamellar myelin whorl seen inside a cavity containing
        a released granule. x 50,000.

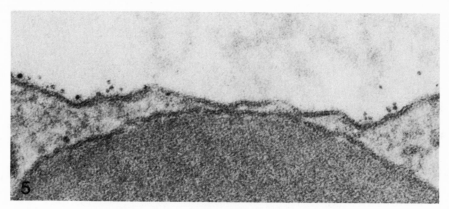

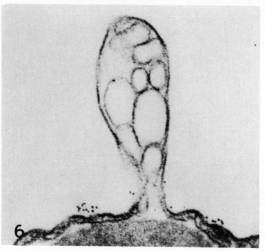

Fig. 5. Degranulating mast cell activated by ConA-FT for 30 min at
37°C showing two granule membranes coming into close
apposition but not yet fused.   The binding of ConA-FT
to the non cytoplasmic surface of the upper granule
membrane indicates that it is exposed to the extracellular
space.   Note the absence of ConA-FT molecules on the
membrane where it is close to the underlying granule
membrane even though cytoplasm still intervenes. x 189,000.

Fig. 6. Mast cell stimulated to degranulate by S anti-Rig-FT for
30 secs at 37°C.   Showing the absence of FT molecules on
an early bleb.

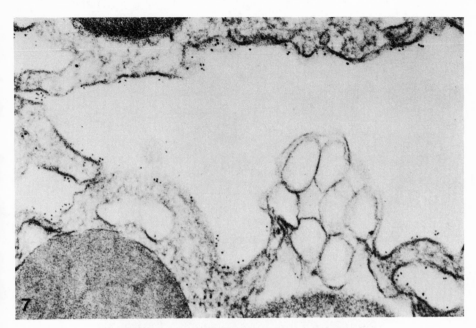

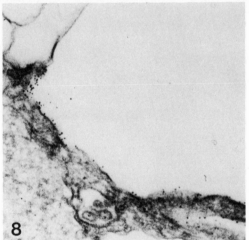

Fig. 7. Plasma membranes of two adjacent mast cells labelled with
monovalent Fab anti-Rig-FT for 30 min at 37°C.   Note the
absence of FAB anti-Rig-FT molecules on the bleb overlying
an altered granule. x 99,000.

Fig. 8. Degranulating mast cell triggeréd by A23187 for 5 min at 37°C
fixed with gluteraldehyde and then labelled with ConA-FT.
Note the absence of label on the bleb and the increased
density of label on the plasma membrane immediately adjacent
to the bleb. x 78,000.

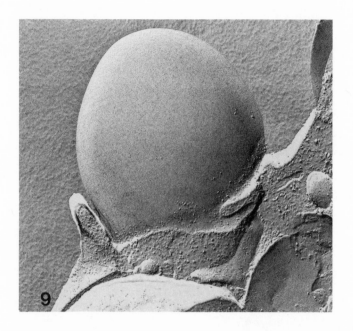

Fig. 9. During the final stages of the blebbing process the particles
are retained by the cell and the bleb is released with almost
entirely smooth fracture faces x 51,500.

REFERENCES

1. Austen, K.F., K.J. Bloch, A.R. Barker, and B.G. Arnason. 1965
    Immunological histamine release from rat mast cells in vitro:
    effect of age of cell donor. Proc. Soc. Exp. Biol. Med. 120:
    542-546.

2. Becker, E.L. and P.M. Henson. 1973. In vitro studies of immuno-
    logically induced secretion of mediators from cells and related
    phenomena. Adv. Immunol. 17: 93-145.

3. Bloom, G.D. and O. Haegermark. 1965. Studies on morphological
    changes and histamine release induced by compound 48/80 in rat
    peritoneal mast cells. Exptl. Cell Res. 40: 637-654.

4. Bloom, G.D. and N. Chakravarty. 1970. Time-course of anaphy-
    latic histamine release and morphological changes in rat
    peritoneal mast cells. Acta Physiol. Scand. 78: 410-419.

5. Farquhar, M.G. and G.E. Palade. 1963. Junctional complexes in
    various epithelia. J. Cell Biol. 17: 375-412.

6. Feltiplace, R., D.M. Andrews, and D.A. Haydon. 1971. The thick-
    ness, composition and structure of some lipid bilayers and
    natural membranes. J. Memb. Biol. 5: 277-296.

7. Foreman, J.C. and J.L. Mongar. 1972. The role of the alkaline
    earth ions in anaphylatic histamine release. J. Physiol. 244:
    753-769.

8. Foreman, J.C., J.L. Mongar, and B.D. Gomperts. 1973. Calcium
    ionophores and movement of calcium ions following physiological
    stimulus to a secretory process. Nature 245: 249-252.

9. Ishizaka, K. and T. Ishizaka. 1968. Immune mechanisms of
    reversed type reaginic hypersensitivity. J. Immunol. 103:
    588-595.

10. Kanno, T., D.E. Cochrane, and W.W. Douglas. 1973. Exocytosis
    (Secretory granule extrusion) induced by injection of calcium
    into mast cells. Can. J. Physiol. Pharmacol. 51: 1001-1004.

11. Keller, R. 1973. Concanavalin A, a model 'antigen' for the in
    vitro detection of cell-bound reaginic antibody in the rat.
    Clin. Exp. Immunol. 13: 139-147.

12. Lagunoff, D., 1973. Membrane fusion during mast cell secretion.
    J. Cell Biol. 57: 232-250.

13. Lawson, D., C. Fewtrell, B. Gomperts, and M.C. Raff. 1975. Anti-immunoglobulin-induced histamine secretion by rat peritoneal mast cells studied by immunoferritin electron microscopy. J. Exp. Med. 142: 391-402.

14. Perera, B.A.V. and J.L. Mongar. 1965. Effect of anoxia, glucose and thioglycollate on anaphylatic and compound 48/80-induced histamine release in isolated rat mast cells. Immunology 8: 519-525.

15. Uvnas, B. 1973. An attempt to explain nervous transmitter release as due to nerve impulse - induced cation exchange. Acta Physiol. Scand. 87: 168-175.

16. Uvnas, B. 1974. Histamine storage and release. Fed. Proc. 33: 2172-2176.

DISCUSSION

COCHRANE: Do you find bleb formation an invariable process in the release of each granule from the surface of a stimulated mast cell?

GOMPERTS: No, we can account for a few bleb from each cell. You may not even find a bleb on a particular thin section of a released cell.

COCHRANE: Exactly what do you mean by the "pinching-off" of the bleb? Could you define this in terms of layers of the bi-lamellar leaflets?

GOMPERTS: The term "pinching off" describes what we see in the electron microscope picture. Presumeably the release of the bleb occurs when its attachment to the cell becomes unstable, possibly due to excessive enlargement due to progressive accretion of lipid from interior granule membranes.

About the mechanism of annealing one cannot say much, except to add that lipid bilayer and membranes do reseal spontaneously when punched, say by a microelectrode. I should have thought that the mechanism of resealing the membrane round the cytosol after the bleb has been shed would be similar.

UVNÄS: Can you explain why you but no others have seen the bleb formation regularly? Any technical tricks?

GOMPERTS: No technical tricks I am sure. Straight forward glutaraldehyde fixation was used throughout our work.

We have attempted osmium fixation for thin section work without success, and we also tried freeze quenching for freeze fracture. Unfortunately you have to work in the absence of cryoprotectants as these release the mast cells, so we were unsuccesful with this approach too.

ANDERSON (Stockholm): As Börje Uvnäs already has said blebs similar to yours were already described in 1965 by Bloom and Haegermark. In our material we find them extremely seldom and I doubt that they have something to do with the histamine release process.

What proofs do you have that the vesicles inside the blebs come from the perigranular membranes?

As far as I see you have just showed apposition of membranes, not a fusion of membranes from a penta-laminar structure to a tri-laminar appearence and a further fusion. Have you any micrographs of such a fusion process?

GOMPERTS: I think the continuity between the plasma membrane and the external membrane of the blebs is clear for all to see. Obviously you can see no continuity of structure between the membranes constituting the internal vesicles and the granule membranes, but it is a fair inference that that is where they originally come from. Otherwise you most face up to the problem of their ultimate destination.

LICHTENSTEIN: What has the morphological pictures you have shown us told us about mechanism. The only new point is that ligand is not part of the bleb which is inconstantly related to degranulation.

GOMPERTS: I would have thought the points are fairly clear and very general.

Fusion occurs through protein depleted membranes.

Electrolyte for granule alteration and histamine release probably enters as the blebs are shed-certainly it seems improbable that the bilayers could admit of a flow of ions.

The mechanism allow the cell to divest itself of an excess of lipid bilayer accrueing to the membrane, which concerving membrane proteins.

BIBERFELD (Stockholm): We have seen under various conditions of fixation "multivesiculated blebs", regularly in mitogen stimulated lymphocytes (Biberfeld, Acta Path. Scand) similar to those, which you are implying as involved in the degranulation of mast cells. It is indeed tempting to speculate that this may reflect a "secretory" event in these metabolically very active lymphoblasts.

We have also observations on myeloma cells by immunoelectrone microscopy in line with your hypothesis of a displacement of membrane proteins and glycoproteins from the surface of the blebs. In contrast to other parts of the plasma membrane "secretory" blebs formed on the surface of human myeloma cells do not react with an anti-Hela cell serum nor with an antiserum to idiotypic myeloma protein antigens.

Can you from your ultrastructural observation exclude that most of the membrane proteins or glycoproteins are actually lost and not displaced from the surface of the blebs?

GOMPERTS: I don't think we can answer your question with absolute certitude. However, as I showed you both in the thin sections and the fracture studies we regularly see an enhanced density of receptor proteins and intercalated particles in the region where the plasma membrane joins the bleb. This probably arises from the lateral displacement of proteins from the fused membranes into this area.

ISHIZAKA, K.: I understand that a smooth area on the cell surface is accompanied by fusion of membranes. When histamine release is inhibited but antigen and antibody reaction occurs on the cell surface, can you then see the smooth area or not?

GOMPERTS: No. The displacement of receptors and of intercalated particles is quite distinct from the patching phenomenon. As I said, fusion with displacement of protein is a calcium

mediated event and you can see it perfectly well with Fab-
ferritin labels in cells triggered with A 23187. Furthermore,
ligand induced aggregation of surface receptors does not appear
to pertent the features of the fracture faces.

BECKER: I found quite interesting your freeze fracture
picture of the movement of intercalated particles away from
fusion zones and your equation of the particle with the various
transport mechanisms of the cell.

This is more than reminiscent of the findings of Berlin
in the neutrophil. He found that during the process of phagocytosis there was exclusion of various transport mechanisms
from the phagocytic vesicle and this exclusion could be prevented by colchicine treatment of the cell. This indicated to
Berlin a function for microtubulea in the exclusion. This
suggests that it might be worth while to look at the effect
of colchicine on the topology of the intercalated particles.

MAST CELL-DERIVED MEDIATORS: STRUCTURAL AND FUNCTIONAL DIVERSITY AND REGULATION OF EXPRESSION[1]

K. Frank Austen, Stephen I. Wasserman[2], and

Edward J. Goetzl[3]

Departments of Medicine, Harvard Medical School and the

Robert B. Brigham Hospital, Boston, Mass. 02120, U.S.A.

Since the mast cell is the only cell type possessing a specific recognition unit, IgE, for a foreign substance and located in the tissues in general rather than in a circulation, hematogenous or lymphatic, the physiologic role of this cell in host defense may be to recruit proteins and cells from the circulation in the absence of appreciable local tissue injury. After immunologic activation the mast cell elaborates mediators that alter the microenvironment so as to achieve the influx of plasma proteins, including immunoglobulins and complement components, and the ingress of phagocytic tissue and peripheral blood cells to the locus of the reaction. The initial or humoral phase of the mast cell response is mediated by substances such as histamine and slow reacting substance of anaphylaxis (SRS-A) and is terminated not only by local controls but also by the constituents of the cellular phase such as the eosinophil. Once the polymorphonuclear leukocytes, attracted by the eosinophil (ECF-A) and neutrophil (NCF-A) chemotactic factors of anaphylaxis have arrived at the reaction site, especially in the presence of complement and specific antibody, local host defense is markedly amplified (Fig. 1). Failure to limit the humoral phase of the mast cell response creates a pathopharmacologic state recognized clinically as urticaria, angioedema, exacerbations of rhinitis or asthma, or systemic anaphylaxis. Similarly, an inability to control the cellular phase permits progression to a local inflammatory state

---

[1] Supported by grants AI-07722 and AI-10356 from the National Institutes of Health.
[2] Postdoctoral Fellow of The Arthritis Foundation.
[3] Investigator, Howard Hughes Medical Institute.

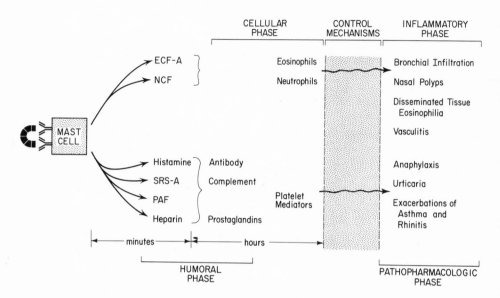

Fig. 1.   Schematic representation of mast cell-dependent humoral and cellular responses.

as observed in histologic studies of nasal polyps and bronchial tissues of atopic allergic persons. Since both IgE and certain IgG subgroups mediate antigen-dependent mast cell reactions, there is ample opportunity for mast cell responses to be directly and indirectly linked to the initiation of the other effector pathways of host resistance and tissue injury.

The formulation that the mast cell represents an antigen-specific sensor or barrier to host penetration is compatible with a location at cutaneous and mucosal surfaces and in connective tissues about venules. The presence of mast cells in the mucosa and lumen of bronchi of the rhesus monkey and the human (Patterson and Suszko, 1971; Orange, 1973), the antigen reactivity of comparable cells from the lumina of bronchi in dogs (Patterson et al, 1974),

and the intraepithelial location of IgE-bearing mast cells in human
tonsils, adenoids, and nasal polyps (Feltkamp-Vroon et al, 1974)
indicates the feasibility of initial mediator release without involvement of interstitial mast cells. Subsequent alterations in
mucosal permeability or entry of antigen into the circulation would
deliver the activating principles to deeper tissue or perivenular
sites. The presence of IgE on the mast cells in human skin and
respiratory tissues has been established by immunofluorescence with
specific anti-human IgE (Feltkamp-Vroon et al, 1974) and by the
generation and release of chemical mediators by anti-IgE from human
lung (Kay and Austen, 1971) and nasal polyp fragments (Kaliner et
al, 1973) and fractionated human lung cells (Paterson et al, 1976).

That the mast cells and its mediators are responsible for at
least a two-phased response is supported by the demonstration of an
early and late diminution in pulmonary function manifested minutes
and hours, respectively, after an aerosol challenge of a sensitive
subject with Aspergillus (Pepys et al, 1968), avian materials
(Hargreave et al, 1966), and grass pollen (Citron et al, 1958).
These same substances (McCarthy and Pepys, 1971; Hargreave and
Pepys, 1972; Taylor and Shivalkar, 1971), upon intracutaneous injection into sensitive persons, elicit an early wheal and flare
that subsides only to be followed in hours at that site by the development of an erythematous, pruritic, somewhat painful, poorly
demarcated swelling. Perhaps most pertinent to the basic mechanism
has been the elicitation of this biphasic reaction in normal subjects by crystalline Bacillus subtilis alpha amylase in the
Prausnitz-Küstner reaction and by the intracutaneous administration
of the $F(ab')_2$ fragment of sheep anti-human IgE (Dolovich et al,
1973). These latter studies establish that IgE-dependent mast cell
activation is sufficient to achieve a clinical local inflammatory
response characterized histologically by mast cell degranulation
and infiltration with eosinophils, neutrophils, and some monocytes
and lacking deposition of immunoglobulins and complement proteins
by immunofluorescent assessment.

STRUCTURAL AND FUNCTIONAL CHARACTERISTICS OF THE CHEMICAL MEDIATORS

The structural and functional properties, tissue and subcellular locations, and synthesis and degradation of the chemical mediators other than histamine are in differing stages of definition
(Table I). Histamine will not be considered in this section because the salient features are well recorded (Riley and West, 1953;
Schayer, 1959; Black et al, 1972). Consideration is also deferred
of secondary mediators such as 5-hydroxytryptamine derived from
platelets by the action of platelet activating factors and prostaglandins formed as perturbated membranes make available substrates
for biosynthesis. The preformed mediators by definition are extractable from tissues and cells before immunologic activation.

TABLE I. PRIMARY CHEMICAL MEDIATORS OF IMMEDIATE HYPERSENSITIVITY

Category	Mediator	Structural Characteristics	Assay(s)	Other Functions	Inactivation
I. PREFORMED	Histamine	β-imidazolyl-ethylamine MW = 111	Contraction of guinea pig ileum; Specific radio-labeling by histamine N-methyl-transferase	Increased vascular permeability; Elevation of cyclic AMP; Enhancement of eosinophil migration	Histaminase; Histamine methyl-transferase
	Eosinophil chemotactic factor of anaphylaxis (ECF-A)	Hydrophobic acidic tetrapeptides MW = 360–390	Chemotactic attraction of eosinophils	Eosinophil deactivation	Aminopeptidase; carboxy-peptidase A
	Neutrophil chemotactic factor (NCF)	Protein MW > 160,000	Chemotactic attraction of neutrophils	Neutrophil deactivation	--
	Heparin	Macromolecular acidic proteoglycan MW ≈ 1 million	Anti-thrombin activation or metachromasia	Anticoagulation	--
II. UNSTORED	Slow reacting substance of anaphylaxis (SRS-A)	Acidic hydrophilic sulfate ester MW ≈ 400	Contraction of antihistamine-treated guinea pig ileum	Contraction of human bronchiole; Increased vascular permeability	Arylsulfatase B
	Platelet activating factors (PAF)	Lipid-like MW 300–500	Release of ^{14}C-5HT from platelets	Aggregation	Phospholipase D (for rat PAF)

The unstored mediators are presumably present in a precursor form
and rendered active by an appropriate stimulus, generally but not
necessarily immunologic in nature. Further, a stimulus that is
subthreshold in releasing preformed mediators may nonetheless induce an appreciable intracellular accumulation of an unstored mediator (Lewis et al, 1974).

Eosinophil Chemotactic Factor of Anaphylaxis (ECF-A)

ECF-A was discovered by Kay, Stechschulte, and Austen (1971)
as a mediator derived by antigen challenge of guinea pig lung slices
prepared with IgG1 and human lung slices sensitized with IgE (Kay
and Austen, 1971). ECF-A was subsequently determined to be present
totally preformed in rat mast cells in association with the granules
(Wasserman et al, 1974a), human leukemic basophils (Lewis et al,
1975), and mast cell-rich tissues such as nasal polyps (Kaliner
et al, 1973) and human lung (Wasserman et al, 1974a). ECF-A obtained by IgE-dependent reactions in human lung slices (Kay and
Austen, 1971) and in purified rat peritoneal mast cells (Wasserman
et al, 1974a) exhibited a molecular weight of approximately 300 to
1000 by gel filtration, and eosinophilotactic material in this size
range was thus extracted from human lung for structural characterization.

Approximately 100 g of human lung fragments derived from surgical specimens were sonicated in butanol:glacial acetic acid
(10:1 v/v) or Tyrode's buffer - 0.1 M Tris HCl, pH 8.6 at 4°C. The
extracts were cleared by centrifugation, lyophilized, resuspended
in 0.1 M acetic acid and applied to a 2 L column of Sephadex G-25
(Pharmacia Fine Chemicals, Inc., Piscataway, N.J.), equilibrated and
eluted in 0.1 M acetic acid. Descending filtration was carried out
with a capillary pump producing flow rates of 3-4% bed volume per
hr at 4°C, and 20 ml fractions were collected. Samples of 0.25 ml
each were assessed for chemotactic activities in a modified Boyden
chamber (Boyden, 1962; Goetzl and Austen, 1972) with two cell suspensions, containing 86% unpurified eosinophils or 92% purified
neutrophils (Böyum, 1968), respectively. The extracts obtained revealed considerable heterogeneity on gel filtration (Fig. 2) and
were quite comparable with the two solvent systems. The net chemotactic response of neutrophils relative to eosinophils was 2.6 in
fraction 36 of the eosinophilotactic peak of greatest apparent size,
0.9 in fraction 60 from the intermediate peak, and 0.3 in fractions
74 and 88, respectively, from the low molecular weight region. The
bimodal nature of the low molecular weight peak was attributed to
the influence of histamine on the bioassay.

Fractions 74 through 88 were pooled, lyophilized, redissolved
in 0.1 M pyridine, and applied to a 32 ml Dowex AG-1 (Bio-Rad Laboratories, Richmond, Calif.) column equilibrated in 0.1 M pyridine.

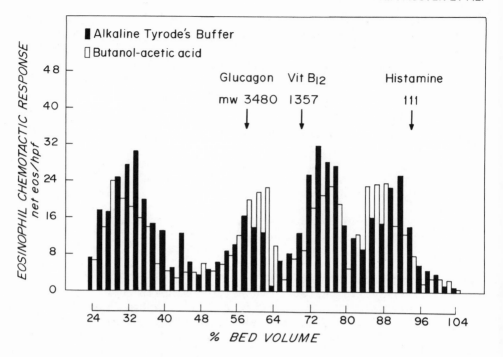

Fig. 2. Sephadex G-25 gel filtration of human lung extract in Tyrode's-0.1 M Tris HCl, pH 8.6 (closed bars) and in butanol-glacial
acetic acid (open bars). Spontaneous migration of eosinophils was
6/hpf and of neutrophils 11/hpf.

For a comparison eosinophilotactic activity released from passively
sensitized human lung fragments upon challenge with antigen E
(Orange et al, 1971) was filtered on Sephadex G-25 and the same low
molecular weight fractions were processed and applied to Dowex AG-1.
The Dowex ion exchange chromatography employed 0.5 L 0.1 M pyridine
and 0.5 L 0.3 M formic acid in a linear gradient of -0.3 pH units
per 4 bed volumes in the pH range from 5 to 2, followed by application of 0.1 M HCl. Fractions of 10 ml each were lyophilized three
times from distilled water and redissolved in 2 ml distilled water;
and 0.2 ml portions were assayed with unpurified eosinophils of 90%
purity. Both extracted and immunologically released ECF-A eluted in

a broad peak at pH 3.1 to 2.1 with no further activity being recognized in the HCl eluate (Fig. 3).

   Subdivision of the eluate from Dowex AG-1 into two regions of equal activity, pH 3.0 - 2.6 and pH 2.6 - 2.2, followed by Sephadex G-10 filtration of each and descending paper chromatography resolved two distinct peptides of low yield but sufficient purity for compositional definition by the method of Spackman et al (1958) as tetrapeptides (Goetzl and Austen, 1975). The amino acid sequence of the purified tetrapeptides was determined by dansylation (Gray, 1967) of the NH$_2$-terminal residue. Subsequent residues were revealed by Edman degradation followed by two-dimensional chromatography of the dansyl-amino acids (Woods and Wang, 1967; Hartley, 1970). The carboxy terminus was established by hydrazinolysis (Fraenkel-Conrat and

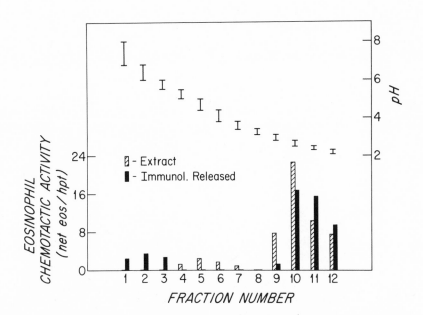

Fig. 3. Dowex AG-1 ion exchange chromatography of fractions obtained at 74-88% bed volume of Sephadex G-25 gel filtration of human lung extract in Tyrode's-0.1 M Tris HCl, pH 8.6 (closed bars) and a diffusate after antigen challenge of passively sensitized human lung fragments (open bars).

Tsung, 1967) or carboxypeptidase A digestion and amino acid analysis, and by selective tritiation, hydrolysis, and chromatographic
identification of the labeled amino acid (Matsuo et al, 1966). The
two tetrapeptides, differing in their N-terminus and being of sequence Val-Gly-Ser-Glu and Ala-Gly-Ser-Glu were then synthesized by
Goetzl and Austen (1975) with solid phase techniques (Stewart and
Young, 1969; Gutte and Merrifield, 1971) and were shown to exhibit
a specificity and potency comparable to natural purified ECF-A.

In order to compare native ECF-A and the synthetic tetrapeptide
further, the eosinophilotactic activity obtained at 74-88% bed volume by Sephadex G-25 gel filtration of a butanol-acetic acid lung
extract was cochromatographed with ^{14}C valyl-tetrapeptide on a 1.5
x 80 cm Sephadex G-10 column equilibrated and run in 0.1 N NH_4OH.
Fraction volumes were 1.4 ml and 0.075 ml portions were assessed for
eosinophilotactic activity with a cell suspension containing 76%
eosinophils. The ^{14}C valyl-tetrapeptide was recovered with native
ECF-A at 36-42% bed volume, clearly separated from the eosinophilotactic activity in the histamine region (Fig. 4).

The synthetic pathway for formation of ECF-A has not been examined, nor has its relationship to the intermediate-sized eosinophilotactic activity been determined. The elaboration of eosinophilotactic peptides of a comparable nature to ECF-A by undifferen-
tiated bronchogenic carcinomas in situ and in tissue culture
(Wasserman et al, 1974b; Goetzl et al, 1976), introduces the possibility that such mediators reside in precursor form in diverse
cells. The inactivation of ECF-A by aminopeptidase M or carboxypeptidase A (Goetzl and Austen, 1975) indicates feasible pathways
for biodegradation, but this point has not yet been examined in
complex systems.

The synthetic tetrapeptides were maximally eosinophilotactic at
concentrations of 10^{-7} to 10^{-6} M or 0.1 to 1.0 nM per chemotactic
chamber (Goetzl and Austen, 1975). Preincubation of eosinophils
with native ECF-A (Wasserman et al, 1975b) or synthetic tetrapeptides at concentrations as low as 10^{-11} to 10^{-10} M prevented their
subsequent directed migration to a chemotactic stimulus, a process
termed deactivation (Ward and Becker, 1968). Deactivation may represent a mechanism by which specifically attracted eosinophils are
held at a site for the purpose of exerting their regulatory functions. The intraperitoneal administration of 0.1 to 1.0 nM synthetic tetrapeptide per guinea pig elicited a preferential influx of
eosinophils followed by neutrophils (Wasserman et al, 1976a), compatible with the in vitro studies showing a preference of the tetrapeptides for eosinophils but a capacity to attract neutrophils as
well (Kay and Austen, 1971; Goetzl and Austen, 1975). No other
functions have been recognized for ECF-A at present. Concentrations
of tetrapeptides as high as 10^{-3} M did not contract the guinea pig
ileum or trachea, the estrous rat uterus, or the gerbil colon and

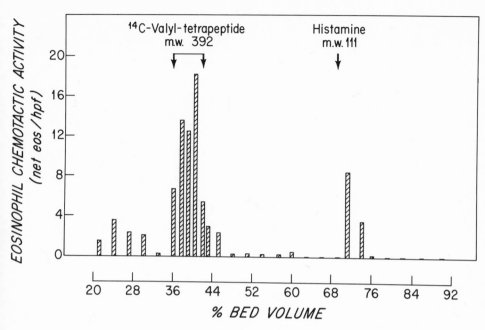

Fig. 4.   Sephadex G-10 gel filtration of fractions obtained at
74-88% bed volume of Sephadex G-25 gel filtration of human lung
extract in butanol-glacial acetic acid (-) and of synthetic
[14]C-valyl-tetrapeptide.   Spontaenous migration was 6 eosinophils/
hpf.

did not alter cutaneous vascular permeability in the guinea pig or
rat.   The intravenous administration of up to 2 nM of synthetic
tetrapeptide to the unanesthetized guinea pig did not alter pulse
rate, blood pressure, or pulmonary mechanics (Wasserman et al,
1976a).

Neutrophil Chemotactic Factor(s) of Anaphylaxis (NCF-A)

NCF-A(s) was initially recognized in an extract of human leukemic basophils as a factor distinct from ECF-A by virtue of its

filtration in the exclusion volume of Sephadex G-25 and its preferential chemotactic activity for neutrophils relative to eosinophils
(Lewis et al, 1975). Extracts of lung, guinea pig and human, and of
purified rat peritoneal mast cells had been known to contain an eosinophilotactic activity with such a filtration characteristic
(Wasserman et al, 1974a), and this fact is again illustrated in
Figure 2 along with the documentation of neutrophil preference.
Purified rat peritoneal mast cells incubated with rabbit antiserum
to rat light chains released not only histamine and ECF-A, but also
a neutrophil chemotactic principle(s) with high molecular weight.
A high molecular weight factor with neutrophil chemotactic activity
has also been released along with histamine and ECF-A into the venous effluent by cold challenge of an upper extremity of patients
with cold urticaria (Wasserman et al, 1976b). The existence in
mast cells of factors that are chemotactic for neutrophils is central to the capacity of the mast cell to mediate host defense or
adverse inflammation.

Heparin

    Sulfated acidic glycosaminoglycans, largely heparin, are re-
sponsible for the metachromasia of mast cell granules (Bloom and
Ringertz, 1961; Lloyd et al, 1967a, b), and heparin has been released from purified rat mast cells by treatment with 48/80 (Fillion
et al, 1970). ^{35}S-labeled, purified rat mast cells challenged with
either calcium ionophore A-23187 or rabbit antiserum to rat light
chains release macromolecular heparin along with the other chemical
mediators. The released and residual heparin, extracted with 0.05 N
NaOH and 1 N NaCl (Fillion et al, 1970), chromatographed together
on Dowex 1 with elution in 3 M NaCl; and both filtered in the exclusion volume of Sepharose-6B (Yurt et al, 1976) as assessed by
specific radioactivity and such additional parameters as uptake of
azure A and augmentation of anti-thrombin activity (Jaques et al,
1949; Odegard et al, 1975). Commercial heparin has the capacity to
augment markedly the inhibitory action of antithrombin on thrombin
(Rosenberg and Damus, 1973), plasma thromboplastin antecedent
(Damus et al, 1973), factor X_a (Yin et al, 1971), and plasmin
(Highsmith and Rosenberg, 1974) and of the inhibitor of the first
component of complement on the activated first component (Rent and
Fiedel, 1975); but comparable studies with macromolecular heparin
are not yet available.

Slow Reacting Substance of Anaphylaxis (SRS-A)

    In contrast to the preformed mediators, SRS-A appears in tis-
sues (Brocklehurst, 1960; Orange, 1974) and cells (Lewis et al,
1974) only after immunologic activation and immediately before its
extracellular release. The mast cell has been presumed to be the

cell source of immunologic generation because the release of SRS-A
follows IgG1-dependent reactions in guinea pig lung slices (Baker
et al, 1964) and IgE-dependent reactions in human lung (Orange
et al, 1971) and nasal polyp (Kaliner et al, 1973) fragments and in
peripheral leukocyte (Grant and Lichtenstein, 1974) and human lung
cell (Lewis et al, 1974; Paterson et al, 1976) suspensions. In
human lung, SRS-A generation continues at a time when the tissue or
cellular content has plateaued and the release of preformed mediators is complete (Lewis et al, 1974), suggesting formation by secondary cell types or by the interaction of antigen with IgE at
sites not linked to the release of preformed mediators. That more
than one cell type and class of immunoglobulin can participate in
SRS-A generation has been documented by the release of SRS-A into
the peritoneal cavity of the rat after either IgE-mast cell (Orange
et al, 1970) or IgGa-neutrophil-complement (Morse et al, 1968)
dependent mechanisms.

The pharmacologic actions of SRS-A, including the contraction
of only certain isolated smooth muscles (Brocklehurst, 1962), impairment of pulmonary mechanics of the intact anesthetized
(Strandberg and Hedqvist, 1975) and unanesthetized (Drazen and
Austen, 1974, 1975) guinea pig, and alterations in cutaneous vascular permeability in the guinea pig (Orange et al, 1969), have been
explored with partially purified preparations. These studies are
subject to reinterpretation once structurally defined material becomes available, but the available data do indicate that the contractile activity characteristic of SRS-A on the guinea pig ileum
occurs at concentrations equal to or less than those required for
a histamine effect.

Both released and extracted cellular SRS-A resist inactivation
at 37°C in 0.2 N NaOH, adhere to Amberlite XAD-2 in water and elute
in 80% ethanol, appear in the ethanol:ammonia:water (6:3:1 v/v)
wash from silicic acid, filter in 80% ethanol with a molecular
weight of 400 to 700 in Sephadex LH-20 (Orange et al, 1973), and
are inactivated by limpet arylsulfatases (Orange et al, 1974).
These characteristics tend to exclude SRS-A from belonging to currently defined mediator classes, and the presence of sulfur in
spark source mass spectrometric analyses of highly purified preparations of rat SRS-A (Orange et al, 1974) suggests a unique structure.

The finding that SRS-A of rat and human origin was inactivated
by limpet arylsulfatase has important implications for the structure of this mediator. Arylsulfatases (EC 3.1.6.1) have been
grouped into type I, which exhibit a preference for substrates
such as p-acetylphenyl sulfate and p-nitrophenyl sulfate and are
inhibited by cyanide but not by phosphate or sulfate ions, and type
II, for which p-nitrocatechol sulfate is the preferred substrate in
a reaction suppressed by sulfate and phosphate but not by cyanide

ions (Roy, 1957). Alternatively, the arylsulfatases were recognized to be soluble (types A and B) or insoluble (type C) in
acetone extracts of tissues and have been further characterized by
physicochemical and functional properties (Dodgson and Spencer,
1957). Type C is microsomal in location and exhibits the substrate
preferences and inhibition characteristics of type I (Dodgson et al,
1955; Dodgson and Spencer, 1957). Arylsulfatases of types A and B
are lysosomal (Dodgson et al, 1955), exhibit a substrate specificity
comparable to type II and are separable by differential electrophoretic mobility on paper (Dodgson et al, 1956) or polyacrylamide
gels (Shapna and Nadler, 1975; Wasserman and Austen, 1976) and by
ion exchange chromatography (Roy, 1971; Harinath and Robins, 1975;
Bleszynski and Roy, 1973; Stevens et al, 1975; Shapna and Nadler,
1975; Wasserman et al, 1975; Wasserman and Austen, 1976). Arylsulfatase A type enzymes from diverse sources have isoelectric points
of 3.6 to 4.0 (Allen and Roy, 1968; Neuwelt et al, 1971; Shapna and
Nadler, 1975), molecular weights in excess of 100,000 (Nichol and
Roy, 1965; Harinath and Robins, 1971; Breslow and Sloan, 1972;
Stevens et al, 1975; Wasserman and Austen, 1976), an ability to
hydrolyze cerebroside sulfate (Mehl and Jatzhewitz, 1968; Jefry and
Roy, 1973), and are inhibited by phosphate and competitively by
sulfate ions (Roy, 1971). Arylsulfatase B type enzymes have isoelectric points in the 8.3 to 8.6 range (Allen and Roy, 1968;
Bleszynski et al, 1969), molecular weights ranging from 25,000 to
66,000 (Allen and Roy, 1968; Harinath and Robins, 1971; Bleszynski
and Roy, 1973; Shapna and Nadler, 1975; Wasserman et al, 1975a;
Wasserman and Austen, 1976), and are inhibited not only by phosphate
and non-competitively by sulfate ions (Roy, 1970, 1971) but also by
chloride ions in the presence of pyrophosphate (Baum et al, 1959).

        In order to confirm the observations with limpet arylsulfatase
(Orange et al, 1974), arylsulfatase B was separated from A in extracts of human lung by anion exchange chromatography and further
purification by gel filtration and cation exchange chromatography
(Wasserman and Austen, 1976); arylsulfatase B, which is the only
arylsulfatase in extracts of human eosinophils, was isolated by
comparable procedures (Wasserman et al, 1975a). Lung and eosinophil
arylsulfatases were subjected to acid disc gel electrophoresis in
6% polyacrylamide gels with a Canalco apparatus (Rockville, Md.).
The entire gel was then incubated in 4.0 ml 0.01 M p-nitrocatechol
sulfate in 0.5 M pH 5.7 sodium acetate buffer for 15 minutes at
37°C; 2.0 ml 1 N NaOH were added and the incubation was continued
for 5 minutes more. A red-orange band (Payne et al, 1974) developed two-thirds of the distance into the gels for both lung and
eosinophil arylsulfatase B, while the band appeared at the loading
point of the gel for arylsulfatase A (Fig. 5). Arylsulfatase B
from both human sources had an apparent molecular weight of 60,000,
a pH optimum for p-nitrocatechol sulfate of 5.5 to 6.0, and a
susceptibility to inhibition by phosphate and sulfate ions and
especially chloride ion in the presence of pyrophosphate. Both

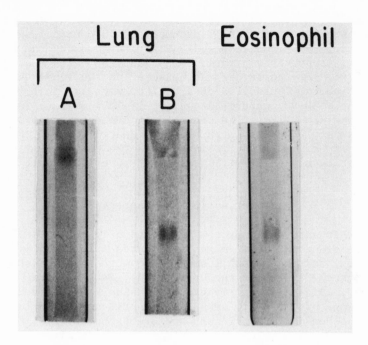

Fig. 5. Acid disc gel electrophoresis of partially purified aryl-sulfatase A and B from human lung tissue and B from human eosino-phils, and development of gel by substrate cleavage and colorimetric detection of the product, p-nitro catechol.

human lung and eosinophil arylsulfatase B inactivated SRS-A of human and rat origin in a linear time-dependent reaction whose rate was determined by the enzyme to substrate ratio. Furthermore, cleavage of p-nitrocatechol sulfate by lung or eosinophil arylsulfatase B was competitively inhibited by SRS-A (Wasserman et al, 1975a; Wasserman and Austen, 1976), consistent with the view that the capacity to inactivate SRS-A represents the intrinsic arylsulfatase activity of the enzymes.

Biodegradation of SRS-A is rapidly accomplished by intact human eosinophils (Wasserman et al, 1975c) but not by comparable concentrations of human neutrophils or mononuclear cells that lack

arylsulfatase activities. Arylsulfatase has been demonstrated in
the lamellar bodies of type II pneumocytes in rabbit lung
(DiAugustine, 1974) and is broadly distributed among the cell types
obtained by isopycnic separation of human lung cells (Paterson
et al, 1976). Arylsulfatase was measured on two separate occasions
in the peripheral leukocytes of a patient with basophil leukemia,
manifested by 80-90% mature basophils, 10-15% immature forms and
0-5% mononuclear cells. Its presence at concentrations of 1.1 and
0.67 units per 10^7 cells at pH 5.7 as compared to 0.52 and 0.28
units per 10^7 cells at pH 5.0 introduces the possibility that some
biodegradation may occur within an SRS-A generating cell type.

                        Platelet Activating Factor(s)

     Platelet activating factor (PAF) was originally recognized as
being released from rabbit mixed leukocytes interacted with specific antigen, and the basophil sensitized with IgE was established
as its source (Siraganian and Osler, 1971; Benveniste et al, 1972;
Benveniste, 1974). PAF activities have also been derived by antigen challenge of passively sensitized rabbit and human lung
(Kravis and Henson, 1975; Bogart and Stechschulte, 1974); IgE-
mediated reversed immunologic reactions of human mixed leukocytes
(Benveniste, 1974) and rabbit and human lung tissue (Kravis and
Henson, 1975; Bogart and Stechschulte, 1974); antigen challenge of
the rat peritoneal cavity passively prepared with hyperimmune rat
antisera predominantly containing IgGa antibody (Kater et al, 1976);
addition of the calcium ionophore A23187 to human leukemic basophils (Lewis et al, 1975); and prolonged incubation of rabbit or
human mixed peripheral leukocytes in alkaline buffer (Benveniste,
1974). Since PAF activity was not recognized in human leukemic
basophils before their stimulation with the calcium ionophore
(Lewis et al, 1975), and its content increased during the incubation of mixed rabbit or human leukocytes in alkaline buffer
(Benveniste, 1974), PAF is apparently not a preformed mediator and
resembles SRS-A in this respect.

     PAF obtained from rabbit or human mixed leukocytes exhibited
cationic characteristics on ion-exchange chromatography, filtered
on Sephadex LH-20 with an apparent molecular weight of 1100 and
chromatographed on silica gel thin layer plates in a region staining with phospholipid-specific indicators (Benveniste, 1974;
Benveniste et al, 1975). Rat PAF activity, purified by a procedure
utilized for SRS-A (Orange et al, 1973), appeared in the ethanol
eluate from Amberlite XAD-2 and in the ethanol:ammonia:water eluate
from silicic acid along with the SRS-A (Kater et al, 1976). This
partially purified rat PAF filtered on Sephadex LH-20 with an
apparent molecular weight of 300-500 and was substantially inactivated by phospholipase D from cabbage or eosinophil sources but
not by proteolytic enzymes, arylsulfatase B, or phospholipases A

or B (Kater et al, 1976). PAF activity is assayed by its capacity
to release ^{14}C-serotonin or other amines from platelets (Benveniste
et al, 1972). Other activities attributed to PAF include the induction of platelet rosettes around rabbit basophils (Benveniste
et al, 1972), and aggregation of platelets in vitro in the presence
of fibrinogen (Benveniste et al, 1975).

NATURAL REGULATION OF MEDIATOR EXPRESSION

The composite events that follow antigen bridging of mast cell
membrane IgE antibody include the biochemical concomitants of membrane perturbation, designated activation, the generation of unstored mediators, and the secretion of newly formed and preformed
mediators of diverse structure and function. An early antigen-
induced event in lung fragments, possibly the activating step,
appears to be the extracellular calcium ion-dependent activation
of a serine esterase (Kaliner and Austen, 1973). The IgE-dependent
generation of unstored mediators in human lung fragments, such as
SRS-A, involves steps distinct from the secretory event, as indicated by the ability of colchicine to suppress mediator release
without decreasing tissue accumulation of SRS-A (Orange, 1974); the
capacity of diisopropyl fluorophosphate (Kaliner and Austen, 1973)
or cytochalasin A or B (Orange, 1974) pretreatment to suppress
SRS-A generation and release without impairment or even augmentation of histamine release; and the potentiality of a cholinergic
agonist to reverse the inhibitory effect of a beta adrenergic
agonist on histamine but not SRS-A release (Kaliner and Austen,
1974a). The opposing actions of beta adrenergic and muscarinic
cholinergic stimuli or of dibutyryl cyclic AMP and 8-bromo cyclic
GMP, respectively, in suppressing and augmenting the IgE-dependent
intracellular accumulation of SRS-A (Lewis et al, 1974), as well
as the release of histamine and SRS-A (Kaliner et al, 1972) from
lung slices, indicates modulation by the levels of cyclic nucleotides at two sites. Studies with purified rat mast cells have
directly demonstrated that elevations in cyclic AMP, achieved
synergistically with PGE_2 and aminophylline, synergistically inhibit histamine release (Kaliner and Austen, 1974b).

The endogenous regulation of mast cell-dependent phenomena occurs at at least four levels, including: intensity of the mast cell
activating event; the action of primary and secondary mediators
upon the concentration of cyclic nucleotides; the receptor binding
and responsiveness of target cells to released mediators; and the
rate at which released mediators undergo biodegradation (Fig. 6).
At the first level, limited IgE-dependent activation of human lung
mast cells can initiate intracellular accumulation of SRS-A without release of either SRS-A or histamine (Lewis et al, 1974). At
the second level, histamine acting via an H_2 receptor to activate
adenylate cyclase can suppress mediator release, as appreciated in

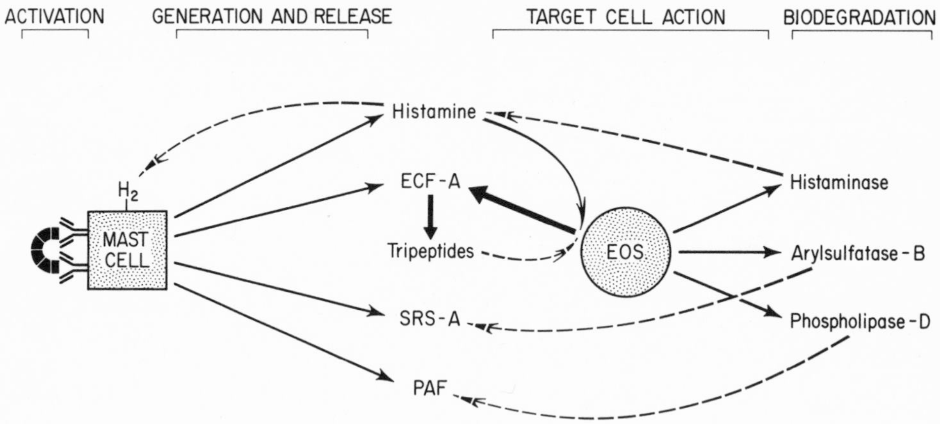

ACTIVATION   GENERATION AND RELEASE   TARGET CELL ACTION   BIODEGRADATION

Fig. 6.   Schematic representation of four levels of natural
regulation of mediator expression.

peripheral blood leukocytes enriched for basophils (Lichtenstein
and Gillespie, 1975); or prostaglandins formed as secondary mediators can decrease or augment histamine release as noted in human
lung fragments with PGE_2 and $PGF_{2\alpha}$ (Tauber et al, 1973).   At the
third level, NH_2-terminal tripeptides of ECF-A block the chemotactic responsiveness of eosinophils by reversible competition for
the target cell binding site, while COOH-terminal tripeptides inhibit irreversibly by deactivating the eosinophils (Goetzl et al,
1976); such tripeptides could be derived from the eosinophilotactic
tetrapeptides (ECF-A) by respective cleavage with carboxypeptidase A and aminopeptidase M (Goetzl and Austen, 1975).   Histamine
in non-chemotactic doses (Clark et al, 1975) facilitates the response of eosinophils to the eosinophilotactic tetrapeptides
(Goetzl and Austen, this volume).   At the fourth level, eosinophils

concentrated by directed migration and deactivation would inactivate released primary mediators such as SRS-A (Wasserman et al,
1975a, c), histamine (Zeiger et al, 1976), and PAF (Kater et al,
1976) because of their content of arylsulfatase B, histaminase,
and phospholipase D, respectively. Eosinophils may also directly
suppress mediator release, as observed with leukocyte suspensions
containing basophils, possibly by elaboration of prostaglandins
(Hubscher, 1975). Biodegradation is not dependent wholly on in-
filtrating cells in that in human lung arylsulfatase B inactivates
SRS-A in a reaction quite comparable to that achieved with the
eosinophil-derived enzyme (Wasserman and Austen, 1976).

SUMMARY

The IgE-dependent activation of mast cells leads to the generation of unstored mediators such as slow reacting substance of
anaphylaxis (SRS-A) and platelet activating factor(s) (PAF), and
their release along with preformed mediators, histamine, macromolecular heparin, eosinophil chemotactic factor of anaphylaxis
(ECF-A), and neutrophil chemotactic factor(s) of anaphylaxis
(NCF-A). Endogenous regulation of mast cell-dependent phenomena
occurs at at least four levels: the intensity and, possibly, the
nature of the activating stimulus; the modulation of mediator generation and release by cellular levels of the cyclic nucleotidases;
the capacity of target cells to bind and respond to primary mediators; and the rate at which mediators undergo biodegradation.
Two areas of recent progress in defining the structural characteristics of mediators that facilitate the appreciation of their
regulation are: the delineation of ECF-A as an acidic tetrapeptide
with two distinct N-terminals (Val/Ala-Gly-Ser-Glu); and the demonstration that SRS-A is inactivated by arylsulfatase B purified from
human lung or eosinophils and by intact resting eosinophils.
Since the mast cell represents an antigen-specific sensor at cutaneous and mucosal surfaces and in connective tissue about venules, it seems likely that the initial or humoral phase of its
response achieves an influx of plasma proteins, such as immunoglobulins and complement components, while the subsequent cellular
phase augments local host defense through the ingress of neutrophils and eosinophils and terminates the humoral phase (eosinophils).

REFERENCES

Allen, E., and Roy, A.B. 1968. The sulfatase of ox liver. XI.
    The isoelectric focusing of a purified preparation of sul-
    fatase B. Biochim. Biophys. Acta 168:243.

Baker, A.R., Bloch, K.J., and Austen, K.F. 1964. In vitro passive sensitization of chopped guinea pig lung by guinea pig 7S antibodies. J. Immunol. 93:525.

Baum, H., Dodgson, K.S., and Spencer, B. 1959. The assay of arylsulfatase A and B in human urine. Clin. Chim. Acta 4:453.

Benveniste, J. 1974. Platelet-activating factor, a new mediator of anaphylaxis and immune complex deposition from rabbit and human basophils. Nature 249:581.

Benveniste, J., Henson, P.M., and Cochrane, C.G. 1972. Leuko-cyte-dependent histamine release from rabbit platelets. The role of IgE, basophils, and a platelet-activating factor. J. Exp. Med. 136:1356.

Benveniste, J., Kamoun, P., and Polonsky, J. 1975. Aggregation of human platelets by purified platelet activating factor from human and rabbit basophils. Fed. Proc. 34:985 (abstract).

Bleszynski, W., Leznicki, A., and Lewosz, J. 1969. Kinetic properties of three soluble arylsulfatases from ox brain, homogeneous in polyacrylamide gel electrophoresis. Enzymologica 37:314.

Bleszynski, W.S., and Roy, A.B. 1973. Some properties of sulfatase B of ox brain. Biochim. Biophys. Acta 317:164.

Black, J.W., Duncan, W.A.M., Durant, C.J., Cannellin, C.R., and Parson, E.M. 1972. Definition and antagonism of histamine H_2-receptors. Nature 236:385.

Bloom, G., and Ringertz, N.R. 1961. Acid polysaccharides of peritoneal mast cells of the rat and mouse. Arkiv för Kemi 16:51.

Bogart, D.B., and Stechschulte, D.J. 1974. Release of platelet activating factor from human lung. Clin. Res. 22:652 (abstract).

Boyden, S. 1962. The chemotactic effect of mixtures of antibody and antigen on polymorphonuclear leukocytes. J. Exp. Med. 115:453.

Böyum, A. 1968. Isolation of leucocytes from human blood, further observations. Scand. J. Clin. Lab. Invest. 21: (Suppl. 97):31.

Breslow, J.C., and Sloan, H.F.   1972.   Purification of arylsul-
    fatase A from human urine.   Biochem. Biophys. Res. Commun.
    46:919.

Brocklehurst, W.E.   1960.   The release of histamine and forma-
    tion of a slow-reacting substance (SRS-A) during anaphylac-
    tic shock.   J. Physiol. 151:416.

Brocklehurst, W.E.   1962.   Slow reacting substance and related
    compounds.   Progr. Allerg. 6:539.

Citron, K.M., Frankland, A.W., and Sinclair, J.D.   1958.   Inhal-
    ation tests of broncho-hypersensitivity in pollen asthma.
    Thorax 13:229.

Clark, R.A., Gallin, J.I., and Kaplan, A.P.   1975.   The selec-
    tive eosinophil chemotactic activity of histamine.   J. Exp.
    Med. 142:1462.

Damus, P.S., Hicks, M., and Rosenberg, R.D.   1973.   Anticoagu-
    lant action of heparin.   Nature 246:355.

DiAugustine, R.P.   1974.   Lung concentric laminar organelle:
    Hydrolase activity and compositional analysis.   249:584.

Dodgson, K.S., and Spencer, B.   1957. Assay of sulfatases.
    Meth. Biochem. Analysis 4:211.

Dodgson, K.S., Spencer, B., and Thomas, J.   1955.   Studies on
    sulfatases.   9. The arylsulfatase of mammalian liver.   Bio-
    chem. J. 59:29.

Dodgson, K.S., Spencer, B., and Wynn, C.H.   1956.   The arylsul-
    fatases of human tissues.   Biochem. J. 62:500.

Dolovich, J., Hargreave, F.E., Chalmers, R., Shier, K.J., Gaul-
    die, J., and Bienenstock, J.   1973.   Late cutaneous aller-
    gic responses in isolated IgE-dependent reactions.   J.
    Allergy Clin. Immunol. 49:43.

Drazen, J.M., and Austen, K.F.   1974.   Effects of intravenous
    administration of slow reacting substance of anaphylaxis,
    histamine, bradykinin, and prostaglandin $F_{2\alpha}$ on pulmonary
    mechanics in the guinea pig.   J. Clin. Invest. 53:1679.

Drazen, J.M., and Austen, K.F.   1975.   Atropine modification of
    the pulmonary effects of chemical mediators in the guinea
    pig.   J. Appl. Physiol. 38:834.

Feltkamp-Vroon, T.M., Stallman, P.J., Analberse, R.C., and
    Reerink-Bronkers, E.E. 1975. Immunofluorescence studies
    on renal tissue, tonsils, adenoids, nasal polyps, and skin
    of atopic and non-atopic patients with special reference to
    IgE. Clin. Immunol. Immunopathol. 4:392.

Fillion, G.M.B., Storach, S.A., and Uvnäs, B. 1970. The re-
    lease of histamine, heparin and granule protein from rat
    mast cells treated with compound 48/80 in vitro. Acta
    Physiol. Scand. 78:547.

Fraenkel-Conrat, H., and Tsung, C.M. 1967. Hydrazinolysis.
    In: METHODS IN ENZYMOLOGY, Vol. XI, p. 151, (C.H.W. Hirs,
    ed.) Academic Press, New York.

Goetzl, E.J., and Austen, K.F. 1972. A neutrophil-immobilizing
    factor derived from human leukocytes. I. Generation and
    partial characterization. J. Exp. Med. 136:1564.

Goetzl, E.J., and Austen, K.F. 1975. Purification and syn-
    thesis of eosinophilotactic tetrapeptides of human lung
    tissue: Identification as eosinophil chemotactic factor
    of anaphylaxis. Proc. Natl. Acad. Sci. 72:4123.

Goetzl, E.J., Rubin, R.H., McDonough, J., Tashjian, A.H., and
    Austen, K.F. 1976. Production of eosinophilotactic pep-
    tides by bronchogenic carcinoma in situ and in vitro.
    J. Clin. Invest (abstract), in press.

Grant, J.A., and Lichtenstein, L.M. 1974. Release of slow re-
    acting substance of anaphylaxis from human leukocytes.
    J. Immunol. 112:897.

Gray, W.R. 1967. Sequential degradation plus dansylation.
    In: METHODS IN ENZYMOLOGY, Vol. XI, p. 469, (C.H.W. Hirs,
    ed.) Academic Press, New York.

Gutte, B., and Merrifield, R.B. 1971. The synthesis of ribo-
    nuclease A. J. Biol. Chem. 246:1922.

Hargreave, F.E., and Pepys, J. 1972. Allergic respiratory re-
    actions in bird fanciers provoked by allergen inhalation
    provocation tests. Relation to clinical features and
    allergic mechanism. J. Allergy Clin. Immunol. 50:157.

Hargreave, F.E., Pepys, J., Longbottom, J.L., and Wraith, D.G.
    1966. Bird breeder's (fancier's) lung. Lancet 1:44.

Harinath, B.C., and Robins, E. 1971. Arylsulfatase in human brain. Separation, purification and certain properties of the two soluble arylsulfatases. J. Neurochem. 18:245.

Hartley, B.S. 1970. Strategy and tactics in protein chemistry. Biochem. J. 119:805.

Highsmith, R.F., and Rosenberg, R.D. 1974. The inhibition of human plasmin by human antithrombin-heparin cofactor. J. Biol. Chem. 249:4335.

Hubscher, T. 1975. Role of the eosinophil in the allergic reactions. I. EDI - An eosinophil-derived inhibitor of histamine release. J. Immunol. 114:1379.

Jaques, L.B., Monkhouse, F.C., and Steward, M. 1949. A method for the determination of heparin in blood. J. Physiol. 109:41.

Jefry, A., and Roy, A.B. 1973. The sulfatase of ox liver. XVI. A comparison of the arylsulfatase and cerebroside sulfatase activities of arylsulfatase A. Biochim. Biophys. Acta 293:178.

Kaliner, M., and Austen, K.F. 1973. A sequence of biochemical events in the antigen-induced release of chemical mediators from sensitized human lung tissue. J. Exp. Med. 138:1077.

Kaliner, M., and Austen, K.F. 1974a. Hormonal control of the immunologic release of histamine and slow reacting substance of anaphylaxis from human lung. In: CYCLIC AMP, CELL GROWTH, AND THE IMMUNE RESPONSE, p. 163, (W. Braun, L.M. Lichtenstein, and C.W. Parker, eds.) Springer-Verlag, New York.

Kaliner, M., and Austen, K.F. 1974b. Cyclic AMP, ATP, and reversed anaphylactic histamine release from rat mast cells. J. Immunol. 112:664.

Kaliner, M., Orange, R.P., and Austen, K.F. 1972. Immunological release of histamine and slow reacting substance of anaphylaxis from human lung. IV. Enhancement by cholinergic and alpha adrenergic stimulation. J. Exp. Med. 136:556.

Kaliner, M., Wasserman, S.I., and Austen, K.F. 1973. Immunologic release of chemical mediators from human nasal polyps. New Engl. J. Med. 289:277.

Kater, L.A., Goetzl, E.J., and Austen, K.F.   1976.   Isolation of
    human eosinophil phospholipase D.   J. Clin. Invest., in
    press.

Kay, A.B., and Austen, K.F.   1971.   The IgE-mediated release of
    an eosinophil leukocyte chemotactic factor from human lung.
    J. Immunol. 107:899.

Kay, A.B., Stechschulte, D.J., and Austen, K.F.   1971.   An
    eosinophil leukocyte chemotactic factor of anaphylaxis.
    J. Exp. Med. 133:602.

Kravis, T.C., and Henson, P.M.   1975.   IgE-induced release of a
    platelet-activating factor from rabbit lung.   J. Immunol.
    115:1677.

Lewis, R.A., Wasserman, S.I., Goetzl, E.J., and Austen, K.F.
    1974.   Formation of SRS-A in human lung tissue and cells
    before release.   J. Exp. Med. 140:1133.

Lewis, R.A., Goetzl, E.J., Wasserman, S.I. Valone, F.H., Rubin,
    R.H., and Austen, K.F.   1975.   The release of four medi-
    ators of immediate hypersensitivity from human leukemic
    basophils.   J. Immunol. 114:87.

Lichtenstein, L.M., and Gillespie, E.   1975.   The effects of the
    H1 and H2 antihistamines on "allergic" histamine release
    and its inhibition by histamine.   J. Pharmacol. Exp. Ther.
    192:441.

Lloyd, A.G., Bloom, G.D., and Balazs, E.A.   1967a.   Evidence for
    the covalent association of heparin and protein in mast-
    cell granules.   Biochem. J. 103:76.

Lloyd, A.G., Bloom, G.D., Balazs, E.A., and Haegermark, O.
    1967b.   Combined biochemical and morphological ultrastruc-
    ture studies on mast-cell granules.   Biochem. J. 103:75.

Matsuo, H., Fujimoto, Y., and Tatsuno, T.   1966.   A novel method
    for the determination of C-terminal amino acid in polypep-
    tides by selective tritium labelling.   Biochem. Biophys.
    Res. Commun. 22:69.

McCarthy, D.S., and Pepys, J.   1971.   Allergic bronchopulmonary
    aspergillosis.   Clinical Immunology: (2) Skin, nasal, and
    bronchial tests.   Clin. Allergy 1:415.

Mehl, E., and Jatzhewitz, H.   1968.   Cerebroside 3-sulfate as a
    physiological substrate of arylsulfatase A.   Biochim. Bio-
    phys. Acta 151:619.

Morse, H.C., III, Bloch, K.J., and Austen, K.F. 1968. Bio-
    logic properties of rat antibodies. II. Time-course of
    appearance of antibodies involved in antigen-induced
    release of slow reacting substance of anaphylaxis
    (SRS-A^{rat}); association of this activity with rat IgGa.
    J. Immunol. 101:658.

Neuwelt, E., Stumpf, D., Austin, J., and Kohler, P. 1971. A
    monospecific antibody to human sulfatase A: Preparation,
    characterization and significance. Biochim. Biophys. Acta
    236:333.

Nichol, L.W., and Roy, A.B. 1965. The sulfatase of ox liver.
    IX. The polymerization of sulfatase A. Biochemistry 4:386.

Odegard, O.R., Lie, M., and Abildgaard, U. 1975. Heparin co-
    factor activity measured with an amidolytic method. Throm-
    bosis Res. 6:287.

Orange, R.P. 1973. Immunopharmacological aspects of bronchial
    asthma. Clin. Allergy 3:(Supplement):521.

Orange, R.P. 1974. The formation and release of slow reacting
    substance of anaphylaxis in human lung tissues. In: PROG-
    RESS IN IMMUNOLOGY II, Vol. 4, p. 29 (L. Brent and J. Hol-
    borow, eds.) North Holland Publishing Co., Amsterdam.

Orange, R.P., Stechschulte, D.J., and Austen, K.F. 1969. Cellu-
    lar mechanisms involved in the release of slow reacting
    substance of anaphylaxis. Fed. Proc. 28:1710.

Orange, R.P., Stechschulte, D.J., and Austen, K.F. 1970. Immun-
    ochemical and biologic properties of rat IgE. II. Capacity
    to mediate the immunologic release of histamine and slow
    reacting substance of anaphylaxis (SRS-A). J. Immunol.
    105:1087.

Orange, R.P., Austen, W.G., and Austen, K.F. 1971. Immunolog-
    ical release of histamine and slow reacting substance of
    anaphylaxis from human lung. I. Modulation by agents in-
    fluencing cellular levels of cyclic 3',5'-adenosine mono-
    phosphate. J. Exp. Med. 134:136s.

Orange, R.P., Murphy, R.C., Karnovsky, M.L., and Austen, K.F.
    1973. The physicochemical characteristics and purification
    of slow reacting substance of anaphylaxis. J. Immunol.
    110:760.

Orange, R.P., Murphy, R.C., and Austen, K.F. 1974. Inactivation of slow reacting substance of anaphylaxis (SRS-A) by arylsulfatases. J. Immunol. 113:316.

Paterson, N.A.M., Wasserman, S.I., Said, J., Kater, L.A., and Austen, K.F. 1976. Mediator release from human lung cells distributed according to density. Fed. Proc. (abstract), in press.

Patterson, R., and Suszko, I.M. 1971. Primate respiratory mast cells. Reactions with ascaris antigen and anti-heavy chain sera. J. Immunol. 106:1274.

Patterson, R., Tomita, Y., Oh, S.H., Suszko, I.M., and Pruzansky, J.J. 1974. Respiratory mast cells and basophiloid cells. I. Evidence that they are secreted into the bronchial lumen, morphology, degranulation, and histamine release. Clin. Exp. Immunol. 16:223.

Payne, W.J., Fitzgerald, J.W., and Dodgson, K.S. 1974. Methods for visualization of enzyme in polyacrylamide gels. Appl. Microbiol. 27:154.

Pepys, J., Turner-Warwick, M., Dawson, P.L., and Hinson, K.R.W. 1968. Arthus (type III) skin test reactions in man. Clinical and immunopathological features. In: ALLERGOLOGY, p. 221, (B. Rose, R. Richter, A. Sehon, and A.W. Frankland, eds.) Excerpta Medica Foundation, No. 162, Amsterdam.

Rent, R., and Fiedel, B. 1975. Effect of heparin on C1-esterase inhibitor (C1-INH). Fed. Proc. 34:964 (abstract).

Riley, J.F., and West, G.B. 1953. The presence of histamine in tissue mast cells. J. Physiol. 120:528, 1953.

Rosenberg, R.D., and Damus, P.S. 1973. Purification and mechanism of action of human antithrombin-heparin cofactor. J. Biol. Chem. 248:6490.

Roy, A.B. 1957. Sulfatase of ox liver. I. Complex nature of the enzyme. Biochem. J. 53:12.

Roy, A.B. 1970. The product inhibition of sulfatase B. Biochim. Biophys. Acta 198:365.

Roy, A.B. 1971. The type II arylsulfatase of the red kangaroo. Biochim. Biophys. Acta. 227:129.

Schayer, R.W. 1959. Catabolism of physiological quantities of histamine in vivo. Physiol. Rev. 39:116.

Shapna, E., and Nadler, H.L. 1975. Purification and some properties of soluble human liver arylsulfatases. Arch. Biochem. Biophys. 170:179.

Siraganian, R.P., and Osler, A.G. 1971. Destruction of rabbit platelets in the allergic response of sensitized leukocytes. I. Evidence of basophil involvement. J. Immunol. 106:1252.

Spackman, D.H., Stein, W.H., and Moore, S. 1958. Automatic recording apparatus for use in the chromatography of amino acids. Anal. Chem. 30:1490.

Stevens, R.L., Fluharty, A.L., Skokut, M.H., and Kihara, H. 1975. Purification and properties of arylsulfatase A from human urine. J. Biol. Chem. 250:2495.

Stewart, J.M., and Young, J.P. 1969. SOLID PHASE PEPTIDE SYNTHESIS, W.H. Freeman and Co., San Francisco.

Standberg, K., and Hedqvist, P. 1975. Airway effects of slow reacting substance, prostaglandin $F_{2\alpha}$ and histamine in the guinea pig. Acta Physiol. Scand. 94:105.

Tauber, A.I., Kaliner, M., Stechschulte, D.J., and Austen, K.F. 1973. Immunological release of histamine and slow reacting substance of anaphylaxis from human lung. V. Effects of prostaglandins on release of histamine. J. Immunol. 111:27.

Taylor, G., and Shivalkar, P.R. "Arthus-type" reactivity in the nasal airways and skin in pollen sensitive subjects. Clin. Allergy 1:407.

Ward, P.A., and Becker, E.L. 1968. The deactivation of rabbit neutrophils by chemotactic factor and the nature of the activatable esterase. J. Exp. Med. 127:693, 1968.

Wasserman, S.I., and Austen, K.F. 1976. Arylsulfatase B of human lung: Isolation, characterization and interaction with slow reacting substance of anaphylaxis. J. Clin. Invest., in press.

Wasserman, S.I., Goetzl, E.J., and Austen, K.F. 1974a. Preformed eosinophil chemotactic factor of anaphylaxis (ECF-A). J. Immunol. 112:351.

Wasserman, S.I., Goetzl, E.J., Ellman, L., and Austen, K.F. 1974b. Tumor associated eosinophilotactic factor. New Engl. J. Med. 290:420.

Wasserman, S.I., Goetzl, E.J., and Austen, K.F.   1975a.   Inacti-
    vation of slow reacting substance of anaphylaxis by human
    eosinophil arylsulfatase.   J. Immunol. 114:645.

Wasserman, S.I., Whitmer, D., Goetzl, E.J., and Austen, K.F.
    1975b.   Chemotactic deactivation of human eosinophils
    by eosinophil chemotactic factor of anaphylaxis. Proc. Soc.
    Exp. Biol. Med. 148:301.

Wasserman, S.I., Goetzl, E.J., and Austen, K.F.   1975c.   Inacti-
    vation of human SRS-A by intact human eosinophils and by
    eosinophil arylsulfatase.   J. Allergy Clin. Immunol.
    55:72 (abstract).

Wasserman, S.I., Boswell, R.N., Drazen, J.M., Goetzl, E.J., and
    Austen, K.F.   1976a.   Functional specificity of the human
    lung acidic tetrapeptides constituting eosinophil chemotac-
    tic factor of anaphylaxis (ECF-A). J. Allergy Clin. Immunol.
    (abstract), in press.

Wasserman, S.I., Soter, N.A., Center, D.M., and Austen, K.F.
    1976b.   Cold urticaria: The appearance in the circulation
    of a neutrophil chemotactic principle during cold challenge.
    Clin. Res. (abstract), in press.

Woods, K.R., and Wang, K.T.   1967.   Separation of dansyl-amino
    acids by polyamide layer chromatography. Biochim. Biophys.
    Acta 133:369.

Yin, E.T., Wessler, S., and Stoll, P.J.   1971.   Identity of
    plasma-activated factor X inhibitor with antithrombin III
    and heparin cofactor.   J. Biol. Chem. 246:3712.

Yurt, R.W., Leid, R.W., Silbert, J.E., Spragg, J., and Austen,
    K.F.   1976.   Immunologic release of heparin from purified
    rat peritoneal mast cells. Fed. Proc. (abstract), in press.

Zeiger, R.S., Yurdin, D.L., and Colten, H.R.   1976.   Histamine
    metabolism: II. Cellular and subcellular localization of
    the catabolic enzymes, histaminase and histamine methyl
    transferase in human leukocytes. J. Allergy Clin. Immunol.,
    in press.

DISCUSSION

MÜLLER-EBERHARD: Is there an inhibitor of the tetrapeptides in serum or other extracellular fluid, or have you found a serum enzyme that destroys their activity, such as aminopeptidase?

AUSTEN: We have not yet studied the natural inactivation mechanisms but presume that an aminopeptidase will be important in some complex biologic fluids. Inactivation by cells is also possible of course.

UVNÄS: Have you any suggestion about the molecular size of your SRS-A?

AUSTEN: The molecular weight is about 400.

UVNÄS: If the mast cell has another function then to respond to IgE, which are the stimulating factors and under which classical conditions do the mast cells respond.

AUSTEN: Other mechanisms of mast cell activation, in addition to IgE dependent, would include some subgroup of IgG as indicated by animal studies. Activation of the classical or alternative complement pathways with generation of C3a and C5a would offer a further mechanism.

Finally even in delayed type hypersensitivity as shown by Mihm and coworkers there can be tissue mast cell degranulation. Thus degranulation can occur in each of the major types of immunologic reaction. It may be primary in immediate and secondary in the others.

STRANDBERG: From the clinical point of view possible control mechanisms operating via tissue accumulation of eosinophils are intriguing. Have you performed any quantitative analyses of the eosinophil enzymes in patients, e.g. asthmatics?

AUSTEN: Such studies are too preliminary for comment.

COCHRANE: Have you injected the ECF-A tetrapeptide into the skin to observe infiltration of cells?

AUSTEN: In monkey skin the tetrapeptides have produced some infiltration but it was not as striking as in the guinea pig peritoneal cavity.

BECKER: Dr. Rivkin has shown that the synthetic peptide, that I will be talking about tomorrow, had no detectable vascular permeability increasing activity, however, the same compounds placed in a plastic sponge in subcutaneous tissue cause an infiltration of neutrophils.

AUSTEN: The sponge may of course alter the microenvironment.

ZETTERSTRÖM (Uppsala): About 15 years ago Prof. Pepys

observed that some patients with allergy to <u>Aspergillus fumiga-</u>
<u>tus</u> had dual skin test reactions. Apart from the immediate
wheal and flare response these patients also showed a strong
edematous, slightly red and warm swelling of the skin which
came 3-8 hours after testing and usually disappeared within
24 hours. This type of dual skin response has now been described after testing with several other allergens.

In my experience the dual skin reaction is seen only in
patients with high titers of specific IgE-antibodies. It is
also possible to passively transfer this skin reaction with
IgE fractions from allergic patients sera. So even the delayed
part of the dual skin response seem to be IgE dependent.

What is your opinion of mediators or mechanisms responsible
for the delayed part of this skin response?

AUSTEN: Such findings are entirely consistent with the formulation that the mast cell activated by IgE dependent mechanism
initiates both the early and late reactions. Such events are
compatible with mediator elaboration capable of directing not
only alterations in vascular permeability but also the ingress
of inflammatory cell types. Thus the mast cell can determine
these events without implicating an Arthus reaction.

GOMPERTS: You omitted from your list of mast cell mediator
the lysosomal enzymes which are certainly released when the cell
is effectively challenged. Do you anticipate that they too play
a specialized role as mediators of mast cell function?

AUSTEN: I am not aware that the lysosomal character of mast
cell constituents has been studied.

UVNÄS: Are eosinophils the only cells capable of destroying
SRS-A?

AUSTEN: As already mentioned, the lung cells possess an
arylsulfatase B which inactivates SRS-A. Furthermore, in leukemi
basophils from one patient there was an arylsulfatase present
that in prelimary studies appears to be an arylsulfatase B. Thus
even the cell type generating SRS-A may have an inactivating
capacity.

PROSTAGLANDINS AND RELATED SUBSTANCES IN ACUTE ALLERGIC REACTIONS

Kjell Strandberg

Department of Pharmacology, Karolinska institutet

S-104 01 Stockholm 60, Sweden

The prostaglandins (PGs) constitute an ever growing family of naturally occurring biologically active carbon 20 unsaturated fatty acids which are synthetized in practically all mammalian tissues studied. They are rapidly deactivated by metabolism in most tissues and there is evicence to suggest that their possible physiological significance is related to local formation and action rather than to a hormone function proper (Piper and Vane 1971). Increased PG formation has been demonstrated in conjunction with a number of physiological and pathophysiological processes, e.g. hormone and nervous activity, smooth muscle contraction, inflammation and hyper-sensitivity reactions (c.f. Piper and Vane 1971, Vane 1974).

With respect to allergic reactions, PGs were shown to appear in the effluents from perfused sensitized guinea-pig lungs during anaphylaxis and in the incubates of passively sensitized human lung fragments exposed to allergen, as determined by thin layer chroma-tography and differential bioassay (Piper and Vane 1969, Piper and Walker 1973). Similarly, addition of allergen to isolated human bronchi sensitized with reaginic serum results in increased PGF_2 formation, as measured by radioimmunoassay (Dunlop and Smith 1975). In a recent study increased plasma levels of the $PGF_{2\alpha}$ metabolite 15-hydroxy-13,14-dihydro $PGF_{2\alpha}$ were found in asthmatic inhaling the aerosolized allergen (Gréen et al. 1975). In human skin PG-like ac-tivity appears as a result of contact dermatitis (Söndergaard and Greaves 1970).

The PGs have potent actions on smooth muscles and cellular re-lease reactions (c.f. Nakano 1973, Kaliner and Austen 1974, Weiss-man et al. 1976). Accordingly, there have been suggestions that in-creased formation of PGs, an imbalance between the PGs formed or a

decreased catabolism of PGs might be of pathophysiological significance in hypersensitivity reactions (Piper and Vane 1969, Horton
1969, Mathé et al. 1973). Some pharmacological actions of the PGs
are compatible with a mediator role, whereas others are not. $PGF_{2\alpha}$
is a bronchoconstrictor agent, while PGE_2 is a less consistent
bronchodilator compound (Cuthbert 1973, Mathé and Hedqvist 1975).
In most vascular beds PGEs are potent vasodilators but in the lung
PGE_2 and $PGF_{2\alpha}$ increase arterial and venous pressure and in the
nasal mucosa they constrict the small vessels (c.f. Nakano 1973).
In human skin intradermal injection of PGE_2 evokes a flare reaction
and itshing, part of which might be mediated by histamine release
(Hägermark and Strandberg 1976).

   In general, PGEs and less potent PGFs stimulate the cellular
build-up of cyclic AMP (cAMP). The findings that an increase in
basophil, mast cell and lung cAMP levels inhibits antigen-induced
histamine release suggest that the tissue levels of PGs, as well
as other events producing changes in cAMP levels, might influence
the allergic release reaction (Lichtenstein and Bourne 1971, Kaliner and Austen 1974, Orange et al. 1971). Interestingly enough,
low concentrations of PGs decrease the cAMP level and enhance the
release reaction in sensitized human lung fragments (Tauber et al.
1973).

   Recently, two PG endoperoxides (PGG_2 and PGH_2), intermediates
in the conversion of arachidonic acid into PGE_2 and $PGF_{2\alpha}$ were isolated (Hamberg and Samuelsson 1973, Hamberg et al. 1974). They are
unstable in aqueous medium ($t_{1/2}$ at 37°C, about 5 min) and following biosynthesis they are enzymatically converted into their end
products. In addition to PGE_2 and $PGF_{2\alpha}$,12L-hydroxy 5,8,10-hepta-
decatrienoic acid (HHT) and 8-(1-hydroxy-3-oxopropyl)-9,12L-dihyd-
roxy-5,10-heptadecadienoic acid (thromboxane B_2) are formed (Hamberg and Samuelsson 1974). Subsequent experiments have demonstrated the formation of a biologically active intermediate product in
the generation of thromboxane B_2 (Hamberg et al. 1976). This substance, designated thromboxane A_2 has a very short half-life in
aqueous solutions (about 30 sec) and is probably identical with
rabbit aorta contracting substance (RCS) discovered by Piper and
Vane (1969). The synthetic pathways recognized on transformation
of arachidonic acid in the guinea-pig lung are presented in fig. 1.
Notably, indomethacin and allied non-steroidal anti-inflammatory
compounds inhibit the fatty acid cyclo-oxygenase but not the fatty
acid dioxygenase (Hamberg and Samuelsson 1974). The PG endoperoxides
were shown to be more potent than PGE_2 and $PGF_{2\alpha}$ on some respiratory and vascular smooth muscles (Hamberg et al. 1975, Tuvemo et
al. 1976) (Table I).

   On superfused human isolated bronchi PGG_2, PGH_2, PGD_2 (isomer
to PGE_2) and $PGF_{2\alpha}$ were about equiactive in producing contraction
whereas a synthetic stable endoperoxide analogue (15S)-hydroxy-
-9 ,11 -(epoxymethano) prosta-5,13-dienoic acid (=EPA) was much more

Table I. Relative contractile effects of PGG_2, PGH_2, PGD_2, PGE_2 and $PGF_{2\alpha}$ on some smooth muscle preparations (from: Hamberg et al. 1975).

Prostaglandin	Gerbil colon (n=5)	Rat stomach (n=5)	Rabbit aorta (n=5)	Guinea-pig trachea (n=7)	Guinea-pig airway insufflation pressure (n=5)
PGG_2	1.5±0.4 (n.s.)	1.9 ± 0.4 (n.s.)	80.4±19.0 (p<0.05)	7.5±1.8 (p<0.05)	8.5±2.4 (p<0.05)
PGH_2	1.2±0.3 (n.s.)	3.3 ± 0.3 (p<0.01)	210.4±41.8 (p<0.01)	9.3±2.2 (p<0.01)	10.8 ± 2.5 (p<0.05)
PGD_2	0.3±0.2 (p<0.05)	1.4 ± 0.8 (n.s.)	—	5.2±0.7 (p<0.01)	5.7 ± 1.1 (p<0.05)
PGE_2	2.9 ± 0.4 (p<0.05)	5.7 ± 0.8 (p<0.01)	I	relaxes[*]	—
$PGF_{2\alpha}$	I	I	—	I	I

[*] Contractions were sometimes seen with concentrations of 2-3 µg/ml.

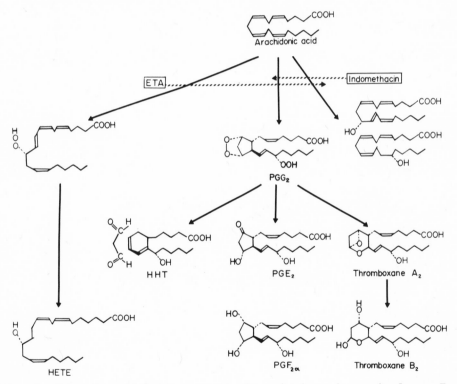

Fig. 1. Transformation of arachidonic acid in guinea-pig lung. Enzymatic reactions inhibited by eicosa-5,8,11,14-tetraynoic acid (ETA) and indomethacin respectively are denoted by discontinuous lines.

active (Strandberg et al., to be published) (fig. 2). Recently, we
have been able to extend this work to thromboxane A_2, which was
found to be considerably more active than the PG endoperoxides in
increasing the airway insufflation pressure in the anaesthetized
guinea-pig (fig. 2) (Svensson et al. to be published). Thromboxane
A_2 was generated by adding arachidonic acid to washed human platelets. Ultrafiltration was immediately started and the filtrate was
used for experiments 30 sec later. 2.5 min after initiating the reaction the biological activity had decreased by about 95%. The high
biological activity and the lability of the active principle in
the ultrafiltrate, the correlation between biological activity and
amounts of thromboxane A_2 determined (Hamberg and Svensson 1976)
and the fact that the biological activity was not antagonized by
an antihistamine (H_1-receptor), a serotonin antagonist or indomethacin provide strong evidence for the view that the biological effects
observed were produced by thromboxane A_2.

These results emphasize that the biological activity following
PG generation depends on the nature of the principles formed. To
elucidate the control mechanisms of the synthetic pathways involved is presently one of the most important obligations in PG research. To monitor the formation of the classical PGs alone might
be misleading with regard to interpretation of the role of PG formation in a particular, biological system. The hazards involved are
further stressed by the rapid tissue catabolism of PGs formed (c.f.
Piper 1973) and the fact that some of the metabolites are biologically active.

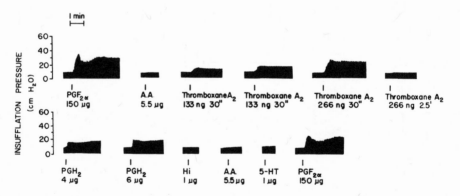

Fig. 2. Effects of intravenous injection of $PGF_{2\alpha}$, arachidonic acid,
thromboxane A_2, PGH_2, histamine and 5-hydroxytryptamine on the airway insufflation pressure in an anaesthetized artificially ventila-
ted guinea-pig pretreated intravenously with 1 mg/kg each of indomethacin, mepyramine and methysergide. The time points set for
thromboxane A_2 refer to the period of time elapsed after generating
the active principle. The intervals between the separate recordings
were 5-10 min.

Thus there are several potential reasons for failures to correlate changes in biological activity with amounts of PGs detected in
the experimental system under study. The problems involved are illustrated by a study of thromboxane formation in perfused guinea-pig
lungs on injection of arachidonic acid in the pulmonary artery
(fig. 3) (Hamberg et al. 1976). Firstly, the output of thromboxane
B_2 was about 7-20 times as high as that of PGE_2 or $PGF_{2\alpha}$. Secondly,
in this experimental system the substantial part of PGE_2 and $PGF_{2\alpha}$
formed will appear in the perfusate as 15-keto-13,14-dihydro metabolites (Mathé and Levine 1973, Liebig et al. 1974). On injection
of ovalbumin in the pulmonary artery, thromboxane B_2 was demonstrated in the perfusates from sensitized guinea-pig lungs showing that
thromboxane A_2 is in fact formed during anaphylaxis in intact guinea-pig lungs (Hamberg et al. 1976). Hence, in addition to $PGF_{2\alpha}$,
thromboxane A_2 and PG endoperoxides must be considered potential
mediators of the anaphylactic reaction in guinea-pig lung. However,
their importance for a mediator function in guinea-pig anaphylaxis,
relative to that of the other candidates may still be questioned.
In a previous study we investigated the effect of indomethacin
pretreatment on the respiratory distress and urinary output of the
major urinary PGF metabolite 5 ,7 -dihydroxy-11-ketotetranor-pros-
tanoic acid in ovalbumin-sensitized guinea-pigs inhaling the antigen (Strandberg and Hamberg 1974). There was an increased output of
PGF metabolites following the anaphylactic reaction (fig. 4). Treatment with indomethacin resulted in a reduced basal output and no
increase was seen on antigen administration. Nonetheless, the animals reacted with anaphylactic shock just as the non-treated guinea-
pigs. Since indomethacin inhibits the fatty acid cyclooxygenase in
the PG synthesis not only the formation of the classical PGs but
also the formation of the PG endoperoxides and thromboxane A_2 is
inhibited (fig. 1). A shift to a predominant biosynthesis of biologically active compounds via fatty acid dioxygenase route is not
likely to make up for the loss of activity as in vivo effects of
arachidonic acid on the respiratory tract and the cardio-vascular
system are abolished by indomethacin pretreatment (Varhaftig et al.
1969). The failure of indomethacin in guinea-pig anaphylaxis seems
surprising in view of the potency of the substances suppressed by
this treatment. Either the PGs and thromboxane A_2 are very rapidly
and efficiently converted into less active compounds once they are
formed thereby excluding a mediator function for them or indomethacin also interferes with enzyme activities normally opposing the
PG system. It has been reported that concomitantly with a decreased
generation of PGs by indomethacin in human lung fragments an increased formation of SRS-A occurs (Walker 1973). Similar observations
were made using the isolated perfused guinea-pig lung and in this
system indomethacin did not inhibit the antigen-induced rise in
perfusion pressure (Liebig et al. 1974). On the other hand, in the
isolated human bronchus the allergen-induced contraction is reduced
by indomethacin (Dunlop and Smith 1975), although attempts to protect asthmatics from bronchoconstriction on exposure to aerosolized

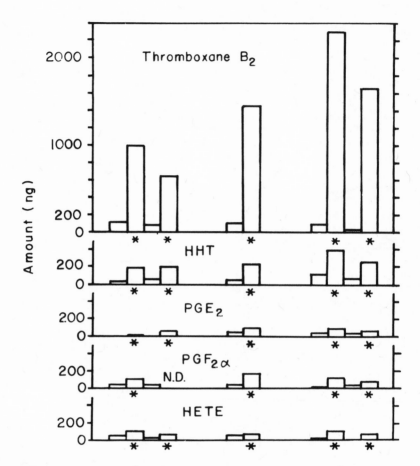

<u>Fig. 3</u>. Efflux of thromboxane B_2, HHT, PGE_2, $PGF_{2\alpha}$ and HETE from perfused guinea-pig lungs. Asterisks indicate injection of 30 ug of arachidonic acid. N.D. = not determined (From: Hamberg et al. 1976).

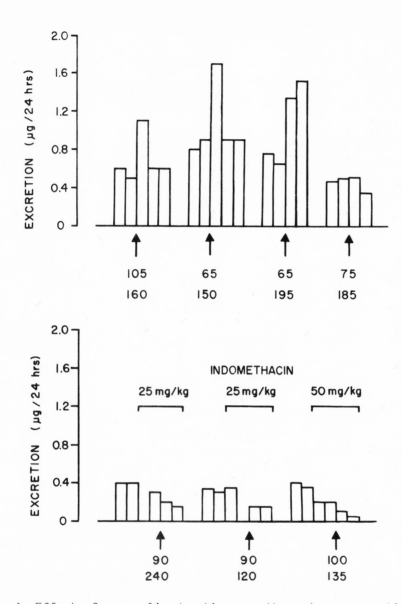

Fig. 4. Effect of aerosolized antigen on the urinary excretion of
5 ,7 -dihydroxy-11-ketotetranor-prostanoic acid in seven unanaesthe-
tized ovalbumin-sensitized guinea-pigs of which three were pretreated with indomethacin. The arrows indicate the day of exposure to
the antigen. The figures below refer to the onset time (sec) for
respiratory distress (upper and convulsions (lower) respectively.

allergen by oral indomethacin in doses that suppress the biosynthesis of PGs have failed (Smith and Dunlop 1975, Svanborg et al.
1976). Admittedly, the concentration of indomethacin in the bio-
phase might have been higher in the in vitro experiments. Notably,
however, the increase in plasma 15-keto,13,14-dihydro $PGF_{2\alpha}$ demonstrated on allergen challenge was anulled by prior treatment with
indomethacin (Svanborg et al. 1976). It seems as final clarification on this point has to await the availability of more selective
prostaglandin synthetase inhibitors.

The cellular origin of the PGs appearing in allergic reactions
is unkown. In experiments with reagin-mediated histamine release
from passively sensitized human lung fragments incubated with birch
pollen allergen there was no quantitative correlation between histamine release and PGE or $PGF_{2\alpha}$ as measured by radioimmunoassay
(Strandberg et al. to be published). Similar results were reported
by Piper and Walker (1973) using bioassay for identification. In
contrast to their finding of a predominant formation of PGE-like
activity we observed about the same percentage increase (about 70
per cent) in PGE and $PGF_{2\alpha}$ release and the absolute amounts of $PGF_{2\alpha}$
formed, as compared to PGE were higher.

The findings that the β-adrenergic stimulating compound isoprenaline and the α-adrenergic blocking compound phentolamine concomitantly inhibit the release of histamine and the appearance of
PGs indicate that the two processes are inter-related (fig. 5). However, although mast cells generate PGE and $PGF_{2\alpha}$, the increased
amounts of PGs found in anaphylaxis do not seem to originate from
the mast cells as antigen-evoked histamine release from mixed pleural cells and isolated rat mast cells was not accompanied by an
increase in the formation of PGs (Strandberg et al. to be published)
(fig. 6). Phosphatidylserine enhanced the histamine release by antigen. The seemingly enhanced formation of PGE by phosphatidylserine
was an artefact due to interference with the radioimmunoassay or generation of immunoreactive material from the phosphatidylserine.
Similarly, in experiments with leucocytes from allergic donors no
increase in PG production was found on addition of the allergen
(Okazaki et al. 1976).

An increased production of PGs secondary to the action of other
mediators set free is an alternative explanation for the appearance
of PGs during anaphylaxis. In preliminary experiments, SRS added to
sensitized human lung fragments has been found to stimulate PG formation. Similarly, perfusion of guinea-pig lungs with histamine or
SRS increased the amounts of PGs in the effluent (Piper and Vane
1969, Liebig et al. 1974, Yen et al. 1976). The findings that PGs
appear on contraction of isolated guinea-pig trachea by acetylcholine and histamine suggest that PGs are formed as a consequence of
smooth muscle activity (Orehek et al. 1973). On the other hand, there
was no significant increase in PG formation when isolated human

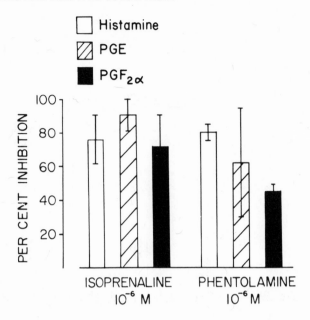

Fig. 5. Inhibition by isoprenaline (mean and standard errors of
the mean, n = 4) and phentolamine (mean and ranges, n = 2) of allergen-induced histamine release and prostaglandin formation in sensitized human lung fragments. Incubation time after addition of allergen 20 min at 37°C. Drugs were added 5 min prior to the allergen.

bronchi were exposed to acetylcholine (Dunlop and Smith 1975) or
histamine and SRS (Yen et al. to be published). Together these data
indicate that the PGs may occur as a result (secondary mediators)
of the release of the primary mediators originating wholly or at
least in part from the mast cells, e.g. histamine and SRS, although
their origin has not convincingly been linked to smooth muscle activity (fig. 7).

    In conclusion, no significant evidence have as yet been presen-
ted to favour a mediator role of the PGs in allergic reactions. Conversely, the possibility must be considered that PG generation
serves the purpose of a control mechanism in such reactions, i.e.
inhibiting further release of chemical mediators from mast cells
and enzymes from polymorphonuclear leucocytes and possibly by regulating the ventilation-perfusion relationship in the lung.

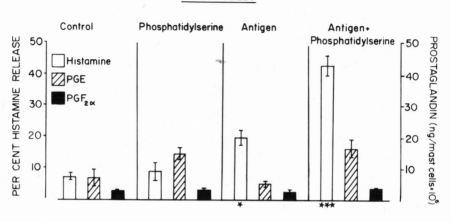

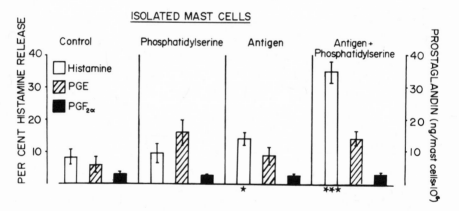

Fig. 6. Histamine release and prostaglandin formation in mixed rat
pleural cells and in Ficoll-isolated rat pleural mast cells exposed
to antigen (ovalbumin, 10 μg/ml) for 10 min at 25°C. Phosphatidylserine, 10^{-4}M. Increased PGE-readings in presence of phosphatidylserine due to interference with the radioimmunoassay. x = p<0.05,
xxx = p<0.001.

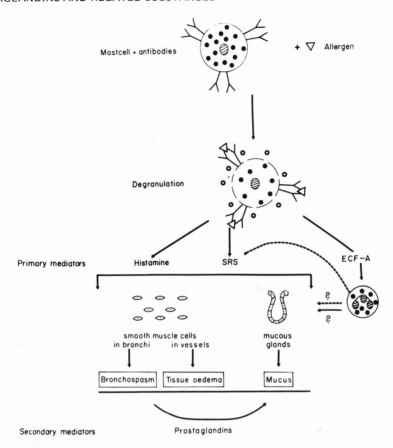

Fig. 7. Tentative scheme for the appearance of prostaglandins in acute allergic reactions. Inhibitory reactions denoted by discontinuous lines.

With regard to the lung, there is presently not much support for this view, since the minimal concentrations of PGs required to inhibit immunologic mediator release from lung tissue are considerably higher than found in these reactions and as to the bronchial effects PGE_2 is a bronchoconstrictor agent in some patients (Walker 1973, Piper and Walker 1973, Mathé and Hedqvist 1975, Strandberg et al. 1976). However, the consequences of PG formation in a particular biological system must ultimately be related to the biological properties of all the substances formed. The existence of several pathways for transformation of the PG precursors along with incomplete knowledge of the factors operating them and the fact that intermediate products in this synthesis as well as metabolites are biologically active underlines the complexity of the PG system and the inherent problems with interpretation of its importance in phy-

siological and pathophysiological reactions. Not even the therape-
utic potentials of the PGs are easily explored. Although aerosolized PGE_1 and PGE_2, for example, have been shown to produce broncho-
dilatation in healthy subjects (Cuthbert 1971) some asthmatics
react with broncoconstriction to PGE_2 (Mathé et al. 1973, Mathé
and Hedqvist 1975). In vitro the longlasting PGE_2 analogue 16,16-
-dimethyl-PGE_2 is consistent constrictor of human bronchi which
further emphasizes the PG receptor specificities in the lung
(Strandberg and Hedqvist 1976).

REFERENCES

CUTHBERT, M.F.: Bronchodilator activity of aerosols of prostaglandins E_1 and E_2 in asthmatic subjects. Proc. R. Soc. Med. 64: 15-16,
1971.

CUTHBERT, M.F.: Prostaglandins and respiratory smooth muscle. In:
The Prostaglandins (Cuthbert, M.F. et al., ed.) Philadelphia,
J.B. Lippincott Co., pp. 253-285, 1973.

DUNLOP, L.S. and SMITH, A.P.: Reduction of antigen-induced contraction of sensitized human bronchi in vitro by indomethacin. Br. J.
Pharmac. 54: 495-497, 1975.

GREEN, K., HEDQVIST, P. and SVANBORG, N.: Increased plasma levels
of 15-keto,13,14-dihydro $PGF_{2\alpha}$ after allergen-provoked asthma in
man. Lancet, 2: 1419-1421, 1975.

HAMBERG, M., SVENSSON, J. and SAMUELSSON, B.: Novel transformations of prostaglandin endoperoxides: Formation of thromboxanes.
In Advances in Prostaglandin and Thromboxane Research (Samuelsson, B.
and Paoletti, R., eds.). Raven Press, New York, in press.

HAMBERG, M., HEDQVIST, P., STRANDBERG, K., SVENSSON, J. and SAMUELS-
SON, B.: Prostaglandin endoperoxides IV. Effects on smooth muscle.
Life Sci. 16: 451-462, 1975.

HAMBERG, M. and SAMUELSSON, B.: Detection and isolation of an endoperoxide intermediate in prostaglandin biosynthesis. Proc. Nat.
Acad. Sci. USA 70: 899-903, 1973.

HAMBERG, M. and SAMUELSSON, B.: Novel transformations of arachidonic acid in guinea-pig lung. Biochem. Biophys. Res. Commun. 61:
942-949, 1974.

HAMBERG, M. and SVENSSON, J.: Biosynthesis and metabolism of prostaglandin endoperoxides and thromboxanes in platelets. Proc. of an
International Symposium on Platelets and Thrombosis. Academic Press
1976.

HAMBERG, M., SVENSSON, J., HEDQVIST, P., STRANDBERG, K. and SAMUELSSON, B.: Involvement of the endoperoxide system in anaphylactic reactions. In Advances in Prostaglandin and Thromboxane Research (Samuelsson, B. and Paoletti, R., eds.). Raven Press, New York, in press.

HAMBERG, M., SVENSSON, J., WAKABAYASHI, T. and SAMUELSSON, B.: Isolation and structure of two prostaglandin endoperoxides which cause platelet aggregation. Proc. Nat. Acad. Sci. USA 71: 345-349, 1974.

HORTON, E.W.: Hypotheses on physiological roles of prostaglandins. Physiol. Rev. 49: 122-166, 1969.

HÄGERMARK, Ö. and STRANDBERG, K.: Pruritogenic activity of prostaglandin E_2. Acta dermatovenereol. (Stockholm), in press.

KALINER, M. and AUSTEN, K.F.: Cyclic AMP, ATP and reversed anaphylactic histamine release from rat mast cells. J. Immunol. 112: 664-674, 1974.

LICHTENSTEIN, L.M. and BOURNE, H.R.: Inhibition of allergic histamine release by histamine and other agents which stimulate adenyl cyclase. In Biochemistry of the Acute Allergic Reactions (Austen, K.F. and Becker, E. L., eds.) Oxford, Blackwell Sci. Publ., pp. 161-174, 1971.

LIEBIG, R., BERNAUER, W. and PESKAR, B.A.: Release of prostaglandins, a prostaglandin metabolite, slow reacting substance and histamine from anaphylactic lungs, and its modification by catecholamines. Naunyn Schmiedeberg's Arch. Pharmacol. 284: 279-293, 1974.

MATHÉ, A.A. and HEDQVIST, P.: Effect of prostaglandins F_2 and E_2 on airway conductance in healthy subjects and asthmatic patients. Amer. Rev. Resp. Dis. 111: 313-320, 1975.

MATHÉ, A.A., HEDQVIST, P., HOLMGREN, A. and SVANBORG, N.: Bronchial hyperreactivity to prostaglandin $F_{2\alpha}$ and histamine in patients with asthma. Br. Med. J. 1: 193-196, 1973.

MATHÉ, A.A. and LEVINE, L.: Release of prostaglandins and metabolites from guinea-pig lung: Inhibition by catecholamines. Prostaglandins 4: 877-890, 1973.

OKAZAKI, T., VERVLOET, D., ATTALLAH, A., LEE, J.B. and ARBESMAN, C.E.: Prostaglandins and asthma: The use of blood components for metabolic studies. J. Allergy Clin. Immunol. 57: 124-133, 1975.

ORANGE, R.P., KALINER, M.A., LARAIA, P.J. and AUSTEN, K.F.: The
immunological release of histamine ad slow reacting substance of
anaphylaxis from human lung. II. Influence of cellular levels of
cyclic AMP. Fed. Proc. 30: 1725-1729, 1971.

OREHEK, J., DOUGLAS, J.S., LEWIS, A.J. and BOUHUYS, A.: Prostaglandin regulation of airway smooth muscle tone. Nature New Biol. 245:
84-85, 1973.

PIPER, P.J.: Distribution and metabolism. In The Prostaglandins
(Cuthbert, M.F., ed.) Philadelphia, J.B. Lippincott Co., pp. 125-150,
1973.

PIPER, P.J. and WALKER, J.L.: The Release of spasmogenic substances
from human chopped lung tissue and its inhibition. Br. J. Pharmac.
47: 291-304, 1973.

PIPER, P.J. and VANE, J.R.: Release of additional factors in anaphylaxis and its antagonism by anti-inflammatory drugs. Nature
223: 29-35, 1969.

PIPER, P.J. and VANE, J.R.: The release of prostaglandin from lung
and other tissues. Ann. N.Y. Acad. Sci. 180: 363-383, 1971.

SMITH, A.P. and DUNLOP, L.: Prostaglandins and asthma. Lancet 1:
39, 1975.

SMITH, M.J.H. and DAWKINS, P.D.: Salicylates and enzymes. J. Pharm.
Pharmacol. 23: 729-744, 1971.

STRANDBERG, K. and HAMBERG, M.: Increased excretion of 5 ,7 -dihydro-
-11-keto-tetranor-prostanoic acid on anaphylaxis in the guinea-pig.
Prostaglandins 6: 159-170, 1974.

STRANDBERG, K. and HEDQVIST, P.: Bronchial effects of some prostaglandin E_1, E_2 and $F_{2\alpha}$ analogues. Acta physiol. scand., in press.

SVANBORG, N., HEDQVIST, P. and GREEN, K.: Aspects on prostaglandin
action in asthma. In Advances in Prostaglandin and Thromboxane
Research (Samuelsson, B. and Paoletti, R., eds.). Raven Press,
New York, in press.

SÖNDERGAARD, J. and GREAVES, M.W.: Recovery of a pharmacologically
active fatty acid during the inflammatory reaction, invoked by
patch testing in allergic contact ekzema. Int. Arch. Allerg. 39:
56-61, 1970.

TAUBER, A.I., KALINER, M., STECHSCHULTE, D.J. and AUSTEN, K.F.:
Immunologic release of histamine and slow reacting substance of anaphylaxis from human lung: V. Effects of prostaglandins. J. Immunol.
111: 27-32, 1973.

TUVEMO, T., STRANDBERG, K., HAMBERG, M. and SAMUELSSON, B.: Formation and action of prostaglandin endoperoxides in the isolated human umbilical artery. Acta physiol. scand., in press.

WALKER, J.L.: The regulatory function of prostaglandins in the release of histamine and SRS-A from passively sensitized human lung tissue. In Advances in the Biosciences. International Conference on Prostaglandins. Pergamon Press. Vieweg, pp. 235-240, 1973.

VANE, J.R.: The contribution of prostaglandins and other mediators to the allergic state. In Allergy '74. Proc. Ninth Europ. Congr. Allergol. Clin. Immunol. (Sanderton, M.A. and Frankland, A.W., eds.) Pitruan Medical Publ. Co. Kent, pp. 79-92, 1974.

VARGAFTIG, B.B., DE MIRANDA, E.P. and LACOUME, B.: Inhibition by non-steroidal anti-inflammatory agents of in vivo effects of slow reacting substance C. Nature 222: 883-885, 1969.

WEISSMAN, G., GOLDSTEIN, I. and HOFFSTEIN, S.: Prostaglandins and the modulation by cyclic nucleotides of lysosomal enzyme release. In Advances in Prostaglandin and Thromboxane Research. (Samuelsson, B. and Paoletti, R., eds.), Raven Press, New York, in press.

YEN, S., SOHN, R.J., MATHÉ, A.A., STRANDBERG, K. and COCHIN, J.: Release of prostaglandins from the guinea-pig lung. Fed. Proc. 35: 458, 1976.

DISCUSSION

GOETZL: I am interested in the time course of release of prostaglandins relative to histamine in your anaphylactic reactions. Does prostaglandin release always follow histamine release confirming your view that it is secondary to an action of histamine?

STRANDBERG: On the average there was a slight delay in the appearance of prostaglandins as compared to histamine. In perfusion experiments using guinea pig lungs there was a definite delay (Mathé and Levine, 1973).

LICHTENSTEIN: Did you define the prostaglandin receptors that you spoke of?

STRANDBERG: No.

MÜLLER-EBERHARD: I noticed in one of your slides that the amount of the major metabolite of prostaglandin F in the urine of sensitized guinea pigs is of the order of a few micrograms per 24 hours. Can this rather small amount be indicative of an involvement of prostaglandins in anaphylaxis?

STRANDBERG: In the anaphylactic reaction there was an increase in the urinary output by about 100 per cent. Over 24 hours this figure is not impressive but if it reflects an instant increase it would certainly be of local pathophysiological importance. In addition, measurements of thromboxane B_2 would be of interest.

AUSTEN: Can you comment about the role of prostaglandins in adverse reactions to non-steroidal anti-inflammatory drugs.

STRANDBERG: There are no conclusive data on this point. It has been suggested that aspirin intolerant asthmatics to a major extent rely on a production of bronchodilator prostaglandin E_2 and develop symptoms when this is cut off by a prostaglandin synthetase inhibitor e.g. aspirin (Szeclic et al.). It would be of interest to determine plasma levels of prostaglandin E metabolites in these patients as compared to other asthmatics.

LICHTENSTEIN: You mentioned that wheal, flare and itch occurred after intradermal injection of prostaglandins. Is this a direct effect of the prostaglandins, i.e. the wheal and itch, or is it due to histamine release?

STRANDBERG: The wheal reaction is minimal and not always seen. We have reasons to believe that part of the skin reactions evoked by prostaglandin E_2 is due to histamine release. Thus antihistamines (anti-H1) reduce the effects and the histamine content in skin drops on injection of prostaglandin E_1 (Söndergaard and Greaves 1971, Hägermark and Strandberg, Acta Dermato-Venereol., Stockholm, in press).

MOVAT: We have no experience with human skin, but E prostaglandins injected intradermally in rabbits and guinea pigs induce hyperemia, which can be quantitated by injecting radiolabelled microspherules intra-arterially. In turn this hyperemia causes a marked accentuation of enhanced vascular permeability induced by mediator such as histamine and bradykinin. In fact, subthreshold doses of the latter have a pronounced effect in the presence of E prostaglandins (Johnston, Hay and Movat "Agents", in press).

STRANDBERG: We have observed an enhancing effect of prostaglandin E_2 on the pruritogenic action of histamine. Similarly, E prostaglandins have been shown to potentiate the actions of other stimuli in a number of other experimental systems.

Generation of
Biologically Active Substances and
Mediator—Target Cell Interactions

THE ANAPHYLATOXINS: FORMATION, STRUCTURE, FUNCTION AND CONTROL

Hans J. Müller-Eberhard

Department of Molecular Immunology
Scripps Clinic and Research Foundation
La Jolla, California 92037

INTRODUCTION

Although present evidence indicates that anaphylaxis due to IgE antibodies does not involve the complement system, it has been established that
complement participates in other forms of acute immunologic reactions as
well as in the inflammatory process. It contributes to both processes by
effecting activation of a variety of cells, including mast cells, basophils,
neutrophils, monocytes, macrophages, platelets and smooth muscle cells.
Complement accomplishes its effects through the interaction of distinct reaction products with constituents of cell membranes. Among the biologically
active reaction products are the activation peptides of C3 and C5, designated C3a and C5a, respectively. For historical reasons they are collec-
tively known as anaphylatoxin (AT). Both peptides are powerful, hormone-
like substances that act on specific cellular receptors. In vitro, C3a and
C5a cause histamine release from mast cells and smooth muscle contraction
and C5a causes directed migration of leukocytes and release of hydrolases.
In vivo, both peptides are phlogogenic.

In the following, the two peptides will be discussed in terms of the most
relevant and recent information on their generation, structure and function.
Because background information has been summarized previously (1-3), this
presentation will emphasize (a) the alternative pathway of complement activation as a mode of AT formation, and (b) the dependence of AT function on
distinct features of their primary and secondary structure.

THE ANAPHYLATOXIN PRECURSORS

C3 and C5 are β-globulins with molecular weights of approximately 180,000. The serum concentration of C3 is 1500 µg/ml and that of C5 75 µg/ml. Both molecules consist of two non-identical polypeptide chains which are linked by disulfide bridges and non-covalent forces. In both molecules the a-chain has a molecular weight of 110,000 and the β-chain of 70,000 (4,5). The two proteins are substrates of interrelated complement enzymes, the C3- and C5-convertases of the classical and the alternative pathways. In each case, attack by the activating enzyme is limited to cleavage of a single peptide bond. The susceptible bond is located in the a-chain of C3 and C5. Dissociation of the arising a-fragments endows the b-fragments with transiently activated binding sites through which attachment to suitable acceptors occurs. The preferential object of attachment of nascent C3b is a biological membrane, that of nascent C5b is C6. Bound C3b exercises immune adherence and opsonic functions, and the C5b,6 complex serves as the condensation point of the membrane attack unit of complement.

ANAPHYLATOXIN FORMATION BY THE CLASSICAL PATHWAY

In molecular terms, the classical complement pathway (3) is well understood and need not be treated here as such. However, the AT-forming enzymes deserve brief consideration. C3 convertase constitutes a fusion product of C2 and C4 (6). More precisely, C4b, the major physiological fragment of C4, functions as the acceptor of C2a, the major physiological fragment of C2. C3 cleaving activity resides in the bimolecular C4b,2a complex. The fragment C4b is made up of three polypeptide chains, a' (88,000 dalton), β (78,000 dalton) and γ (33,000 dalton). The fragment C2a consists of a single polypeptide chain with a molecular weight of 85,000 dalton. Accordingly, the quaternary structure of C3 convertase comprises four chains and the calculated molecular weight of the enzyme is 284,000 dalton. The active site of the enzyme resides in the C2a subunit as evidenced by the fact that C2a, dissociated from the complex, hydrolyses N-acetyl-glycyl-lysine methyl ester (AGLME) and that AGLME inhibits cleavage of C3 by the C4b,2a complex (7). The enzyme is a serine esterase as it is inhibitable by diisofluorophosphate (8). Fragmentation of C2 upon activation had been inferred from the molecular weight difference between C2a and its precursors (9,10). The activation fragment C2b, however, could not be demonstrated. Recently, it has been possible to visualize C2b on sodium dodecyl sulfate polyacrylamide gel electrophoresis. According to this study (11) C2 consists of a single polypeptide chain (120,000 dalton) which upon activation of C2 is cleaved into two fragments, C2a (85,000 dalton) and C2b (35,000 dalton).

C5 convertase is a condensation product of the C4b,2a complex and of C3b, the major physiological fragment of C3. In the trimolecular complex, C3b modulates C2a such that it acquires the ability to act on C5. Since C3b consists of two chains, a' (101,000 dalton) and β (70,000 dalton), the quaternary structure of C5 convertase comprises six polypeptide chains and the total molecular weight of the enzyme is 455,000 dalton (12).

C2 thus represents the essential zymogen of the classical pathway for the AT-forming process. In its activated form (C2a) it is modulated first by C4b to express C3 convertase activity, and then by C4b and C3b to express C5 convertase activity. As will be seen, the structural and functional analogies of the classical convertases to their counterparts in the alternative pathways are striking.

ANAPHYLATOXIN FORMATION BY THE ALTERNATIVE PATHWAY

Until very recently this pathway was not well understood. However, it was believed that the serum protein properdin is recruited in the initial reaction of the pathway and that properdin activation is a prerequisite of the formation of the C3 and C5 convertases of the pathway. This view is no longer tenable, because it could be shown that the properdin pathway may be initiated in serum entirely depleted of properdin (13). It was further shown that the initial events depended on the presence of a novel serum protein, termed the initiating factor. Earlier observations in our laboratory showed that proactivator (Factor B), C3b and proactivator convertase (Factor D) form a C3 convertase which exerts a positive feedback (14). In analogy to the cobra venom factor (CVF) dependent C3 convertase (15), this enzyme was proposed to have the composition C3b,Bb, where Bb represents the major physiological fragment of proactivator (16). Fearon, Ruddy and Austen (17) extended these findings by demonstrating that this enzyme may be formed on C3b bearing cells (EC3b) and that under appropriate conditions the cell bound enzyme could initiate lysis of the cell by the late acting complement components. This development afforded precise quantitation of the activity of the enzyme.

On the basis of a large body of experimental evidence accumulated in our laboratory and furnished by other investigators (reviewed in full elsewhere (18)), a comprehensive concept of the molecular dynamics of the properdin pathway was put forth recently by Medicus, Schreiber, Götze and Müller-Eberhard (13). At least five proteins participate in the reactions of the pathway: the critical zymogen of the entire pathway, proactivator or Factor B; a second enzyme, proactivator convertase or Factor D; and the modulators, C3/C3b, initiating factor or Factor I (IF) and properdin (P).

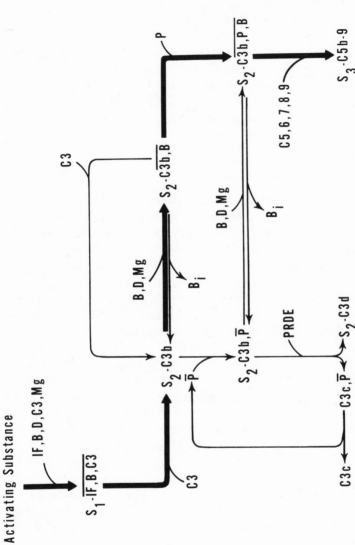

FIGURE 1 – Schematic representation of the molecular dynamics of the properdin pathway. S_1 represents the site of initiation at which the properdin receptor forming enzyme is generated. S_2 denotes the site of attachment of C3b doublets, which serve as properdin receptor. S_2 also is the site of formation of the properdin activating principle which acts as the $\bar{P}$-C5 convertase. S_3 refers to the site of binding of the C5b–9 membrane attack complex. The properdin receptor destroying enzyme (PRDE) acts on several different sites. (From: Medicus, Schreiber, Götze and Müller–Eberhard (13)).

Initiating factor is a heat stable pseudoglobulin which appears to consist of two identical polypeptide chains of 85,000 dalton each (19). The precursor form has, at pH 8.6, the electrophoretic mobility of a β-globulin. Proactivator is a thermolabile β_1-glycoprotein which has pseudoglobulin characteristics. It consists of a single polypeptide chain of 93,000 dalton which on enzymatic activation of the molecule is cleaved into two fragments, Ba (30,000 dalton) and Bb (63,000 dalton) (20). The 63,000 dalton fragment contains the active site; it hydrolyses AGLME (16,21). The enzyme belongs to the group of serine esterase as it is inhibitable by diisofluorophosphate (8). The molecule can also undergo reversible activation without proteolytic cleavage when modulated by activated properdin and native C3 in presence of proactivator convertase (22). The components C3 and C3b are familiar proteins and have been briefly described above. Proactivator convertase is an α-globulin with a molecular weight of 24,000 dalton which consists of a single polypeptide chain (20). The natural substrate of the enzyme is the proactivator. Properdin is a very cationic protein with a molecular weight of 180,000. It is a tetramer which may be dissociated by guanidine hydrochloride into four 45,000–50,000 dalton subunits (23,20).

The flow of events as envisaged by us is schematically depicted in Figure 1. Throughout the pathway, the essential enzymatic site resides in Factor B which initially is in complex with native C3 and IF and later with bound C3b and properdin (P). The initial C3 convertase is generated on the surface of the activating particle (animal, bacterial or fungal cell) without the involvement of P. Experimental evidence suggests that IF establishes contact with chemical structures of the activating particle (S_1) and then interacts with Factors B, D and native C3 to form a loose complex which is endowed with C3 cleaving activity. The enzyme deposits C3b molecules on the particle surface at sites (S_2) located in the vicinity of the enzyme. Binding of Factor D-activated Factor B to C3b results in generation of the bound, labile C3 convertase, C3b,B. By increasing the multiplicity of bound C3b molecules, the enzyme converts itself to the labile C5 convertase, suggesting that the latter consists of at least two critically oriented and closely spaced C3b molecules in complex with Factor B. The labile C3/C5 convertase, which also acts on C3, constitutes the properdin activating principle. Upon collision of native P with the complex, P undergoes a transition to its bound form P̄. Activated P confers an increased degree of stability on C3b,B, converting it to the C3b,P,B enzyme (which was independently demonstrated by Fearon and Austen (24)). The properdin stabilized C5 convertase, as the labile C5 convertase, effects cleavage of C5 and self-assembly of the membrane attack complex C5b-9. Native C3 does not participate in this enzymatic reaction. When present, C3 is turned over and the enzyme is disassembled at a rate greater than that characteristic for its spontaneous decay. Reverse assembly of the enzyme may commence with uptake of P̄ by S_2, C3b and is completed upon incorporation of activated Factor B into the complex. Action of a serum enzyme, the P receptor destroying enzyme (PRDE) on $S_2,C3b$ abrogates its receptor function, and action of the enzyme on $S_2,C3b,\bar{P}$ releases P possibly in association with a C3b fragment. Properdin is recruited late in the sequence rather than early as was previously assumed. Its sole function appears to be that of a stabilizer of the key enzyme of the properdin system.

The AT-forming enzymes of the alternative pathway are the C3 convertase $\overline{C3b,B}$, which generates C3a and the C5 convertase, tentatively denoted $\overline{(C3b)_2,B}$, which generates C5a. The C3 convertase functions as soluble enzyme or in particle-bound form. The C5 convertase apparently occurs only when assembled on a solid phase. A derivative of the enzyme is the properdin stabilized C5 convertase. Formalistically the alternative convertases resemble their classical pathway counterparts. The first C3b molecule fulfills a function analogous to that of C4b in the classical enzymes, while the second C3b molecule fulfills a function analogous to that of C3b in the $\overline{C4b,2a,3b}$ complex. Factor B functions like C2 (Table 1).

That C3a AT can be formed by soluble $\overline{C3b,B}$ was demonstrated by the appearance of C3a activity on incubation of serum with epsilon amino caproic acid (EACA). This compound inhibits serum carboxypeptidase B and the C3b inactivator and thus allows formation of the alternative C3 convertase and active C3a. For generation of C5a AT a solid phase was required (particulate inulin or zymosan) in addition to EACA (25). The use of EACA in conjunction with alternative pathway activators has allowed generation and isolation of the ATs in amounts sufficient for structural studies (26).

Table 1

Composition of the Anaphylatoxin Forming Enzymes

	C3 Convertases	C5 Convertases
Classical	$\overline{C4b,2a}$	$\overline{C4b,2a,3b}$
Alternative	$\overline{C3b,Bb}$	$\overline{C3b,Bb,3b}$

STRUCTURE AND FUNCTION OF THE ANAPHYLATOXINS

The ATs have the following characteristics in common: Both peptides are derived from the α-chain of their respective precursors by restricted proteolysis (4,5). Both peptides have arginine in COOH-terminal position which is essential to their AT activity (27,28). They are composed of a similar number of amino acid residues (28,29). They contain α-helical structure (30,31). Both release histamine from mast cells and cause smooth muscle contraction (32). Intradermally they cause the formation of an immediate wheal and erythema reaction (33).

The two ATs differ in their pharmacological potency and biological specificity, C5a being more potent than C3a and each peptide apparently addressing its own receptor. They are absolutely distinct with respect to leukotactic activity, C5a being active and C3a inactive (34). (The earlier report of chemotactically active C3a produced from isolated C3 by either $C\overline{4,2}$ or trypsin (35) is reproducible and requires further investigation.) Further, C5a contains a carbohydrate moiety and C3a does not (28,29).

C3a is derived from the NH_2-terminal end of the α-chain of C3 by cleavage of the bond between residues 77 and 78 (29). The bond is selectively attacked by the C3 convertase of either the classical or the alternative pathway. The NH_2-terminal position is occupied by serine and the COOH-terminus by arginine (27,29). The molecular weight of the peptide is 8900 dalton (29) and its electrophoretic mobility, at pH 8.6, is $+2.1 \times 10^{-5}$ cm^2 V^{-1} sec^{-1}. Earlier molecular weights, which were based on physical measurements, indicated a lower value (7200 dalton) (27). The present value is based on the known covalent structure of the molecule. The minimal effective concentration that causes contraction of guinea pig ileum in an organ bath is 1.3×10^{-8} M (25) and the minimal dose that causes wheal and erythema formation in the human skin is 2×10^{-12} mol (33).

Hugli (29) recently elaborated the amino acid sequence of the 77 residue peptide. The molecule contains three methionine, two tyrosine and six half-cystine residues and it lacks tryptophan, carbohydrate and free sulfhydryl groups. This very basic peptide possesses two clusters of cationic side chains, one between positions 7 to 21 and the other between positions 64 and 77. Two cysteinylcysteine sequences were found which are joined by a single disulfide bond. One cysteine residue from each of the cysteinylcysteine sequences is disulfide linked to one of the two remaining cysteinyl residues. Thus, all six half-cystine residues which occur in positions 22, 23, 36, 49, 56 and 57 are interlinked, forming a disulfide knot. Such disulfide arrangements are a rare occurrence in small peptides, but have been described for certain pituitary hormones as reviewed by Hugli (29). The circular dichroism spectrum of C3a exhibited pronounced minima at 208 and 222 nm. From the negative mean residue ellipticity it was calculated that C3a contains 40–45% α-helical structure (31).

Two essential structural requirements have been recognized to date for the expression of C3a biological activity: The COOH-terminal arginine and the ordered secondary structure. Removal of the arginine residue by carboxypeptidase B results in total loss of biological activity (27). Treatment with guanidinium chloride and mercaptoethanol also leads to inactivation and loss of negative ellipticity. Upon removal of the denaturing agents, full activity and the typical circular dichroism spectrum are restored (31).

C5a is derived from the α-chain of C5 by C5 convertase of either pathway (4). Its molecular weight had been reported to be approximately 16,000 dalton on the basis of physical measurements (25). Recently, amino acid and COOH-terminal analysis of human C5a performed in our laboratory by Fernandez and Hugli (28) indicated the presence of 73 residues and a molecular weight of 9000 dalton for the peptide moiety. The discrepancy in molecular weight measurements could be explained by Fernandez and Hugli who demonstrated that, unlike C3a, C5a contains a sizable carbohydrate moiety. They found 4 glucosamine, 3–4 neuraminic acid and 7–11 neutral hexose residues per molecule of C5a. Since the total carbohydrate content is 30%, the total molecular weight is estimated to be 12,000 dalton. The COOH-terminus is occupied by arginine, removal of which abrogates AT activity (25,28). Like C3a, the C5a AT has a substantial content of α-helical structure, approximately 40%. Treatment of C5a with mercaptoethanol progressively diminishes the ellipticity at 208 and 222 nm and reduces its AT activity to limiting values. Removal of the reducing agent restores both the characteristic circular dichroism spectrum and the biological activity (30).

The minimal effective concentration of C5a in causing contraction of the guinea pig ileum in an organ bath is 7.5×10^{-10} M (25), the minimal effective dose for causing a cutaneous wheal and erythema is 1×10^{-15} mol (36). The peptide evokes chemotaxis of polymorphonuclear leukocytes at 7×10^{-9} M. Fernandez, Henson and Hugli (34) showed that $C5a_{desArg}$, which is inactive as AT, retained potential leukotactic activity and that expression of this activity required the presence of serum. Some of the properties of the human ATs are listed in Table 2.

Porcine C5a differs from human C5a with respect to the susceptibility of the COOH-terminal residue to carboxypeptidase B (CPB). Porcine C5a generated in absence of EACA has leucine at the COOH-terminus, while arginine is found in this position when EACA was present during incubation of serum. C5a(arg) was active at 3×10^{-10} M, C5a(leu) at 7×10^{-9} M, suggesting that

Table 2

Properties of the Human Anaphylatoxins

	C3a	C5a
Electrophoretic mobility	+2.1	-1.7
Diffusion coefficient	—	12.1
Frictional ratio	—	1.05
Molecular weight:		
Gel filtration	8700	17,500
Gel electrophoresis	7200	16,500
Amino acid analysis	8900	9,000
Carbohydrate content	none	30%
Total molecular weight	8900	12,000
Amino acid residues	77	73
COOH-terminus	arginine	arginine
Activity:		
Ileum contraction	1.3×10^{-8} M	4×10^{-10} M
Leukotaxis	inactive	7×10^{-9} M
Wheal and flare	2×10^{-12} mol	1×10^{-15} mol

C5a(leu) is 90% inactivated (37). Porcine C5a, which contained COOH-terminal arginine was resistant to CPB and its arginine could only be removed by CPB after boiling of the peptide. It is proposed therefore that nascent C5a in porcine serum is susceptible to inactivation by serum CPB, and that due to a subsequent conformational change, the residual, active C5a becomes resistant to the enzyme and remains active.

CONTROL

Both C3a and C5a are controlled by serum CPB, which is an α-globulin with a molecular weight of 300,000 (38). It is responsible for total suppression of C3a AT and C5a AT activity in human serum and C3a AT activity in porcine serum. It inactivates these peptides by highly efficient removal of their COOH-terminal arginine residue. Inhibition of the enzyme with EACA allows demonstration of C3a and C5a activity in whole human serum following complement activation (25).

CONCLUSION

Our knowledge of the biochemistry and biology of the anaphylatoxins has been significantly advanced in recent years. Four enzymes are responsible for the release of the anaphylatoxins from their precursors: The C3 and C5 convertases of the classical and the alternative complement pathways. These four enzymes utilize two zymogens, C2 and Factor B. Three of the enzymes also utilize C3b as an essential subunit. The fragment C3b is a product of the very parent molecule from which C3a AT is derived.

Both ATs are potent biological effectors. On a molar basis C5a is approximately twenty times as active as C3a. However, human serum contains twenty times more C3a precursor than C5a precursor, and the turnover of C3 by the C3 convertases is more than twenty times greater than the turnover of C5 by the C5 convertases. The latter are exceedingly slow enzymes. These quantitative considerations appear to balance the relative biological significance of C3a and C5a.

Both peptides exhibit differences and similarities in structure and function. It is probable that a comparison of their covalent structure, when it becomes possible, will reveal certain common characteristics that will account for their partially similar function. The fact that one peptide contains a sizable carbohydrate moiety while the other does not may explain some of their differential functional properties.

The biological potency of the peptides demands rigid regulation of their activity. This regulation is exercised by the enzyme serum carboxypeptidase B, which removes the COOH-terminal arginine residue from both C3a and C5a, thereby effecting abrogation of AT activity. Serum carboxypeptidase B appears to be geared primarily towards the ATs because its AT inactivating efficiency far exceeds its inactivating action on the kinins. In spite of the control which the high molecular weight enzyme exercises within the vasculature, the ATs can express their biological activities in the extravascular space as the results of their intradermal injection have shown. More work is needed to define the functions of these highly potent and highly regulated peptides in vivo.

This is publication number 1124. This work was supported by Grants AI 07007 and HL 16411 from the National Institutes of Health. Dr. Müller-Eberhard is the Cecil H. and Ida M. Green Investigator in Medical Research, Scripps Clinic and Research Foundation.

REFERENCES

1. Müller-Eberhard, H.J., and Vallota, E.H., In: Biochemistry of the Acute Allergic Reactions, Second Intl. Symposium. K.F. Austen and E.L. Becker, Eds., Blackwell Scientific Publications, Oxford, 1971, p. 217.

2. Vogt, W., Pharmacol. Rev., 26, 125, 1974.

3. Müller-Eberhard, H.J., Ann. Rev. Biochem., 44, 697, 1975.

4. Nilsson, U.R., Mandle, R.J., Jr., and Mapes, J.A., J. Immunol., 114, 815, 1975.

5. Bokisch, V.A., Dierich, M.P., and Müller-Eberhard, H.J., Proc. Nat. Acad. Sci. USA, 72, 1989, 1975.

6. Müller-Eberhard, H.J., Polley, M.J., and Calcott, M.A., J. Exp. Med., 125, 359, 1967.

7. Cooper, N.R., Biochemistry, 14, 4245, 1975.

8. Medicus, R.G., Götze, O., and Müller-Eberhard, H.J., Manuscript in preparation.

9. Stroud, R.M., Mayer, M.M., Miller, J.A., and McKenzie, A.T., Immunochemistry, 3, 163, 1966.

10. Polley, M.J., and Müller-Eberhard, H.J., J. Exp. Med., 128, 533, 1968.

11. Müller-Eberhard, H.J., Manuscript in preparation.

12. Müller-Eberhard, H.J., In: Proteases and Biological Control. E. Reich, D.B. Rifkin, and E. Shaw, Eds., Cold Spring Harbor Laboratory, 1975, p. 229.

13. Medicus, R.G., Schreiber, R.D., Götze, O., and Müller-Eberhard, H.J., Proc. Nat. Acad. Sci. USA, 73, 612, 1976.

14. Müller-Eberhard, H.J., and Götze, O., J. Exp. Med., 135, 1003, 1972.

15. Cooper, N.R., J. Exp. Med., 137, 451, 1973.

16. Götze, O., and Müller-Eberhard, H.J., J. Exp. Med., 134, 90s, 1971.

17. Fearon, D.T., Austen, K.F., and Ruddy, S., J. Exp. Med., 138, 1305, 1973.

18. Götze, O., and Müller-Eberhard, H.J., Adv. Immunol., 23, 1976, In Press.

19. Schreiber, R.D., Götze, O., and Müller-Eberhard, H.J., Fed. Proc., 35, 253, 1976.

20. Götze, O., In: Proteases and Biological Control. E. Reich, D.B. Rifkin, and E. Shaw, Eds., Cold Spring Harbor Laboratory, 1975, p. 255.

21. Cooper, N.R., In: Progress in Immunology. B. Amos, Ed., Academic Press, New York, Vol. 1, 1971, p. 567.

22. Schreiber, R.D., Medicus, R.G., Götze, O., and Müller-Eberhard, H.J., J. Exp. Med., 142, 760, 1975.

23. Minta, J.O., and Lepow, I.H., J. Immunol., 111, 286, 1973.
24. Fearon, D.T., and Austen, K.F., J. Exp. Med., 142, 856, 1975.
25. Vallota, E.H., and Müller-Eberhard, H.J., J. Exp. Med., 137, 1109,
      1973.
26. Hugli, T.E., Vallota, E.H., and Müller-Eberhard, H.J., J. Biol.
      Chem., 250, 1472, 1974.
27. Budzko, D.B., Bokisch, V.A., and Müller-Eberhard, H.J., Biochem-
      istry, 10, 1166, 1971.
28. Fernandez, H.N., and Hugli, T.E., Fed. Proc., 35, 1976, In Press.
29. Hugli, T.E., J. Biol. Chem., 250, 8293, 1975.
30. Morgan, W.T., Vallota, E.H., and Müller-Eberhard, H.J., Biochem.
      Biophys. Res. Comm., 57, 572, 1974.
31. Hugli, T.E., Morgan, W.T., and Müller-Eberhard, H.J., J. Biol.
      Chem., 250, 1479, 1974.
32. Johnson, A.R., Hugli, T.E., and Müller-Eberhard, H.J., Immunology,
      28, 1067, 1975.
33. Wuepper, K.D., Bokisch, V.A., Müller-Eberhard, H.J., and Stoughton,
      R.B., Clin. Exp. Immunol., 11, 13, 1972.
34. Fernandez, H.N., Henson, P.M., and Hugli, T.E., J. Immunol., 1976,
      In Press.
35. Bokisch, V.A., Müller-Eberhard, H.J., and Cochrane, C.G., J. Exp.
      Med., 129, 1109, 1969.
36. Vallota, E.H., and Müller-Eberhard, H.J., Fed. Proc., 31, 624, 1972.
37. Vallota, E.H., Hugli, T.E., and Müller-Eberhard, H.J., J. Immunol.,
      1976, In Press.
38. Bokisch, V.A., and Müller-Eberhard, H.J., J. Clin. Invest., 49, 2427,
      1970.

DISCUSSION

MOVAT: I wonder if you could comment on the biological activity of anaphylatoxins. In the 1950s Rocha and Silva, Hahn
and other showed that the effect of classical anaphylatoxin
(presumably C5a) was partially suppressed by antihistamines in
the guinea pig.

Subsequently Dias da Silva and Lepow were able to demonstrate degranulation of rat mast cells by C3a. In addition, however, Vogt and others demonstrated non-histamine mediated effects of anaphylatoxins.

What then is the mode of action of anaphylatoxins in addition to the direct effect, i.e. does C5a act on guinea pig mast
cells, releasing histamine and C3a on rat mast cells? Can you
estimate how much of the activity is due to the direct effect
and how much is due to histamine release?

MÜLLER-EBERHARD: Both human C3a and C5a release histamine

from rat mast cells, as was shown by Dr. Alice Johnson in our
laboratory. Their histamine releasing ability is comparable,
which is in contrast to their considerably different potency
in the contraction of guinea pig ileum. C5a is approximately
20 times more active than C3a.

C3a has also been shown to degranulate human cutaneous
mast cells following intradermal injection of the peptide. In
addition to acting via histamine, both peptides appear to have
a direct effect on smooth muscle. The relative contribution of
direct and histamine-mediated action is not known.

DIAMANT: Would it be possible to get activation of the
complement system in an in vitro system consisting of sensitized
lung tissue after challenge with antigen in the absence of added
serum?

MÜLLER-EBERHARD: In absence of serum which contains the
anaphylatoxin precursors this possibility appears remote. However, given the proper antibody and complement components, anaphylatoxin should arise in sensitized lung tissue.

LICHTENSTEIN: There is nor evidence, nor much likelihood,
that IgE mediated mast cell reactions lead to release of anaphylatoxin. Moreover, work by Petersson et al., Grant and Siraganian have shown that in the basophils histamine release caused by C5a seems to operate by a mechanism different to that induced by antigen; cells desensitized by antigen are still fully
responsive to C5a and vice versa.

MÜLLER-EBERHARD: Certainly, neither C3a nor C5a render the
ileum of a sensitized guinea pig unresponsive to antigen and
vice versa.

GOETZL: How does the peaks of chemotactic activity of C5a
des Arg and serum compare to the optimal chemotactic concentration of native C5a and what is your explanation for the ability
of serum to restore chemotactic activity to C5a des Arg?

MÜLLER-EBERHARD: We have no information on the nature of
the serum factor or factors that render C5a des Arg leukotacti-
cally active.

BECKER: Would not a further possible explanation be that
there is a further degradation of the inactive des-arginine
derivative which leads to a chemotactically active component.

MÜLLER-EBERHARD: This is a distinct possibility.

LICHTENSTEIN: Is there much likelihood, with the control
systems present in man, that C3a or C5a are activated in vivo?

MÜLLER-EBERHARD: There is every reason to believe that C3a
and C5a are generated in vivo. Their rapid inactivation by serum
carboxypeptidase B does not preclude their acting effectively
in a tissue microenvironment, where the concentration of serum
carboxypeptidase B is probably rather low due to its high molecular weight (300,000). That the anaphylatoxins can in fact act
in the tissues is shown by their effect in the skin.

COCHRANE: In response to Dr. Lichtenstein's question concerning possible in vivo activity of C3a or C5a I would like

to add that we have seen that rapid activation of C3a in rabbits
by i.v. injection of cobra venom factor (CoF) brings about a
short lasting but distinct hypotensive episode.

That this effect is related to C3 and terminal components
(perhaps the anaphylatoxins) was supported by experiments in
which C3 was removed 1-2 days before infusion of CoF i.v.
and no hypotensive effect was observed.

UVNÄS: From what sera do you isolate your anaphylatoxins?
Does any species specificity exist?

MÜLLER-EBERHARD: We isolate C3a and C5a from both human
and porcine serum after treatment with zymosan or particulate
inulin. It is important, however, that 1M epsilon amino caproic
acid is present to inhibit the serum carboxypeptidase B. We
have not been able to detect species specificity with respect
to biological activity.

AUSTEN: In the fluid phase, can the activation be initiated by C3, B, $\overline{D}$, and $\overline{P}$?

MÜLLER-EBERHARD: The reaction can in fact be initiated by
a soluble C3 convertase of the alternative pathway. More incubation of serum with 1 M ε-amino caproic acid results in proactivator dependent accumulation of active C3a, but not of C5a.

It is probable that the $\overline{P}$-stabilized fluid phase C3 convertase also leads to C3a anaphylatoxin production.

SOME INTERRELATIONS AMONG CHEMOTAXIS, LYSOSOMAL ENZYME SECRETION AND PHAGOCYTOSIS BY NEUTROPHILS [*]

Elmer L. Becker

Department of Pathology, University of Connecticut

Health Center, Farmington, CT 06032 U.S.A.

A number of acute allergic responses e.g. the Arthus reaction, experimental nephrotoxic nephritis etc involve the chemotaxis, lysosomal enzyme secretion and phagocytosis of neutrophils. In these reactions, chemotactic factors liberated at the site causes infiltration of neutrophils and the secretion of lysosomal enzymes from these cells induced by actual or frustrated phagocytosis of the antigen-antibody complexes initiating the reaction induces the tissue damage (1). These functions of the neutrophil are not completely independent and unrelated. There are a number of similarities and differences in the biochemical requirements for each of these functions (2). In addition all the chemotactic factors tested, C5a, pronase sensitive and pronase insensitive fractions from E. coli culture filtrates and synthetic peptides are capable of inducing not only chemotaxis but lysosomal enzyme release (3, 4) and if these same factors are presented to the neutrophil at the same time as the particle, EAC423 they also will inhibit erythrophagocytosis (5).

However, we are still quite ignorant as to how the chemotactic factors or any other stimulus initiate any of these functions. The size, complexity and unknown structure of most chemotactic factors have prevented drawing any firm inferences as to the nature of the primary interaction of chemotactic agents with the neutrophil surface. Recently Schiffmann et al reported that simple N-formyl methionyl peptides enhanced the migration of neutrophils and were

[*] Supported by N.I.H. grant A109648 and N.I.H. contract NIDR-N-01-DE-52477.

presumably chemotactic $\overset{2}{\vee}$ (6). Based on this finding, my colleagues
and I have begun a systematic study of the relation of the structure of simple peptides, to their ability to stimulate neutrophil
movement, to induce lysosomal enzyme secretion (7) and to enhance
phagocytosis(vide infra). In what follows I shall briefly summarize the results we have obtained so far, describe the inferences drawn concerning the nature of the primary interaction of
chemotactic peptide and neutrophil surface and then indulge in some
speculations as to the possible general interrelationships among
random locomotion, chemotaxis and lysosomal enzyme secretion and
phagocytosis suggested by these and other findings.

STRUCTURE-ACTIVITY RELATIONS OF SYNTHETIC PEPTIDES

Over 24 peptides mostly di and tripeptides have been synthesized and tested for their activity. All but two of them are methionyl or N-formyl methionyl derivatives. Rabbit peritoneal neutrophils were used throughout. The assay of the relative migratory
activity of the peptides employed the penetration into the filter
of a modified Boyden chamber as described previously (8).

Various substances induce increased penetration of cells into
the filter of a Boyden chamber system either by enhancing their
random locomotion or their response to a chemical gradient of the
substance (chemotaxis) or both. Zigmond and Hirsch (9) have described a technique for determining if the movement of the cell
into the filter of a Boyden chamber system under the influence of
different gradients is greater than could be expected on the basis
of increased rates of random locomotion and to that extent is due
to a true chemotactic response. Their technique was used to test
two representative synthetic peptides, F-Met-Leu-Phe and F-Met-Met-
Met over the range of 6 x 2 x 10^{-12}M to 5 x 10^{-10}M and 10^{-9}M to
10^{-6}M respectively. Over these ranges of concentration,the effects
of the two peptides were rapid and largely reversible, the basic
conditions for the appropriate application of the technique. Both
peptides were found to stimulate random movement of the neutrophil.
In addition, the neutrophils under the influence of a positive concentration gradient of the peptides moved into the filter significantly farther than predicted on the basis of a random walk process

$\overset{2}{\vee}$ The Boyden chamber system measures enhanced migration due to
either an increase in random migration or directed migration (chemotaxis). In the interests of terminological precision, in what
follows, I have used the non-committal terms "enhanced migration"
or "stimulated movement" etc. to describe results obtained by the
Boyden chamber system except under where the author(s) has experimentally demonstrated the nature of the movement.

in which the only variable was the rate of random locomotion and not as far as predicted when the concentration gradient was negative (7). Thus, at least part of the movement induced by the class of peptides under discussion is chemotactic.

The migration enhancing activities of the various peptides were measured by plotting the stimulated locomotory activity against the logarithm of the concentration of peptide. The resulting sigmoid dose response curves were parallel in their linear portions and had the same maximum (7, 10). It was therefore possible to validly describe the activities of the different peptides in terms of their ED_{50}'s, the concentration of chemotactic factor giving 50% of the maximum activity.

Like other chemotactic factors (11, 12), the peptides in the presence of 5 μg/ml cytochalasin B induce the release of the lysosomal enzymes, β glucuronidase and lysozyme but cause no release of the cytoplasmic marker enzyme, lactic dehydrogenase, LDH. Parallel sigmoid log dose response curves were obtained for the release of β glucuronidase and lysozyme allowing the ability of a given peptide to induce secretion of the two enzymes to be expressed as its ED_{50} for each enzyme.

Fig. 1, adapted from (7) shows a comparison of the ED_{50}'s of the migration enhancing activity and the secretory inducing activity for lysozyme and β glucuronidase for the 19 peptides that were sufficiently active to induce both chemotaxis and secretion. Each value for the ED_{50} seen in Fig. 1 is the mean of three separate experiments.

Fig. 1, makes apparent both the activity of certain of the peptides and the wide spread in their activities. The peptide with the highest activity, F-Met-Leu-Phe, (#3, Fig. 1), had an ED_{50} for migration enhancement of $7.0 \times 10^{-11}M$ and for lysozyme and for β glucuronidase release of $2.4 \times 10^{-10}M$ and 2.6×10^{-10} respectively; the corresponding ED_{50}s for the peptide of the lowest activity, Met-Met-Met (14, Fig. 1) are 1.0×10^{-4}, 8.8×10^{-4} and $7.2 \times 10^{-4}M$, respectively. The difference between the activities of the two peptides is over a million fold. The migratory enhancing activity of F-Met-Leu-Phe can be easily detected at $1 \times 10^{-11}M$ and with sufficiently active cells at $1 \times 10^{-12}M$. The number of cells used in the assay of migration enhancement is 2.5×10^{6}. At a concentration of $10^{-11}M$ this corresponds to approximately 2000 molecules of peptide per cell; the number of molecules at the leading edge of the gradient is obviously less than this. F-Met-Leu-Phe is probably not the most active peptide obtainable. This suggest the possibility that only one or a few molecules per cell of the most active compound might be sufficient to stimulate movement.

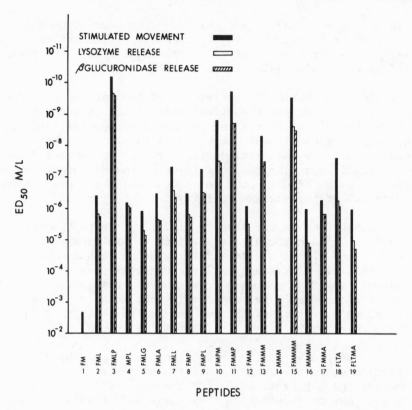

1. The relation between the structure and activity (ED_{50}) of different peptides in stimulating movement and inducing secretion of lysozyme or β glucuronidase. 1. F-Met, 2. F-Met-Leu, 3. F-Met-Leu-Phe, 4. Met-Leu-Phe, 5. F-Met-Leu-Glu, 6. F-Met-Leu-Ala, 7. F-Met-Leu-Leu, 8. F-Met-Phe, 9. F-Met-Phe-Leu, 10. F-Met-Phe-Met, 11. F-Met-Met-Phe, 12. F-Met-Met, 13. F-Met-Met-Met, 14. Met-Met-Met, 15. F-Met-Met-Met-Met, 16. Met-Met-Met-Met, 17. F-Met-Met-Ala, 18. F-Leu-Trp-Met, 19. F-Leu-Met-Arg. These are a partial summary of the results reported in (7).

There are striking regularities and a very great specificity in the relation of the structure of the synthetic peptides to their activity (Fig. 1), the activity of a peptide depends not only on its constituent amino acids but on the position of a given amino acid in the peptide chain. The latter can be seen by considering the structural requirements for optimal activity starting at the NH_2-terminal end of the peptide.

In confirmation of the findings of Schiffmann et al (6)

blocking the positively charged NH_2-terminal group greatly increases activity. For example, the ED_{50} for Met-Leu-Phe (Fig. 1, 4) is $6.7 \times 10^{-7}M$, whereas, the ED_{50} of F-Met-Leu-Phe (Fig. 1, 3) is $7 \times 0^{-11}M$, a 10,000 fold increase in activity. The increases in activity on N-formylating Met-Met-Met (Fig. 1, 14) or Met-Met-Met-Met (Fig. 1, 16) to form F-Met-Met-Met(Fig. 1, 13) and F-Met-Met-Met (Fig. 1, 15) respectively, are of the same order of magnitude.

Schiffmann et al (6) reported that F-methionine is required in the amino terminal position for migration enhancing activity. The activity of F-Leu-Trp-Met (Fig. 1, 18), with an ED_{50} of 5.7×10^{-8} and F-Leu-Trp-Met-Arg, with an ED_{50} of $1.1 \times 10^{-5}M$ indicate that there is no absolute requirement for methionine in the amino terminal position.

The three dipeptides F-Met-Leu (Fig. 1, 2), F-Met-Phe (Fig. 1, 8) and F-Met-Met (Fig. 1, 12), have essentially the same activity. The positively charged F-Met-His and negatively charged F-Met-Glu were found to be distinctly less active than F-Met-Leu (6). These findings suggest that the only requirements for maximum activity in the second position from the amino terminal end is that the amino acid be neutral and sufficiently non-polar.

Although leucine, methionine and phenylalanine are essentially equivalent in the second position of the F-Met dipeptides, this is not the case when they are in the third position of the F-Met tripeptides. Phenylalanine in the third position contributes much more to the activity than either methionine or leucine. F-Met-Leu-Phe (Fig. 1, 3) is 500 times more active than F-Met-Leu-Leu (Fig. 1, 7), and F-Met-Met-Phe (Fig. 1, 11) is approximately 20-30 times more active than F-Met-Met-Met (Fig. 1, 13). Methionine, leucine and phenylalanine affect activity to approximately the same extent when they are in the second position of a tripeptide: the ED_{50} for chemotaxis of F-Met-Phe-Leu (Fig. 1, 9) is $5.4 \times 10^{-8}M$, that of F-Met-Met-Leu (Fig. 1, 6) is $4.8 \times 10^{-8}M$; the ED_{50} of F-Met-Phe-Met (Fig. 1, 10) is 1.5×10^{-9} and that of F-Met-Met-Met (Fig. 1, 13) is 5.1×10^{-9}. Thus, phenylalanine when in the second position of a di or tripeptide, is approximately equivalent to leucine or methionine, however in the third position, phenylalanine is much more active than the other two amino acids. Whether the specific effect of phenylalanine in the third position of the tripeptides is due to its aromatic character or its structural specificity is not known. Neither is it known whether the high activity of phenyl -- alanine is due to its being in the third position of a tripeptide or because it is terminal.

Another striking aspect of Fig. 1 is the closeness with which the migration enhancing activity of the various peptides correlates with their ability to induce lysozyme and β glucuronidase secretion. The correlation coefficients obtained when the logarithms of the

ED_{50}s for migration enhancing activity are plotted against the logarithms of the ED_{50}s for β glucuronidase or lysozyme are both 0.98 (7) and this close correlation is over a million fold range in concentrations. When the logarithm of the ED_{50}s are plotted against the logarithms of the ED_{50}s for either β glucuronidase or lysozyme release the slopes of the straight lines that are obtained are both indistinguishable from 1.0 (7), indicating that the enzyme releasing and migration enhancing activity of the peptides are linearly related to each other.

Inspection of Fig. 1 also reveals that higher concentrations of peptide are required to give lysosomal enzyme release than a corresponding migration enhancing response. On the average, rabbit neutrophils require approximately 7.5 times more peptide for lysozyme release and 9.3 times more for β glucuronidase than for migration enhancement (7).

THE NATURE OF THE PRIMARY INTERACTION OF PEPTIDE CHEMOTACTIC FACTOR WITH THE NEUTROPHIL SURFACE

Wilkinson has suggested that although non-polar side chains are of key importance in chemotactic recognition, as long as this requirement is met there is no real necessity for a structurally specific interaction of cell and chemotactic factor (13). The results just described support the idea that non-polar side chains are of importance in activity but do not agree with the hypothesis that the only key factor is the hydrophobicity of the chemotactic agent. Rather they show also the critical importance of structural specificity. This is demonstrated by the very large contribution to activity of the terminal phenylalanine; the manner in which the quantitative nature of the contribution of phenylalanine depends on its position in the peptide chain; the difference in activity between formyl-methionyl and acetyl-methionyl peptides reported by Schiffmann et al (6); the fact that F-Met-Leu-Phe is 500 times more active than F-Met-Phe-Leu and F-Met-Met-Phe is 10 times more active than F-Met-Phe-Met even though in these latter instances one would not expect the pairs of compound to differ very much in their hydrophobicity.

The simplest hypothesis explaining the nature of the relationships between the structure of the peptides and their acitivty is that the peptides bind to a structurally specific receptor on the neutrophil surface. This hypothesis is in accord with the extremely great specificity of the structural requirements and, even more, the manner in which the activity depends not only on the nature of the amino acids but also on their position in the peptide chain.

The wide variety of agents reported to be chemotactic (reviewed in 13) suggests the possibility that other chemotactic receptors on the neutrophil exist in addition to the one postulated for the synthetic peptides. Moreover, we cannot preclude the additional possibility that one or more of these are not structurally specific. Admittedly, however, this openmindedness is more a tribute to our ignorance of the structural requirements for activity than an acknowledgment of the neutrophils' tolerance of diversity.

There is some evidence that both random locomotion and chemotaxis may result from the interaction of the chemotactic agents with the same putative receptor. In the relatively few instances where this has been looked at, the peptides and other chemotactic agents induce increased random locomotion and chemotaxis in the same range of concentrations (7, 9).

As already pointed out, there is an essentially exact correlation between the migration enhancing and enzyme secreting activities of synthetic peptides. This strongly suggests that the same primary interaction of peptide with neutrophil surface initiates both phenomena i.e. that not only random locomotion and chemotaxis but the secretion of lysozyme and of β glucuronidase can be triggered by the same neutrophil receptor.

All chemotactic agents so far tested, including the synthetic peptides, when added to neutrophil and erythrocyte are able to inhibit in an apparent competitive fashion the initial rates of erythrophagocytosis (5). More direct evidence of an ability of chemotactic factors to affect phagocytosis is seen in Fig. 2. Fig. 2 shows that F-Met-Leu-Phe adsorbed to latex spherules (0.81 μm diameter) greatly enhances their ingestion by rabbit peritoneal neutrophils. This finding is in agreement with the mention by Henson of unpublished work showing that C5a adsorbed to latex particles enhances their phagocytosis (15). The data concerning the ability of chemotactic factors to affect phagocytosis are all preliminary; no structure-activity studies have been attempted, although these are planned. Nevertheless, the results obtained so far make clear that in addition to the other capabilities of the chemotactic peptides, they also can enhance phagocytosis. A reasonable hypothesis, currently guiding our work is that the peptides interact with the same putative receptor to induce phagocytosis as well as the other neutrophil functions.

Hook et al have demonstrated that certain of the F-methionyl peptides also induce non-cytotoxic histamine release from human basophils (2). No structure activity comparisons have been made. Dr. Sheldon Taubman of the Department of Pathology, University of Connecticut Health Center, has shown in unpublished work that none of the synthetic peptides tested, including the most active are able to release histamine from rat peritoneal mast cells.

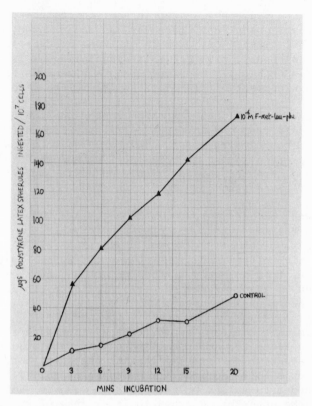

2. The ability of F-Met-Leu-Phe when adsorbed to latex spherules
to enhance their ingestion by rabbit peritoneal neutrophils. Latex
particles (0.81 mμ diameter, 20 mg 11.2 ml)incubated with 10^{-6}M
F-Met-Leu-Phe for one hour at 37° washed once and resuspended to
original volume. 10^{-7} neutrophils with 0.5 mg / ml particles incubated for designated times and ingestion measured as described
in (14).

THE LIKELIHOOD THAT THE VARIOUS NEUTROPHIL FUNCTIONS
RESULT FROM PARALLEL BIOCHEMICAL SEQUENCES

Assuming that the combination of peptide with the same neutrophil receptor induces random and directed movement, lysosomal enzyme
secretion and phagocytosis (and probably other responses) one can
imagine that these various responses are effected in one of two general ways. The first is that the peptide-receptor combination triggers a single series of biochemical steps one or another part of
which is responsible for causing each of the various neutrophil
functions. The second view is that the peptide receptor interaction
initiates a series of parallel but coordinated and interdependent

biochemical sequences which are responsible for the various neutrophil functions. What evidence we have suggests that it is the
latter which is more likely to be correct.

The various neutrophil functions can be dissociated from each
other in a variety of ways which make it improbable that these functions are responses to parts of a single sequence (reviewed in 2).
In addition, there need not be a rigid coupling of stimulated random and directed locomotion with all substances and under all conditions. Agents such as K^+ (16) and ascorbic acid (17) are not
chemotactic although they enhance random locomotion. Approximately
one third of the lysozyme comes from primary granules, the remain-
der from secondary granules; all of the β glucuronidase resides in
the primary granule (18). The average maximum release of lysozyme
by the peptides is over 80 percent of the total neutrophil lysozyme (7); there is a close correlation between the releasing activities of the synthetic peptide for both enzymes. Thus, the stimulation of the same putative receptor may induce release from both primary and secondary granules. Nevertheless, approximately 25 percent more peptide is required to release 50 percent of the total
β glucuronidase than to release the same proportion of β glucuronidase (7). This implies that the release of the two enzymes is not
rigidly coupled, and in fact, it has been found that, under at least
some circumstances, the release of two enzymes may proceed more or
less independently (3, 19, Becker and Showell unpublished information, 17).

SPECULATIONS CONCERNING THE NATURE OF THE INTERRELATIONS
OF THE EFFECTOR MECHANISMS OF CHEMOTAXIS, RANDOM LOCOMOTION
LYSOSOMAL ENZYME SECRETION AND PHAGOCYTOSIS

I have not forgotten the warning of Calvin Webb about
imaginative insight having to stop short of delerium;
but defeatism is a crime too. The Healing Hand. G. Majno.

All of the neutrophil functions just discussed involved some
form of movement, either of the whole cell as in chemotaxis and
random locomotion; movement of a cell organelle,the granule, from
the cell interior to the plasma membrane, as in lysosomal enzyme
secretion; or movement of a portion of the cell membrane and con-
tiguous structures around the particle, as in phagocytosis. It is
reasonable, therefore in trying to understand how the chemotactic
factors can induce or enhance these various functions to consider
the mechanisms of cell movement which might be involved. The two
systems currently postulated to be concerned in movement of the
neutrophil are the micro-tubules and micro-filaments (2, 21). I wish
now to consider in summary fashion what is known or suspected about

the involvement of these two systems in the cell functions of the neutrophil.

There is evidence that microfilaments are required in random locomotion, chemotaxis and phagocytosis but probably not in induced lysosomal enzyme secretion. A patient subject to recurrent infections possessed neutrophils deficient in random locomotion, chemotaxis and ingestion but with enhanced lysosomal degranulation (22). Associated with these functional defects was a decrease in the number of microfilaments and a lessened ability of actin isolated from the neutrophils to polymerize in vitro. Cytochalasin B which inter alia interferes with microfilament function, inhibits random locomotion and chemotaxis (23, 24, 25) and phagocytosis (25, 26) but enhances lysosomal enzyme release (11, 27).

A number of workers have suggested that microtubules superimpose direction or orientation to leukocyte movement but are not required for movement itself (28 – 31). There is conflicting evidence that microtubules are required in lysosomal enzyme secretion from neutrophils and the bulk of the evidence suggests that they are not required for phagocytosis.

C5a, a chemotactic factor induces the transient assembly of microtubules in the presence of cytochalasin B (32) and a more prolonged assembly in its absence (33). Colchicine and other anti-microtubule agents although not affecting or even enhancing random locomotion (11, 30, 34, 35) inhibit stimulated movement (11, 30, 34-38). However, different investigators have reported wide variations in the concentrations required for inhibition. In addition, trimethyl colchicinic acid, which has no effect on microtubules, inhibits the response to chemotactic agents, although higher concentrations are required than colchicine (37).

A defect in microtubule assembly is reported to be the basic deficiency in the neutrophils of mice with Chediak-Higashi syndrome (39). The response to chemotactic factors of the neutrophils of patients with this syndrome is defective although random locomotion is reportedly unaffected (40, 41); see, however (42).

There is a large variation in the reported effects of colchicine and other anti-microtubule agents on lysosomal enzyme secretion. In many cases, these substances are reported to inhibit secretion (11, 43) but frequently at concentrations above those presumably required to inhibit microtubule function, and in some instances no inhibition was obtained (44, 45). A difficulty with most of these studies is that no ultra-structural studies were done to actually demonstrate that the anti-microtubule agents actually had the effect presumed. Hofstein et al correlated microtubule assembly with lysosomal enzyme release under a variety of conditions and concluded that microtubule assembly was a necessary but not sufficient condition for lysosomal enzyme secretion (46). Neutrophils of patients with Chediak-Higashi syndrome are reported to be defective in their ability to degranulate (42, 47).

At this time it is, therefore, necessary to conclude that although there is suggestive evidence that microtubules are required in neutrophil lysosomal enzyme release more work is necessary before this conclusion can be whole heartedly accepted.

Colchicine and other anti-microtubule agents either have no effect on phagocytosis (48) or inhibit it at concentrations far beyond those required to affect microtubules (49). The only exception is the report of Stossel et al (50) who found that colchicine gave a dose-dependent reduction in the rate of phagocytosis. The degree of inhibition except at the very highest concentrations was not impressive. However the conditions were probably not optimum for colchicine to act on microtubules. The neutrophils of patients with Chediak-Higashi syndrome phagocytize oil droplets more rapidly than normally (47), in accord with the hypothesis of a non-requirement for microtubules in phagocytosis.

The evidence, thus, suggests that there is no absolute need for microtubule involvement in phagocytosis. If the zipper hypothesis of the mechanism of phagocytosis (50) applies to neutrophils,the movement of the membrane around a particle to form a phagosome would be directed by the stimulation afforded by the successive interaction of particle and neutrophil surface and would not require the direction by microtubules.

The very tentative conclusions that arise from this brief and incomplete survey are summarized in Table 1. In Table 1 we see that random locomotion results from the activation of the microfilament system; activation of the microtubule system superimposes direction (chemotaxis) upon the movement. Phagocytosis requires microfilaments but questionably does not require the microtubule system, although the latter may play an adjunct role. Lysosomal enzyme secretion does not appear to require microfilaments, and in fact they may impede secretion. There is conflicting evidence that microtubule function is required.

TABLE 1

	Microfilaments	Microtubules
Random Locomotion	+	−
Chemotaxis	+	+
Phagocytosis	+	− ?
Lysosomal Enzyme Secretion	−	+ ?

SUMMARY

A series of synthetic di and tripeptides, most of them formyl methionyl peptides, are chemotactic, and stimulate random locomotion and lysosomal enzyme secretion by neutrophils. The high degree of activity of the peptides, their specificity and the nature of the structural requirements strongly suggest that the primary interaction of peptide and neutrophil is a binding of the peptide with a stereo-specific receptor on the neutrophil surface. Whether all chemotactic factors act through the same putative receptor is unknown.

An essentially exact correlation exists between the concentration of synthetic peptides required to induce migration and their ability to induce release of lysozyme or β glucuronidase. One of the peptides, F-Met-Leu-Phe when adsorbed to a latex particle enhances its phagocytosis.

The overall hypothesis suggested by these and other findigns is that a synthetic peptide of the proper structure (and possibly other agents) interacts with a single type of structurally specific receptor on the neutrophil surface to initiate a series of parallel but coordinated and interdependent biochemical sequences leading to microfilament and microtubule activation in addition to other processes. Depending on how the stimulus is presented to the cell this may result in phagocytosis, random locomotion, chemotaxis and/ or lysosomal enzyme secretion (see also 15).

REFERENCES

1. Cochrane, C.G.,1968. Immunologic tissue injury mediated by neutrophilic leukocytes. Adv. Immunol. 9:97-163.

2. Becker, E.L. and P.M. Henson, 1973. In vitro studies of immuno-logically induced secretion of mediators from cells and related phenomena. Adv. Immunol. 17:93-193.

3. Becker, E.L., P.M. Henson, H.J. Showell and L.S. Hsu, 1974. The ability of chemotactic factors to induce lysosomal enzyme release 1. The characteristics of the release, the importance of surfaces and the relation of the release to chemotactic responsiveness. J. Immunol. 112:2047-2054.

4. Goldstein, I.M., M. Brai, A.G. Osler and G. Weissmann, 1973. Lysosomal enzyme release from human leukocytes: Mediation by the alternate pathway of complement activation. J. Immunol. 109:33-37.

5. R. Musson and E.L. Becker, 1975. The effect of chemotactic
    factors on erythrophagocytosis by human neutrophils. Fed.
    Proceed. 34:1019.

6. Schiffmann, E., B.A. Corcoran and S.M. Wall, 1975. Formyl-
    methionyl peptides as chemoattractants for leucocytes . Proc.
    Nat. Acad. Sci. U.S.A. 70:2916 - 2918.

7. Showell, H.J., R.J. Freer, S.H. Zigmond, E. Schiffmann, S.
    Aswankumar, B. Corcoran and E.L. Becker, 1976. The structure
    activity relations of synthetic peptides as chemotactic fac-
    tors and inducers of lysosomal enzyme secretion for neutrophils.
    J. Exp. Med. In press.

8. Becker, E.L. and H.J. Showell, 1972. Effects of Ca^{2+} and Mg^{2+}
    on the chemotactic responsiveness of rabbit polymorphonuclear
    leukocytes. Z. Immunitätsforsch. 143:466-476.

9. Zigmond, S.H. and J. G. Hirsch, 1973. Leukocyte locomotion and
    chemotaxis. New method for evaluation and demonstration of cell-
    derived chemotactic factor. J. Exp. Med. 137:387-410.

10. Schiffmann, E., H.J. Showell, B.A. Corcoran, P.A. Ward, E. Smith,
    and E.L. Becker, 1975. The isolation and partial characteriza-
    tion of neutrophil chemotactic factors from E. coli. J. Immunol.
    114:831-837.

11. Becker, E.L., and H.J. Showell, 1974. The ability of chemo-
    tactic factors to induce lysosomal enzyme release II. The
    mechanism of the release. J. Immunol. 112:2055-2062.

12. Zurier, R.B., S. Hoffstein and G. Weissmann, 1973. Cytochala-
    sin B: Effect on lysosomal enzyme release from human leukocytes.
    Proc. Nat. Acad. Sci. U.S.A. 70:844-845.

13. Wilkinson, P.C., 1974. Chemotaxis and Inflammation,Churchill
    Livingstone, Edinburgh and London.

14. Roberts, J. and J.H. Quastel, 1963. Particle uptake by poly-
    morphonuclear leucocytes and Ehrlich Ascites-Carcinoma Cells.
    Biochem. J. 89:150-156.

15. Henson, P.M., 1974. Mechanisms of activation and secretion by
    platelets and neutrophils. Progress in Immunology II, L. Brent
    and J. Holborow (Eds) North-Holland, Amsterdam-Oxford, pp.
    95-105.

16. Showell, H.J. and Becker, E.L., 1976. The effects of external
    K^+ and Na^+ on the chemotaxis of rabbit peritoneal neutrophils.
    J. Immunol. 116:99-105.

17. Goetzl, E.J., S.I. Wasserman, I. Gigli and K.F. Austen, 1974.
     Enhancement of random migration and chemotactic response of
     human leukocytes by ascorbic acid. J. Clin. Investig. 53:
     813-818.

18. Baggiolini, M., J.G. Hirsch and C. de Duve, 1969. Resolution
     of granules from rabbit heterophil leukocytes into distinct
     populations by zonal sedimentation . J. Cell Biol. 40:529-
     541.

19. Goldstein, I.M., J.K. Horn, H.B. Kaplan and G. Weissmann, 1974.
     Calcium-induced lysozyme secretion from human polymorphonuclear
     leukocytes. Biochem. Biophys. Research. Commun. 60:807-812.

20. Hook, W.A., E. Shiffmann, S. Aswanikumar and R.P. Siraganian,
     1976. Histamine release from basophils by formyl-methionine
     peptides. Fed. Proceed. In press.

21. Stossel, T.P., 1974. Phagocytosis. New Eng. J. Med. 290:717-
     723, 1974.

22. Boxer, L.A., E.T. Hedley-Whyte and T.P. Stossel, 1974. Neu--
     trophil actin dysfunction and abnormal neutrophil behavior.
     New.Eng. J. Med. 291:1093-1099.

23. Becker, E.L., A.T. Davis, R.D. Estenson and P.G. Quie, 1972.
     Cytochalasin B IV Inhibition and stimulation of chemotaxis
     of rabbit and human and polymorphonuclear leukocytes. J.
     Immunol. 108:396-402.

24. Borel, J.F. and Stählein, H., 1972. Effects of cytochalasin
     B on chemotaxis and immune reactions. Experentia 28:745.

25. Zigmond, S.H. and J.G. Hirsch, 1972. Effects of cytochalasin B
     on polymorphonuclear leucocyte locomotion, phagocytosis and
     glycolysis. Exp. Cell Res. 73:383-393.

26. Canarozzi, N.A. and S.E. Malawista, 1973. Phagocytosis of hu-
     man blood leukocytes measured by the uptake of ^{131}I-labelled
     human serum albumin: inhibitory and stimulatory effects of cy-
     tochalasin B. Yale J. Biol. and Med. 46:177-189.

27. Zurier, R.B., Hoffstein, S. and Weissmann, G., 1973. Cyto-
     chalasin B: effect on lysosomal enzyme release from human
     leukocytes. Proc. Nat. Acad. Sci. U.S.A. 70:844-848.

28. Bhisey, A.N. and J.J. Freed, 1971. Altered movement of endo-
     somes in colchicine-treated cultured macrophages. Exp. Cell
     Res. 64:430-438.

29. Allison, A.C., P. Davis and S. de Petris, 1971. Role of con-
    tractile micro-filaments in macrophage movement and endocytosis.
    Nature New Biol. 232:153-155.

30. Bandmann, U., L. Rydgren and B. Norberg, 1974. The difference
    between random movement and chemotaxis. Exp. Cell Res. 88:63-
    73.

31. Russel, R.J., P.C. Wilkinson, F. Sless and D.M.V. Parrot, 1975.
    Chemotaxis of lymphoblasts. Nature 256:646-648.

32. Goldstein, I., S. Hoffstein, J. Gallin and G. Weissmann, 1973.
    Mechanisms of lysosomal enzyme release from human leukocytes:
    microtubule assembly and membrane fusion induced by a compo-
    nent of complement. Proc. Nat. Acad. Sci. U.S.A. 70:2916-2920.

33. Gallin, J.I. and A.S. Rosenthal, 1974. Divalent cation re-
    quirements and calcium fluxes during human granulocyte che-
    motaxis. J. Cell Biol. 62:594-606.

34. Ramsey, W.S. and A. Harris, 1973. Leukocyte locomotion and
    its inhibition by antimitotic drugs. Exp. Cell Res. 82:262-
    270.

35. Edelson, P.J. and H.F. Fudenberg, 1973. Effect of vinblastine
    on the chemotactic responsiveness of normal human neutrophils.
    Infection and Immunity 8:127-129.

36. Caner, J.E., 1965. Colchicine inhibition of chemotaxis. Arth.
    and Rheum. 8:757-764.

37. Phelps, P. and D.J. McCarty, Jr., 1969. Crystal induced ar-
    thritis. Postgraduate Medicine 45:87-93.

38. Ward, P.A., 1971. Leukotactic factors in health and disease.
    Am. J. Path. 64:521-530.

39. Oliver, J.M., R.B. Zurier and R.D. Berlin, 1975. Concanava-
    lin A cap formation on polymorphonuclear leukocytes of normal
    and beige (Chediak-Higashi) mice. Nature 253:471-473.

40. Gallin, J.I., J.S. Bujack and S. M. Wolff, 1974. Granulocyte
    function in the Chediak-Higashi syndrome of mice. Blood 43:
    201-206.

41. Clark, R.A. and H.R. Kimball, 1972. Defective granulocyte
    chemotaxis in the Chediak-Higashi syndrome. J. Clin. Investig.
    51:649-665.

42. Gallin, J.I., J.A.Klimerman, G.A. Padgett and S.M. Wolff, 1975. Defective mononuclear leukocyte chemotaxis in the Chediak-Higashi syndrome of humans, mink and cattle. Blood 45:863-870.

43. Weissmann, G., I. Goldstein, S.Hoffstein and P.K. Tsung, 1975. Reciprocal effects of cAMP and cGMP on microtubule-dependent release of lysosomal enzymes. Ann. N.Y. Acad. Sci. 253:750-762.

44. Henson, P.M, 1972. Pathologic mechanisms in neutrophil-mediated injury. Am. J. Path. 68:593-612.

45. Hawkins, D., 1972. Inhibition of neutrophil lysosomal release Fed. Proceed 31:748.

46. Hoffstein, S., 1975. Microtubule assembly and secretion in human polymorphonuclear leukocytes. Fed. Proceed 34:868.

47. Stossel, T.P., R.K. Root and M. Vaughn 1972. Phagocytosis in chronic granulomatous disease and the Chediak-Higashi syndrome. New. Eng. J. Med. 286:120-123.

48. Malawista, S.E., 1975. Action of colchicine in acute gouty arthritis. Arth. Rheum 18:835-846.

49. Lehrer, R.I., 1973. Effects of colchicine and chloramphemicol on the oxidative metabolism and phagocytic activity of human neutrophils. J. Infect. Dis. 127:40-48.

50. Stossel, T.P., R.J. Mason, J. Hartwig and M. Vaughn, 1972. Quantitative studies of phagocytosis by polymorphonuclear leukocytes: use of emulsions to measure the initial rate of phagocytosis. J. Clin. Investig. 51:615-625.

51. Griffin, F.M. Jr., J.A. Griffin, J.E. Leider and S.C. Silverstein, 1975. Studies on the mechanism of phagocytosis 1. Requirements for circumferential attachment of particle-bound ligands to specific receptors on the macrophage plasma membrane. J. Exp. Med. 142:1263-1282.

DISCUSSION

GOETZL: Does a prior exposure of the rabbit polymorpho-nuclear leukocyte to low concentrations of synthetic peptide influence the response upon rechallenge with an active concentration of peptide in any of your assays?

BECKER: We can get "deactivation" of the neutrophil by prior exposure to the peptide but this requires chemotactic or inhibitory concentrations.

GOMPERTZ: Is the neutrophil "aware" of the peptide concentration gradient along its dimension (this must be very small indeed). Or does the induced random movement allow the cell to search for the concentration gradient over a greater unit dimension?

Maybe the method of chemotactic measurement actually perturb the nature of the gradient, by locking the cells on the membrane filter at the point of much higher gradient: or does the method of analysis which you described (Hirsch?) take account of this.

BECKER: Dr. Sally Zigmond has shown that the neutrophil detects the concentration gradient along its dimensions.

In regard to the second part of the question, there is no direct evidence bearing upon this point.

MOVAT: In collaboration with Ranadive we studied the role of IgG receptors in lysosomal enzyme release (Ranadive et al. Int. Arch. Allergy, 1973; Sojnani et al., Lab. Investig. in press). Among other things we used latex particles, which per se, although they were ingested, did not cause lysosomal enzyme release, unless they were IgG or Fc coated.

When you adsorb the peptides to the polysterene particles and obtain enhanced phagocytosis, do you get lysosomal enzyme release?

BECKER: I do not know at present.

LICHTENSTEIN: How is the enzyme release by the peptides modulated? I refer to the differences in mechanisms between peptide induced histamine release (C5a) which is fast and not cAMP dependent compared to IgE bridging. The latter is similar to the phagocytic release of lysosomal enzyme as described by Wersman, Henson and Cochrane.

BECKER: With cytochalasin B, the release by peptides, as other chemotactic factors is very rapid being completed within a minute. When the release is carried out in the absence of cytochalasin B on surfaces, the release is much slower. Thus, one can obtain either mode of release depending on circumstances.

COCHRANE: Have you tried to inactivate the neutrophils by exposing to peptide activator under conditions unfavorable to a particular activity? For example can you expose the cells to peptide at 10°C, then wash, and find if the cells are fully responsive to C5a or some other, presumably unrelated activator? This would support your thoughts of specific receptor sites.

BECKER: We have done inactivation studies but generally at 37°C.

COCHRANE: Are the effects of peptide activation of neutrophils blocked by DFP?

BECKER: We have not tested the effect of peptide activation with DFP.

AUSTEN: In establishing a chemotactic gradient across the dimension of the cell, what is the role of binding as distinct from activation?

BECKER: I do not know but I guess both are necessary.

DIAMANT: Are the effects you have studied calcium and energy dependent?

BECKER: Ca^{2+} and Mg^{2+} are required in chemotaxis. Phagocytosis, from the work of Stossel apparently requires divalent cations. Release, which occurs in the precence of cytochalasin B, is only inhibited to a limited extent by EDTA. If it occurs on appropriate surfaces Ca^{2+} is an absolute requirement. All the functions are energy dependent.

DIAMANT: Have you been able to block one of the effects without disturbing the appearance of the others?

BECKER: Cytochalasin B for example inhibits random locomotion, chemotaxis and phagocytosis but enhances stimulated secretion.

THE HAGEMAN FACTOR SYSTEM: MECHANISM OF CONTACT ACTIVATION

John H. Griffin, Susan D. Revak, and Charles G. Cochrane

Scripps Clinic and Research Foundation
Department of Immunopathology, 476 Prospect Street
La Jolla, California 92037

The role of the components of the Hageman factor system in the pathogenesis of inflammation is poorly understood. In order to examine the potential participation of the system in inflammation, abundant work has been performed in the past several years to delineate the component proteins and examine their mechanisms of interaction. In this paper, we wish to review the state of knowledge of the system, including the latest information available regarding the activation of Hageman factor, and to summarize the inflammatory properties attributed to its members.

The components of this system, outlined in Fig. 1, consist of a series of proenzymes that, upon activation, act sequentially to generate three distinct processes: the generation of kinins, fibrin, and fibrinolysis.

Activation of components of the three pathways is associated with limited proteolytic cleavage of each component. This may be exemplified by the action of activated Hageman factor on its substrates prekallikrein and factor XI. In each case, the substrate is cleaved into two subunits as activation takes place. The subunits appear upon reduction of the activated molecule. Similarly with Hageman factor, as will be shown below, the activation in plasma is accompanied by cleavage, although reduction of the molecule is not necessary to demonstrate cleavage.

While not understanding the mechanisms by which the Hageman factor system participates in the development of inflammation, ample evidence indicates that each cardinal sign of the inflammatory process can be expressed by activity of the system. Inflammatory activities mediated by components of the systems are listed in Table I.

371

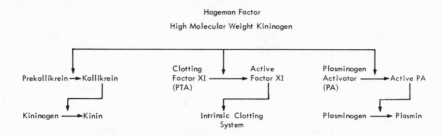

Fig. 1. The schematic representation of the Hageman factor system.

Table I. Inflammatory activities associated with the Hageman factor system.

Inflammatory Activity	Components Responsible
Increased vascular permeability	Bradykinin Histidine-rich peptide of High MW Kininogen Fibrinogen fragment E Active Hageman factor (PF/dil)
Pain	Bradykinin
Hypotension	Bradykinin
Chemotaxis of neutrophils	Kallikrein Plasminogen activator Fibrinogen fragment D C3 cleaved by plasmin
Smooth muscle contraction	Bradykinin
Fibrin formation (coagulation)	Combined activity of Hageman factor, High MW Kininogen, kallikrein and factor XI (intrinsic clotting system) Active Hageman factor→ factor VII (extrinsic clotting system)
C1 (Complement) activation	Plasmin

Permeability Factor of Dilution (PF/dil)

One of the notable examples of an association between the Hageman factor (HF) system and inflammation involves a permeability-inducing substance that develops when diluted plasma contacts glass. The generation of this activity has been demonstrated in the plasma of several animal species (1-6). Generation of PF/dil has been shown to require the presence of HF (6-8) and prekallikrein (9-11). However the nature of the PF/dil molecule has remained unknown. It has been postulated that PF/dil is a constituent of plasma that is activated by HF and which, in turn, activates prekallikrein (6-8,12). However, studies in which purified active HF were shown to convert purified prekallikrein to an active form mitigate against the possibility that PF/dil is an intermediate between HF and prekallikrein (13-16).

In an attempt to link HF and PF/dil Kellermeyer and Ratnoff (17) treated normal human plasma with antibodies to HF before dilution which prevented generation of PF/dil, while treatment after dilution did not prevent the permeability effect of already generated PF/dil, suggesting that something other than HF was responsible for the actual permeability effect. More recently, employing immunadsorption techniques on a solid matrix, it was found that activated PF/dil could be removed from solution by insolubilized antibodies to HF, but not with other antibodies (11). This indicated that PF/dil shared immunologic specificity with HF and was most likely identical. The inability of soluble antibody to HF to block PF/dil activity in other studies (17) could be explained if the antibodies were not directed to the enzyme site of the HF molecule. The same antibodies could block activation of HF in whole plasma, however, by sterically inhibiting contact with glass. These possibilities have not been verified experimentally. The association of PF/dil and the presence of HF in chromatographic and electrophoretic fractions of plasma has recently been shown (18).

The means by which PF/dil or activated HF induce permeability of blood vessels is not certain. Presumably bradykinin and/or peptides derived from high MW kininogen (19) is generated in the recipient animal although there is no evidence for this. Antihistamines do not block the permeability. It is of interest that intradermal injections of activated HF produce a latent (60 minute) reaction of permeability (20) and that one of the activated products of HF i.e., plasmin, when similarly injected yields permeability reactions that are not inhibited by antihistamine (21). The latter observation suggests the permeability resulting from infused plasmin does not derive from activated complement components, namely anaphylatoxins.

Participation of the Hageman Factor System in Acute Anaphylaxis

The role of the HF system in particular diseases remains obscure. While activation or consumption of certain components has been associated with particular diseases of human beings, the data are incomplete in virtually all of these. A definite participation of the HF systems in the pathogenesis of the disease has therefore escaped rigorous proof. It is for this reason that it is essential to understand the biochemistry of the components and conduct critical experiments establishing requirement for certain components or groups of components in the pathogenesis of a given form of inflammatory injury.

One disease in which a number of studies have suggested that activation of the HF system is associated with development of injury is anaphylaxis. Abundant experimental data has accumulated to support this. Beraldo (22) observed an increase in bradykinin in the blood of dogs during anaphylactic shock. In immunized guinea pig and rabbits, Brockelhurst and Lahiri (23) measured bradykinin in the blood following injection of antigen intravenously. Employing isolated, perfused lung of immunized guinea pigs, Brockelhurst and Lahiri (24) observed release of a kinin-forming activity, presumably kallikrein, upon infusion of specific antigen. Jonasson and Becker (25) in similar studies perfused antigen intravascularly in isolated, sensitized guinea pig lung, and measured release of kallikrein activity. The kallikrein was identical to plasma kallikrein in molecular size and charge and in its sensitivity to inhibitors. The process was also elicited by infusion of ellagic acid, a known activator of Hageman factor. More recently, Halonen and Pinckard (26,27) have shown loss of Hageman factor and activity of several components of the intrinsic clotting system following IgE-induced anaphylaxis in rabbits. It is probable that activation of the Hageman factor system in these cases is secondary to the immunologic event in that immunologic aggregates, including those consisting of IgE molecules, fail to bind or activate Hageman factor in vitro (28).

It is apparent from the interesting experimental leads that additional studies might demonstrate a pathogenic role of the HF system in anaphylaxis. This state is similar to the possible contribution of the HF system to several other diseases such as the hypotensive shock associated with bacteremic states, disseminated intravascular coagulation, certain forms of glomerulonephritis, nephrotic syndrome and arthritis, and other diseases as well. Analytical data in which the components of the HF system are closely followed through their activation and consumption in association with the disease state must be obtained, along with evidence that activation occurs at the target site or that activated components reach the target site. Inhibition of the active components or prevention of their activation must then be performed to establish a role of the components of the HF system in the pathogenic process. Such data are not yet at hand in any of the diseases in question.

Knowledge of the relationship of components of the Hageman factor pathways to development of tissue injury has been handicapped by an inability to follow the individual molecules as they participate in the reactions. In order to accomplish this it has been essential to purify the molecules, and prepare the purified proteins labeled with radioactive iodine. In addition, it is essential to have a firm understanding of the molecular mechanisms of activation of each component of the various pathways and of the molecular interactions involved in the activation. Different laboratories have devoted considerable attention to these problems and data have emerged that have expanded our understanding. Several reviews on these topics have previously appeared (29-32). In this presentation, we will focus attention on the mechanisms of the contact phase of activation of the HF system, taking into consideration the participation of four principle molecules: Hageman factor (HF), high molecular weight kininogen (HMWK), prekallikrein (PK) and clotting factor XI (plasma tromboplastin antecedent).

The Structure of Human Hageman Factor

The HF zymogen can be isolated as a single polypeptide chain of 76,000 to 80,000 MW determined on polyacrylamide gels in the presence of sodium dodecyl sulfate (33). Proteolytic activation of HF by kallikrein, plasmin, or trypsin yields a 28,000 MW species which contains the enzymatic active site (14,15,34-37) and 48,000 MW or 40,000 MW fragments which bind avidly to negatively charged, activating surfaces but which do not contain an active site (37).

Activation of Human Hageman Factor

Studies of the mechanisms of surface-dependent activation of HF can best be performed using purified proteins and a model activating surface, such as kaolin. Hypotheses based on such studies can then be tested in vitro in plasma as well as in vivo using as activating agents materials which are more biologically relevant than kaolin.

The importance of prekallikrein to the activation of HF was recognized when it was shown that kallikrein could proteolytically activate HF (36), that rabbit kallikrein could stimulate clotting of rabbit plasma (38), and that Fletcher plasma, deficient in prekallikrein (9,10), exhibits abnormal surface-activated reactions (39,40). More recently, plasma deficient in high MW

kininogen (HMWK) (41), known as Fitzgerald (42,43), Williams (44), or
Flaujeac trait (41) has been shown to be incapable of contact activation of
HF. HMWK had also been studied under the name of "contact activation cofactor" (45,46). These observations led to the following series of experiments
based upon which an hypothesis for the mechanism of surface activation of HF
was advanced (47).

The activation of HF can be conveniently determined using clotting
assays to measure the ability of activated HF, denoted as HF_a, to generate
factor XI_a. The ability of various combinations of purified HF, HMWK,
prekallikrein, and kaolin to activate partially purified factor XI in an incubation mixture was studied by measuring the factor XI_a formed during an
8 min incubation at 37°. The results seen in Table II show that efficient
conversion of factor XI to factor XI_a requires HF, HMWK, prekallikrein, and
kaolin. For example, omission of either prekallikrein or HMWK gave 10-fold
less activation of factor XI.

Further studies showed that a mixture of purified HF, HMWK, prekallikrein and kaolin gave the same rapid rate of activation of purified factor XI
as an equivalent aliquot of factor XI-deficient plasma. This suggested that
potent, surface-mediated activation of factor XI in plasma is explicable in
terms of HF, HMWK, and prekallikrein (47).

The same experimental system as described in Table II was used to demonstrate that HMWK exerted its effect on the activation of HF in a stoichio-
metric, rather than a catalytic, manner. It was observed that optimal effects
of HMWK in stimulating activation of HF occured when nearly equal quantities of the two proteins were present on the kaolin. On this basis, it was
suggested that HF and HMWK form stable, surface-bound complexes with each
other.

With the observation that HMWK is essential for the rapid activation of
HF on kaolin, it was important to determine the mechanism by which this stimulation was exerted. Considering that a combination of HF, prekallikrein and
HMWK were essential to activate HF on the surface, experiments were designed to find: a) if HMWK stimulated the action of active kallikrein on
surface-bound HF; b) if surface-bound, active HF, i.e., HF_a, activated prekallikrein more rapidly in the presence of HMWK; and c) if HMWK promoted
the activation of factor XI by surface-bound HF_a.

a) A role of HMWK in stimulating the enzymatic action of kallikrein on
surface-bound Hageman factor. Evidence that HMWK augments the rate of
cleavage of HF by kallikrein came from a study of the proteolytic activation
of 125I-HF by kallikrein. The kinetics of cleavage of kaolin-bound 125I-HF

Table II. Activation of factor XI by mixtures of Hageman factor (HF), high MW kininogen (HMWK), prekallikrein (PK) and kaolin* (from Griffin and Cochrane, ref. 47)

REAGENTS				Factor XI$_a$ Generated (Clotting Units per ml)
Kaolin	HF	HMWK	PK	
+	+	+	+	0.34
+	−	−	−	0†
−	+	+	+	0.001
+	−	+	+	0.001
+	+	−	+	0.026
+	+	+	−	0.030
+	+	−	−	0.006
+	−	−	+	0.005
+	−	+	−	0.007

*The + or − sign indicates the presence or absence of the indicated reagent in a mixture containing factor XI at 0.83 units per ml which was incubated 8 min. at 37° and then assayed for factor XI$_a$ activity. The concentrations of HF, HMWK, and prekallikrein, when present in the mixture, were 18, 14, and 6 μg/ml respectively. Kaolin was 3.6 mg/ml. The solution contained 0.10M NaCl, 0.05 Tris-Cl, pH 7.4. The observed clotting times varied from >300s for factor XI alone to 118s for 0.34 clotting units per ml.
†The background activity for factor XI alone plus kaolin was 0.006 clotting units/ml and this value was subtracted from each value in order to define the net activation of factor XI.

by kallikrein in the presence or absence of HMWK were defined using SDS gels to separate the 28,000 MW and 48,000 MW HF cleavage products from the native 76,000 MW molecule. The integrated radioactivity of each MW species as a function of reaction time is seen in Fig. 2. These data show that HMWK increases 11-fold the rate of cleavage of HF by kallikrein.

b) A role of HMWK in the activation of prekallikrein by surface-bound active Hageman factor. Since active HF is known to activate prekallikrein by limited specific proteolysis, the effect of HMWK on the kinetics of the activation of prekallikrein by kaolin-bound trypsin-activated HF_a was studied. The amount of kallikrein activity at various times was determined by measuring the rate of hydrolysis of a tripeptide substrate of kallikrein, Bz-Pro-Phe-Arg-paranitroanilide (47). The data in Fig. 3 show that the activation of prekallikrein proceeds at least 20-times more rapidly in the presence of HMWK than in its absence. Significantly, the total final amount of prekallikrein which was activated was not affected by HMWK.

c) A role of HMWK in the activation of factor XI by surface-bound HF_a. The importance of HMWK for the activation of factor XI by surface-bound, trypsin-activated HF_a was demonstrated when it was shown that such HF_a could activate factor XI in the presence but not in the absence of HMWK (47).

Thus, the importance of HMWK to surface-dependent HF reactions is not limited to only one particular reaction. Rather, HMWK promotes the proteolytic activation of HF as well as the proteolytic activation of both prekallikrein and factor XI by HF_a.

Binding and Cleavage of HF in Human Plasma

Plasma containing ^{125}I-HF was subjected to contact activation in glass tubes, and the binding of ^{125}I-HF in plasma to the activating glass surface as well as the cleavage of the ^{125}I-HF during contact activation were studied (48). The kinetics of cleavage of ^{125}I-HF in normal, prekallikrein-deficient (Fletcher), and HMWK-deficient (Fitzgerald) plasma are seen in Fig. 4. In normal plasma, rapid cleavage of HF occurs and is complete within 5 min, plateauing in Fig. 4 at 60%. The remaining 40% of HF molecules which were not cleaved were shown to be in the supernatant (48). That is, when there is a limiting amount of surface, binding of HF to the surface is a prerequisite for cleavage. In contrast to the rapid cleavage of HF seen in normal plasma, plasmas deficient in prekallikrein or HMWK do not exhibit rapid cleavage of HF (Fig. 4), though a slow cleavage over a long period of time is evident.

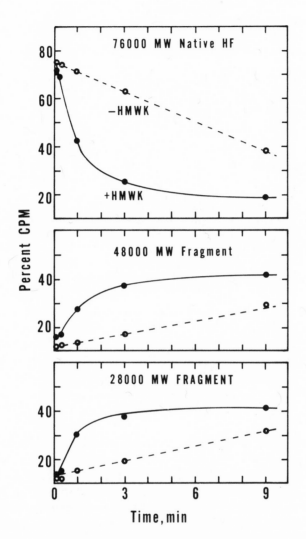

Fig. 2. Kinetics of cleavage of kaolin-bound ^{125}I-HF by kallikrein in the presence or absence of high MW kininogen (HMWK) (from ref. 47).

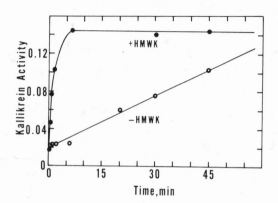

Fig. 3. Kinetics of activation of prekallikrein by kaolin-bound, trypsin-activated HF$_a$ in the presence and absence of HMWK (from ref. 47).

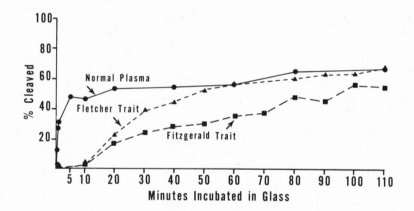

Fig. 4. Rate of cleavage of ^{125}I-HF in normal, prekallikrein-deficient (Fletcher), and HMWK-deficient (Fitzgerald) plasma in glass tubes. 20 μl aliquots of plasma (diluted 1:6) were shaken in glass tubes at 20°, and the extent of cleavage of ^{125}I-HF was measured using SDS gel electrophoresis (from ref. 48).

The failure of the HF to be cleaved rapidly in glass tubes in plasmas deficient in prekallikrein or HMWK is not, however, due to a failure to bind to the activating surface. Fig. 5 shows the kinetics of binding and of cleavage of ^{125}I-HF during the first 120 seconds of incubation, expressed as the percent of total Hageman factor present which is cleaved or bound. The kinetics of binding of HF is the same for normal, prekallikrein-deficient, and HMWK-deficient plasmas. Cleavage as shown in Fig. 4 is rapid in normal plasma, but is not observed in the deficient plasmas. Cleavage of factor XI deficient plasma occured at a rate equal to that in normal plasma.

Reconstitution of the respective deficient plasmas with prekallikrein and HMWK restored the rapid rate of cleavage of ^{125}I-HF upon exposure of the plasma to glass (48).

In summary, these studies (48) showed that the rapid cleavage of HF in plasma requires binding to an activating surface and the presence of prekallikrein and HMWK. The failure of plasmas deficient in either of these proteins to exhibit rapid cleavage of HF in spite of the observed binding may help to explain the clotting, kinin generation and fibrinolytic abnormalities they exhibit, and it suggests that the activation of HF in plasma is associated with its cleavage.

Hypothetical Mechanism for Surface-Dependent Activation of Hageman Factor

The surface-dependent activation of HF has previously generally been discussed in terms of nonproteolytic activation of HF due to conformational changes associated with binding to the activating surface. In contrast to such previous concepts and based on the observations summarized above, an hypothesis emphasizing proteolytic activation of HF was advanced (47) describing the mechanism of activation of surface-bound HF. Fig. 6 depicts schematically the proposed mechanism. Exposure of HF in plasma to an activating surface leads to the formation of a complex between HF and HMWK on the surface which thereby places HF into a conformation which is very susceptible to proteolytic cleavage, that is, activation. This yields surface-bound HF_a. The bound HMWK:HF_a complex is a potent activator of factor XI and of prekallikrein. The newly generated kallikrein reciprocally activates more HF in other surface-bound HF·HMWK complexes thereby augmenting the amount of HF_a and, consequently, the activation of factor XI, prekallikrein, and plasminogen proactivator.

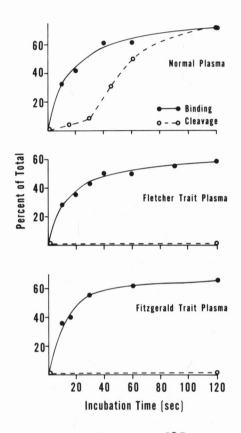

Fig. 5. Kinetics of binding and cleavage of ^{125}I-HF in normal, prekallikrein-deficient, and HMWK-deficient plasmas in glass tubes. The solid lines denote binding while the dashed lines indicate cleavage (from ref. 48).

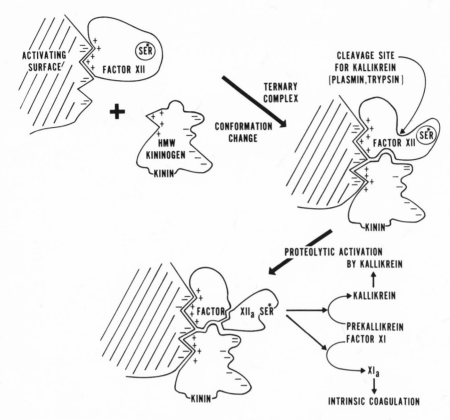

Fig. 6. Schematic mechanism of activation of surface-bound HF.

The reciprocal proteolytic activation involving HF and prekallikrein is a key element of this proposal. While this scheme may explain the activation pathway for the majority of HF molecules, the question remains of what molecules provide the triggering proteolytic action for the HF-HF_a-prekallikrein-kallikrein cycle. The possibility of low levels of non-proteolytically activated HF_a or kallikrein must be addressed. Further experiments to test and to expand this hypothesis are clearly warranted.

This is publication no. 1141 from the Department of Immunopathology, Scripps Clinic & Research Foundation, 476 Prospect Street, La Jolla, CA 92037. This work was supported by U.S. Public Health Service grant AI-07007 from the National Institute of Allergy and Infectious Diseases, program project grant HL-16411 from the National Heart and Lung Institute, NR105837 contract from the Office of Naval Research, Council of Tobacco Research #764-D, and J. H. Griffin's Research and Career Development Award K04 HL-00192.

REFERENCES

1. MacKay, M.E., A.A. Miles, C.B. Schacter, and D.L. Wilhelm, 1953, Susceptibility of the guinea pig to pharmacological factors from its own serum. Nature 172:714.

2. Mill, P.J., J.M. Elder, A.A. Miles, and D.L. Wilhelm, 1958, Enzyme like globulins from serum reproducing the vascular phenomena of inflammation. VI. Isolation and properties of permeability factor and its inhibitor in human plasma. Br. J. Exp. Pathol. 39:343.

3. Stewart, R.B. and J.Q. Bliss, 1957, The permeability increasing factor in diluted human plasma. Br. J. Exp. Pathol. 38:462.

4. Elder, J.M. and D.L. Wilhelm, 1957, Enzyme-like globulins from serum reproducing the vascular phenomena of inflammation. V. Active permeability factor in human serum. Br. J. Exp. Pathol. 39:23.

5. Margolis, J., 1958, Activation of a permeability factor in plasma by contact with glass. Nature 181:635.

6. Margolis, J., 1958, Activation of plasma by contact with glass. Evidence for a common reaction which releases plasma kinin and initiates coagulation. J. Physiol. 144:1.

7. Ratnoff, O.D. and A.A. Miles, 1962, Activation of a vascular permeability increasing factor in human plasma incubated with purified activated Hageman factor. J. Lab. Clin. Med. 60:1009.

8. Ratnoff, O.D. and A.A. Miles, 1964, The induction of permeability increasing activity in human plasma by activated Hageman factor. Br. J. Exp. Pathol. 45:328.

9. Wuepper, K.D., 1972, Biochemistry and biology of components of the plasma kinin-forming system. In Inflammation: Mechanisms and Control, I.H. Lepow and P.A. Ward, eds., New York, Academic Press, pp. 93-117.

10. Wuepper, K.D., 1973, Prekallikrein deficiency in human plasma. J. Exp. Med. 138:1345.

11. Johnston, A.R., C.G. Cochrane, and S.D. Revak, 1974, The relationship of PF/dil and activated human Hageman factor. J. Immunol. 113:103-109.

12. Webster, M.E. and O.D. Ratnoff, 1961, Role of Hageman factor in the activation of vasodilatory activity in human plasma. Nature 192:180.

13. Nagasawa, S., H. Takahashi, M. Koida, T. Suzuki, and J.G.G. Schoenmakers, 1968, Partial purification of bovine plasma kallikreinogen, its activation by the Hageman factor. Bioch. Biophys. Res. Comm. 32:644-649.

14. Cochrane, C.G. and K.D. Wuepper, 1971, The first component of the kinin forming system in human and rabbit plasma. Its relationship to clotting factor XII (Hageman factor). J. Exp. Med. 134:986.

15. Kaplan, A.P. and K.F. Austen, 1971, A prealbumin activator of prekallikrein. II. Derivation of activators of prekallikrein from active Hageman factor by digestion with plasmin. J. Exp. Med. 133:696.

16. Eisen, V. and H.G. Smith, 1970, Plasma kinin formation by complexes of aggregated γ-globulin and serum proteins. Br. J. Exp. Pathol. 51: 328.

17. Kellermeyer, R.W. and O.D. Ratnoff, 1967, Abolition of permeability enhancing properties of Hageman factor by specific antiserum. J. Lab. Clin. Med. 70:365-371.

18. OhIshi, S. and W.E. Webster, 1975, Vascular permeability factors (PF/nat and PF/dil: Their relationship to Hageman factor and the kallikrein-kinin system.) Biochem. Pharmacol. 24

19. Matheson, R.T., D.R. Miller, Y.N. Han, S. Iwanaga, H. Kato, and K.D. Wuepper, 1976, Delineation of a new permeability-enhancing peptide released by plasma kallikrein from HMW-kininogen (Flaujeac factor). Clin. Res., in press.

20. Graham, R.C. Jr., R.H. Ebert, O.D. Ratnoff, and J.M. Moses, 1965, Pathogenesis of inflammation. J. Exp. Med. 121:807-818.

21. Ratnoff, O.D., 1965, Increased vascular permeability induced by plasmin. J. Exp. Med. 122:905-921.

22. Beraldo, W.T., 1950, Formation of bradykinin in anaphylactic and peptone shock. Am. J. Physiol. 163:283.

23. Brockelhurst, W.E. and S.C. Lahiri, 1962, The production of bradykinin in anaphylaxis. J. Physiol. 160:159.

24. Brockelhurst, W.E. and S.C. Lahiri, 1962, Formation and destruction of bradykinin during anaphylaxis. J. Physiol. 165:39 P.

25. Jonasson, O. and E.L. Becker, 1966, Release of kallikrein from guinea pig lung during anaphylaxis. J. Exp. Med. 123:529.

26. Halonen,M. and R.N. Pinckard, 1975, Intravascular effects of IgE anti-body upon basophils, neutrophils, platelets and blood coagulation in the rabbit. J. Immunol. 115:525.

27. Pinckard, R.N., C. Tanigawa, and M. Halonen, 1975, IgE-induced blood coagulation alterations in the rabbit. Consumption of coagulation factors XII, XI, IX in vivo. J. Immunol. 115:519.

28. Cochrane, C.G., K.D. Wuepper, B.S. Aiken, S.D. Revak, and H.L. Spiegelberg, 1972b, The interaction of Hageman factor and immune complexes. J. Clin. Invest. 51:2736.

29. Magoon, E.H., J. Spragg, and K.F. Austen, 1974, Human Hageman factor dependent reactions. Adv. in Biosciences 12, Schering Symp. on Immunopathology, 225.

30. Cochrane, C.G., S.D. Revak, K.D. Wuepper, A. Johnston, D.C. Morrison, and R. Ulevitch, 1974, Activation of Hageman factor and the kinin forming, intrinsic clotting and fibrinolytic systems. Adv. in Biosciences 12, Schering Symp. On Immunopathology, 237.

31. Cochrane, C.G., S.D. Revak, R. Ulevitch, A. Johnston, and D.C. Morrison, 1976, Hageman factor: Characterization and mechanism of activation. Conference on Chemistry and Biology of the Kallikrein-Kinin System in Health and Disease, In press.

32. Kaplan, A.P. H. Meier, L.W. Heck, and L. Yecies, 1976, Conference on Chemistry and Biology of the Kallikrein-Kinin System in Health and Disease,   In press.

33. Revak, S.D., C.G. Cochrane, A. Johnston, and T. Hugli, 1974, Structural changes accompanying enzymatic activation of Hageman factor. J. Clin. Invest. 54:619.

34. Wuepper, K.D., 1972, Biochemistry and biology of components of the plasma kinin-forming system. In Inflammation: Mechanisms and Control. I.H. Lepow, and P.A. Ward, eds. New York, Academic Press. pp.93.

35. Kaplan, A.P., and K.F. Austen, 1970, A prealbumin activator of pre-kallikrein. J. Immunol. 105:802.

36. Cochrane, C.G., S.D. Revak, and K.D. Wuepper, 1973, Activation of Hageman factor in solid and fluid phases. J. Exp. Med. 138:1564.

37. Revak, S.D., and C.G. Cochrane, 1976, The relationship of structure and function in human Hageman factor. The association of enzymatic and binding activities with separate regions of the molecule. J. Clin. Invest. 57:852.

38. Wuepper, K.D. and C.G. Cochrane, 1972, Effect of plasma kallikrein on coagulation in vitro . Proc. Soc. Exp. Biol. Med. 141:271.

39. Hathaway, W.E., L.P. Belhasen, and H.S. Hathaway, 1965, Evidence for a new plasma thromboplastin factor: I. Case report, coagulation studies and physicochemical properties. Blood J. Hematol. 26:521.

40. Hattersby, P.G., and D. Hayse, 1970, Fletcher deficiency: a report of three unrelated cases. Br. J. Haematol. 18:411.

41. Wuepper, K.D., D.R. Miller, and M.J. Lacombe, 1975, Deficiency of human plasma kininogen. J. Clin. Invest. 56:1663.

42. Saito, H., O.D. Ratnoff, R. Waldmann, and J.P. Abraham, 1975, Deficiency of a hitherto unrecognized agent, Fitzgerald factor, partici-pating in surface-mediated reactions of clotting, fibrinolysis, generation of kinins, and the property of diluted plasma enhancing vascular permeability (PF/DIL). J. Clin. Invest. 55:1082.

43. Donaldson, V.H., H.I. Glueck, M.A. Miller, H.Z. Movat, and F. Habal, 1976, Kininogen deficiency in Fitzgerald trait: role of high molecular weight kininogen in clotting and fibrinolysis. J. Lab. Clin. Med. 87:327.

44. Colman, R.W., A. Bagdasarian, R.C. Talamo, C. F. Scott, M. Seavey, J.A. Guimaraes, J.V. Pierce, and A.P. Kaplan, 1975, Williams Trait. Human kininogen deficiency with diminished levels of plasminogen pro-activator and prekallikrein associated with abnormalities of the Hageman factor-dependent pathways. J. Clin. Invest. 56:1650.

45. Schiffman, S. , and P. Lee, 1974, Preparation, characterization, and activation of a highly purified factor XI: Evidence that a hitherto unrecognized plasma activity participates in the interaction of factors XI and XII. Br. J. Haematol. 27:101.

46. Schiffman, S., and P. Lee, 1975, Partial purification and characterizatior of contact activation cofactor. J. Clin. Invest. 56:1082.

47. Griffin, J.H., and C.G. Cochrane, 1976, Involvement of high molecular weight kininogen in surface dependent reactions of Hageman factor. Fed. Proc. 35:692, and Proc. Nat. Acad. Sci. USA, in press.

48. Revak, S.D., C.G. Cochrane, and J.H. Griffin, 1976, Plasma proteins necessary for the cleavage of human Hageman factor during surface activation. Fed. Proc. 35:692.

DISCUSSION

MÜLLER-EBERHARD: Did I understand correctly that Hageman factor on binding to kaolin is cleaved and the e-fragment is subsequently released? If so, is this enzymatic cleavage autocatalytic or does prekallikrein express proteolytic activity?

COCHRANE: Cleavage of Hageman factor, bound to kaolin, occurs only after exposure to enzymes. In the case of plasma, the principle enzyme is kallikrein. There is no evidence of autocatalysis.

AUSTEN: What is the relationship of high molecular weight (HMW) to low molecular weight (LMW) kininogen in genetic, functional and antigenic terms?

COCHRANE: Of the five kininogen deficient plasmas so far observed, four are deficient in both high and low molecular weight kininogen, while one, Fitzgerald plasma, is only partly deficient in LMW kininogen while totally deficient in HMW.

In terms of restoration of the capacity to activate Hageman factor, the deficient plasmas are reconstituted only by addition of HMW kininogen.

AUSTEN: Do both plasmin and kallikrein activate C1 to C$\bar{1}$?

COCHRANE: Plasmin was first observed to activate C1s by Ratnoff and his colleagues. We have been able to repeat the observation, testing C$\bar{1}$s activity by its consumption of C4.

MOVAT: If you add to your negatively charged surface shown on the board, prekallikrein in addition to factor XII and HMW kininogen, is there an inhibition of the activated XII (or XII fragments) by DFP?

COCHRANE: Activation of Hageman factor on the surface by kallikrein led to susceptibility to DFP.

MOVAT: Are you still unable to demonstrate a biologically

active fragment intermediate between factor XII (mol. weight approx. 80,000) and prekallikrein activator (mol. weight approx. 28,000)?

COCHRANE: Using purified Hageman factor we have never observed active fragments of Hageman factor other than those of 52,000, 40,000 and 28,000 mol. weight as noted in the talk. This has been true whether the Hageman factor was activated in isolated form or in whole plasma. It has been difficult to understand where the reported intermediate mol. weight Hageman factor fits into the current scheme.

MÜLLER-EBERHARD: Do you propose that HMW kininogen acts as a modulator on Hageman factor rendering it more susceptible to kallikrein?

In that case this modulation of substrate by non-enzymatic proteins could be analogous to the effect of C3b on proactivator of the alternative complement pathway. Without binding to C3b, proactivator is not susceptible to cleavage by proactivator convertase.

COCHRANE: As you say, the HMW kininogen does indeed appear to act as a modulator of Hageman factor function, increasing its capacity to interact with prekallikrein, kallikrein and Factor XI.

NEUTROPHIL GENERATION OF PERMEABILITY ENHANCING PEPTIDES FROM PLASMA SUBSTRATES

H.Z. Movat, J.O. Minta, M.J. Saya, F.M. Habal, C.E. Burrowes, Safia Wasi and Esther Pass

Division of Experimental Pathology, Department of Pathology, University of Toronto, Toronto M5S 1A8, Canada

INTRODUCTION

Wherever antigen–antibody complexes are deposited in tissues, there is fixation of complement, generation of chemotactic substances, accumulation of PMN-leukocytes, phagocytosis of the complexes by these cells, followed by release of phlogistic agents, which cause tissue injury and inflammation (Movat, 1976).

Two and one-half years ago we presented evidence (Movat et al., 1973) that during incubation of antigen–antibody (immune) complexes with PMN-leukocytes there is (a) phagocytosis of the immune complexes, phagolysosome formation and degranulation of the cells, which are neutrophils (Fig. 1) and (b) release of lysosomal enzymes which contain a kinin-generating protease (Table I). As shown in Table I when the cells are fractionated the kinin-forming and ß-glucuronidase activities are recovered mainly in the 16,000g or granule fraction. Table I shows furthermore, that the cell lysate, although containing the highest concentration of the lysosomal marker ß-glucuronidase, contains less kinin-generating activity than the material released by the phagocytosing cells or the 16,000g pellet. This observation could be attributed to a kininase or kinin-inactivating enzyme, detectable in the cytosol fraction or 16,000g supernatant (Movat et al., 1973). The cytoplasmic marker lactic dehydrogenase was not released during interaction of the cells with the immune complexes, but was detectable in the whole cell lysate and in the 16,000g supernatant. It was also shown that cytochalasin B markedly enhanced the release of lysosomal enzymes and this procedure was used in all subsequent experiments dealing with the isolation

391

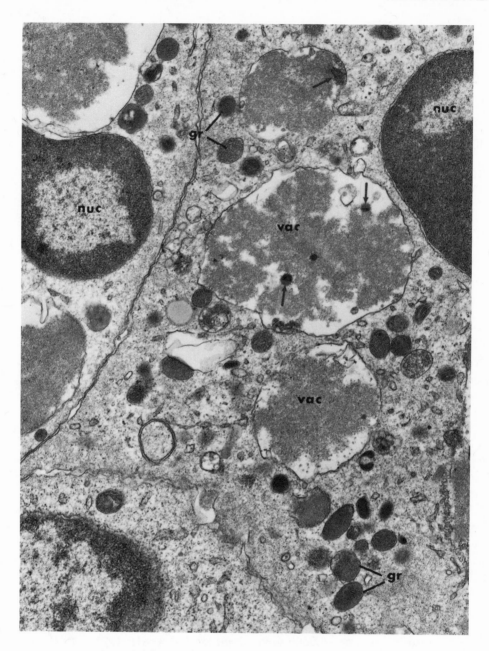

FIG. 1

Electron micrograph of portions of 3 human neutrophil leukocytes
incubated with immune complexes. nuc = nucleus; gr = granules;
vac = vacuoles; arrows = fragmented granules.

TABLE I

Kinin-forming, hydrolase and lactic dehydrogenase activity of PMN-leukocyte fractions and of material released upon interaction of leukocytes and antigen–antibody precipitates

Sample	ß-glucuronidase μg phenolphthalein/ hr/ml/sample	Kinin μg/ml sample	Lactic dehydrogenase units/ml/sample
Cells + Ag–Ab	135	1.3	35
Cells + Tyrode	17	0	19
Cell lysate	362	0.68	5150
400g pellet	79	0.57	370
16,000g pellet	207	1.1	126
16,000g supernatant	55	0	5510

The final concentration of PMN-leukocytes was 10^8/ml. In the kinin assay 0.1 ml kininogen (2.05 mg protein) was incubated at 37° for 1 hour with 0.1 ml of the various samples and the reaction stopped by immersing the tubes for 10 minutes in boiling water. After dilution with de Jalon solution the reaction mixtures were tested on the estrous rat uterus standardized with synthetic bradykinin.

and characterization of the protease. Phagocytosis per se is not a sine qua
non for lysosomal enzyme release. In fact immune complexes formed "in
situ" on the leukocyte surface constitute a better stimulus for lysosomal
enzyme secretion than do preformed ingested complexes (Sajnani et al.,
1976).

PROTEASES OF HUMAN NEUTROPHIL LEUKOCYTES

Human PMN-leukocytes, the majority of which are neutrophils, contain
a large number of proteolytic enzymes, or at least enzymes can be demonstrated which degrade various proteins (Janoff, 1972). In recent years some
of these have been characterized physico-chemically. Among these are an
elastase first described by Janoff and Scherer (1968) and further characterized in recent years (Janoff, 1973; Ohlsson and Olsson, 1974; Schmidt and
Havemann, 1974; Taylor and Crawford, 1975; Feinstein and Janoff, 1975a),
a collagenase (Lazarus et al., 1968; Ohlsson and Olsson, 1973) and a chymotrypsin-like enzyme (Rindler-Ludwig and Braunsteiner, 1975; Schmidt and
Havemann, 1974; Feinstein and Janoff, 1975b). The latter, together with
the elastase, is capable of degrading cartilage chondromucoprotein (Malemud and Janoff, 1975).

The protease described in the introduction was first identified as a highly
basic protein with an approximate molecular weight of 21,000 by gel filtration through Sephadex G-100 in an aqueous medium (Movat, 1974). The
elution pattern showed an overlap of caseinolysis, kinin-generation and
alanine esterase activity. Subsequently, the protease was isolated by cation
exchange chromatography on SP-Sephadex, gel-filtration through Sephadex
G-75 and rechromatography on the cation exchanger. When the lysosomal
lysate is first chromatographed on the cation exchanger the protease elutes
with 0.25-0.4M NaCl, whether a gradient is used (Movat et al., 1975) or
steps (Movat et al., 1976). This is illustrated in Figure 2. The purified protease consists of five bands (Fig. 3). However, when the electrophoresis is
done with DFP treated highly purified protease in SDS disc gels, only a
single band is demonstrable. Such DFP treated protease still has the five
band pattern in acid gels and since they form a family of parallel lines when
electrophoresed at various gel concentrations, they probably represent charge
isomers (Fig. 4) (Hedrik and Smith, 1968). Furthermore, antibody against
the material shown in Figure 3 gives a single precipitin line by immunoelectrophoresis (see Inhibition Studies below).

The molecular weight was estimated to be 28,000-29,000 by gel filtra-
tion of the radioiodinated protein through Sepharose 6B in guanidine HCl
(Movat et al., 1975) and 26,000-27,000 by SDS disc gel electrophoresis
(Movat et al., 1976). Both these values were obtained with DFP-inactivated

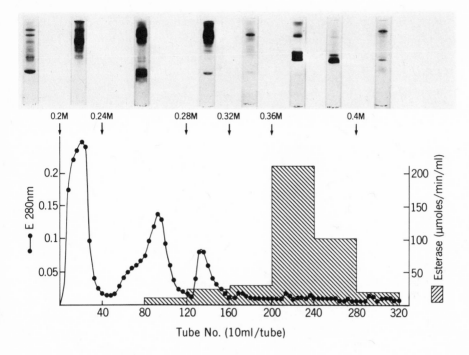

FIG. 2

Chromatography of lysosomal lysate (215 ml; total O.D. 280:
1290; esterolysis: 62.0 μmoles/min/ml) on a 2.5 x 12 cm
column of SP–Sephadex C–50, equilibrated with 0.01M phosphate buffer, pH 6.0. Elution was carried out by increasing
stepwise the NaCl concentration. Activity is expressed as
μ–moles of p–nitrophenol, i.e. the hydrolysis of the synthetic
ester t–butyl–oxycarbonyl–L–alanine–p–nitrophenol.

protease, since the enzyme undergoes autodigestion in the dissociating
media. The highly purified protease focussed in the range of 10.0 to 11.8.
However, the crude enzyme had a pI range of 8.0–11.5. By sucrose density
gradient a sedimentation coefficient of 2.7 was determined.

As shown by sucrose density gradient ultracentrifugation, the bulk of
the protease had an S–value of 2.7, but some of the material, binding less
firmly to the cation exchanger had a sedimentation coefficient of 4.6–4.7S
(Movat et al., 1975). This latter was referred to as "minor PMN–protease

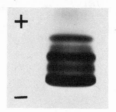

FIG. 3

Electrophoretic pattern of highly purified PMN-protease

activity" and since gel filtration in an aqueous medium indicated a wide
molecular weight range (40,000-60,000) i.e. twice or three times the value
obtained for the "major PMN-protease", it was postulated to represent polymerization (Movat et al., 1976). Recent studies have shed new light on
these findings. When the material released by the neutrophil leukocytes is
immediately inactivated with DFP it has different physico-chemical properties. The availability of monospecific antibody made it possible to monitor
the elution of the protease from SP-Sephadex and Sephadex G-75. The bulk
of such DFP inactivated protease eluted not with 0.36M NaCl, as did the
uninactivated (see Fig. 2), but between 0.24 and 0.28M NaCl. When this
material was passed through a 2.5 x 100 cm column of Sephadex G-75 (0.1M
phosphate; pH 6.0; 0.15M NaCl) the estimated molecular weight of the protease was just over 80,000 (Fig. 5). The purification procedures carried out
until now with the native protease were facilitated by the fact that the
highly basic protease constituted over 80% of the protein eluting with 0.36-
0.4M NaCl during the initial SP-Sephadex chromatography. Because the
protease apparently undergoes autodigestion, not only in dissociating, but
also in aqueous media, it will be essential to examine the physico-chemical
properties of the DFP-inactivated protease. To purify this material eluting
together with a large number of other proteins will be much more difficult,
although essential if one intends to characterize the protease. It is our con-
tention that we are dealing with the leukocyte elastase, which has been isolated by affinity chromatography (Janoff, 1973; Ohlsson and Olsson, 1974;
Feinstein and Janoff, 1975a). These procedures however, are unsuitable for
the purification of the DFP-inactivated protease, which can be purified
probably only with the aid of an immunoabsorbent column. In the meantime,

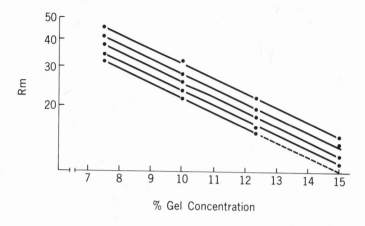

FIG. 4

Plot of relative mobility of the five bands comprising the
PMN-protease against gel concentration.

we have preliminary data on the gel filtration behaviour of the inactivated
protease in the presence of the dissociating solvent 4M guanidine HCl, which
tends to confirm the data obtained by Sephadex G-75.

The native protease is not inhibited by SH-protease inhibitors, the trypsin
inhibitor tosyl-lysine-chloromethyl ketone, but readily inactivated by certain
elastase inhibiting alanine-chloromethyl ketone inhibitors (Fig. 6).

Of the plasma proteinase inhibitors, α_1-antitrypsin, α_2-macroglobulin
and antithrombin III inhibit the protease, the antithrombin requiring trace
amounts of heparin as a cofactor (Movat et al., 1976). With the inhibitors
the enzyme forms complexes, demonstrable by immunoelectrophoresis (Fig. 7).
Thus there are natural inhibitors which are probably responsible for homeo-
stasis.

When injected intradermally the protease produces both enhancement of
vascular permeability and hemorrhage (Movat et al., 1975).

EFFECT OF THE PMN-PROTEASE ON PLASMA-DERIVED SUBS-
TRATES: GENERATION OF PHLOGISTIC CLEAVAGE PRO-
DUCTS

As indicated already in the introduction the crude lysosomal lysate

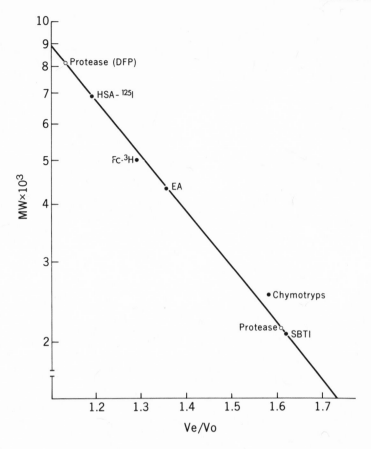

FIG. 5

Gel filtration on Sephadex G-75. Plot of elution (Ve/Vo)
vs. molecular weight. The PMN-protease was passed
through the column untreated and DFP-inactivated. The
inhibition with DFP was carried out immediately after release from the cells. HSA = human serum albumin; EA =
egg albumin; SBTI = soybean trypsin inhibitor.

generates kinin when added to kininogen. The kininogen used in these
studies was highly purified. Both high and low molecular weight kininogens
were used (Habal et al., 1974; 1975; Habal and Movat, 1976). Our initial
studies indicated that the peptide generated by a lysosomal lysate from purified kininogen was bradykinin, with traces of a meth-lys-bradykinin-like

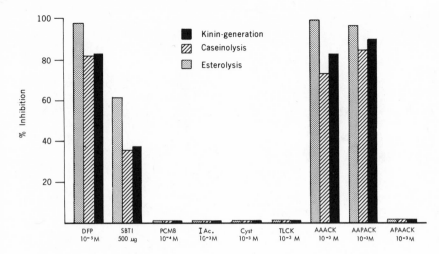

FIG. 6

Inhibition of kinin-generating, caseinolytic and alanine esterase activities by PMN-protease. DFP = diisopropylfluorophosphate; SBTI = soybean trypsin inhibitor; PCMB = p-chloromercuribenzoate; IAc = iodoacetic acid; Cyst = cysteine; TLCK = tosyl lysine-chloromethyl ketone; AAACK = N-acetyl-(L-ala)$_3$ chloromethyl ketone; AAPACK = N-acetyl-L-ala-L-ala-L-pro-L-ala chloromethyl ketone; APAACK = N-acetyl-L-ala-L-pro-L-ala-L-ala chloromethyl ketone. For details see original reference (from H.Z. Movat et al. - Int.Arch. Allergy, 50, 257, 1976).

peptide (Movat and Habal, 1976). However, we became aware of the fact that certain granules of human leukocytes contain an aminopeptidase (Folds et al., 1972). Plasma and certain tissue aminopeptidases cleave the Lys-Arg bond in the decapeptide (lysyl-bradykinin or kallidin) or undecapeptide (methionyl-lysyl-bradykinin), as described by Erdős et al. (1976). According to Behal and Folds (1967) certain heavy metal salts inhibit the aminopeptidase of PMN-leukocytes. Thus blocking the aminopeptidase with zinc chloride or using the highly purified neutrophil protease gave rise to the meth-lys-bradykinin-like peptide exclusively (Fig. 8). The separation of the peptides was done by the highly reproducible CM-cellulose method of Habermann and Blennemann (1964). The property of the peptide was further characterized by passage through Sephadex G-15 (Fig. 9). Pharmacologically, the order of potency of the peptide on smooth muscle preparations was:

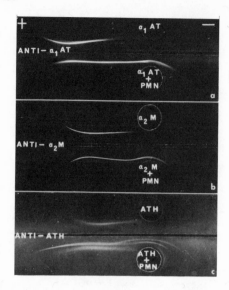 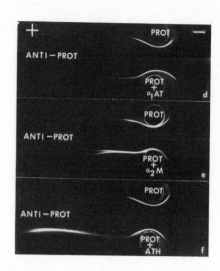

FIG. 7

Immunoelectrophoresis of α_1-antitrypsin, α_2-macroglobulin
and antithrombin III with and without lysosomal lysate
(PMN), developed with antibody against the appropriate
inhibitor (a-c). Immunoelectrophoresis of purified PMN-
protease (Prot) with and without inhibitors and developed
with monospecific antibody (anti-Prot) against the protease
(d-f) (from H.Z. Movat et al. - Int. Arch. Allergy , 50,
257, 1976).

rat uterus > rat duodenum > guinea pig ileum. The aminopeptidase elutes in
the excluded peak when a crude PMN-leukocyte lysosomal lysate is passed
through SP-Sephadex (see Fig. 2). This crude aminopeptidase was further
purified by rechromatography on SP-Sephadex, passage through QAE-Sephadex and Sephadex G-200 (Pass and Movat, 1976). Using pharmacological
techniques (Reiss et al., 1971) (bioassay on the guinea pig ileum or rat
uterus) it was possible to demonstrate a three to four-fold increase in activity on the rat uterus and approximately ten to fifteen-fold increase in
activity on the guinea pig ileum when the undecapeptide was bioassayed
after incubation with the aminopeptidase. The aminopeptidase increased
also the activity of the PMN-protease generated kinin, when incubated and

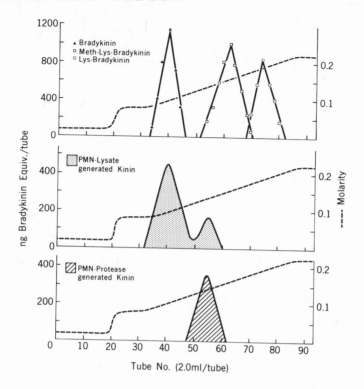

FIG. 8

Chromatography of kinins on a 1.4 x 8.0 cm column of
CM-cellulose equilibrated with 0.02 M formate
(pH 4.8): The upper third shows the elution of the
synthetic kinins. The middle third that of the kinins
generated when kininogen is incubated with a lysosomal lysate and the lower third the kinins generated
when kininogen is incubated with the purified PMN-
protease.

tested by bioassay (Fig. 10). The material shown in the lower panel of
Figure 8 acquires the charge and elution characteristics of bradykinin after
treatment with the aminopeptidase.

Our working hypothesis is that the kinin generated by the PMN-protease
(elastase) is either meth-lys-bradykinin or has one additional amino acid

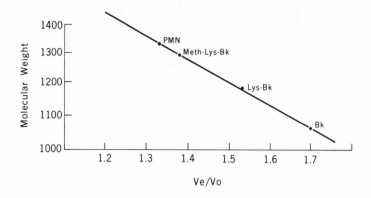

FIG. 9

Gel filtration of the PMN-protease generated kinins
on two interconnected columns of (1.6 x 80 and 1.6
x 92 cm) of Sephadex G-15 equilibrated with 0.2M
formate buffer (pH 4.0). The column was calibrated
with synthetic kinins.

and thus a molecular weight between 1,288 and 1,500. Its amino acid
sequence and the nature of the di-or tripeptide cleaved by the aminopeptidase remains to be elucidated; likewise, the vascular permeability
enhancing effect of the PMN-generated kinin. Preliminary data indicate
that, compared to bradykinin, its phlogistic potency is greater than its
smooth muscle contracting capacity (Table II).

Another plasma-derived substrate on which the PMN-protease acts is the
third component of complement.

C3 was highly purified from resolubilized euglobulin precipitates by
passage through QAE-Sephadex and CM-Sephadex and then interacted with
trypsin, plasmin, or the PMN-protease (Saya, 1975). Only the data with
the leukocyte lysosomal enzyme will be described here.

Conversion of C3 into a more anodally migrating component could be
demonstrated by immunoelectrophoresis (Fig. 11). The degree of conversion
depended on the amount of protease used and on the time of incubation. The
purity of the C3 preparation is shown in Figure 12a (alkaline gel). Figure 12

TABLE II

Vascular permeability induced in guinea pig skin with PMN-protease generated kinin (CPM/Lesion)

Dilution of kinin	1/4	1/8	1/16	1/32	1/64	1/128
with Trypsin	25,100	18,500	12,400	13,600	6,100	4,600
with PBS	36,600	28,000	20,400	17,500	9,300	6,100

PMN-protease generated kinin obtained by CM-cellulose chromatography was concentrated to yield approximately 6.0 μg/ml of bradykinin equivalents, when tested on the rat uterus. One aliquot (0.8 ml) was incubated for 5 minutes with 100 μg of trypsin (0.1 ml) and the latter neutralized with 120 μg of lima bean trypsin inhibitor (0.1 ml). Another aliquot (0.8 ml) was mixed with 0.2 ml PBS.

The guinea pigs received intravenously Evans blue and ^{125}I-labelled human serum albumin (20 μc/kg) and intradermally serial two-fold dilutions of the treated or untreated kinin (0.1 ml).

One tenth μg synthetic bradykinin induced a lesion with 9,700 CPM.

The data represent the average obtained in 3 guinea pigs.

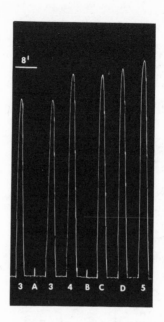

FIG. 10

Kymograph tracing of contractions of the estrous rat
uterus (5 ml bath). The numerals represent synthetic
meth-lys-bradykinin in ng/ml. At "A" the PMN-
protease generated kinin was applied to the bath,
chosen to be just subthreshold; at "B" the aminopeptidase (0.1 ml) was applied; at "C" and "D" the
kinin was preincubated with aminopeptidase for 5 and
15 minutes respectively before adding to the bath.

also shows in acid gels (b, c, d) the pattern of C3, the protease (used in
catalytic amounts) and the product of incubation of C3 and the protease.
Incubation of protease with a fixed amount of C3 for 10 minutes caused
fragmentation; the higher the concentration of the protease the less catho-
dal were the fragments. The same was true with increasing the time of incubation of the two reactants (Fig. 13).

Subthreshold doses of protease, which by themselves caused no enhancement of vascular permeability, induced such enhancement when first incuba-

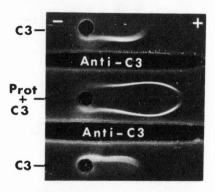

FIG. 11

Immunoelectrophoresis of C3 and neutrophil protease
treated C3. Twenty µg C3 was incubated for 15
minutes at 37° C with 2.2 µg of protease and the
reaction stopped with α_1-antitrypsin (3.0 µg). C3 in
upper and lower wells, C3 and protease reaction mixture in center well and anti-C3 in troughs.

ted with C3. Alternatively, the C3 could be incubated with varying concentrations of protease or for varying lengths of time and the protease inactivated with α_1-antitrypsin (Figs. 14 and 15). With radiolabelled C3 a
small peak with an S-value smaller than that of soybean trypsin inhibitor
(2.3S) was demonstrable by sucrose density ultracentrifugation when C3 was
incubated with the protease. Vascular permeability enhancing fractions
corresponded to the < 2.3S peak, but trailed into fractions with higher sedimentation velocity (Fig. 16).

The fragments obtained with C3 lacked chemotactic activity, both in
vitro and in vivo.

When C3 was incubated with protease for 5 or 10 minutes a contraction
of the guinea pig ileum was induced (Fig. 17), which lead to tachyphylaxis.
No contraction was induced with reactants incubated for 30 minutes. The
IgG fraction (DFP treated to inactivated traces of kallikrein) of rabbit anti-
C3 preincubated with C3 prevented the production of the spasmogen.

As indicated, these studies were performed with C3 prepared initially as
a euglobulin precipitate. No C5 could be demonstrated in the final product
by immunodiffusion.

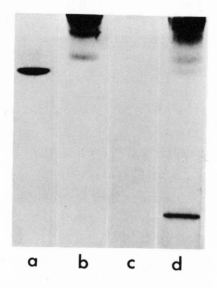

FIG. 12

Disc gel electrophoresis of C3 and of neutrophil protease
treated C3. Gel "a" shows homogeneity of the C3 preparation used in this run in an alkaline gel (pH 8.6). Gel
"b" represents the same C3 preparation in an acid gel (pH
4.5). Gel "c" shows the gel to which the same amount of
protease was applied as to gel "d"; the latter representing the incubation mixture of protease (4.4 µg) and C3
(300 µg), incubated for 10 minutes and the reaction
stopped with α_1-antitrypsin (12 µg).

Cleavage of complement components by PMN-leukocyte lysosomal lysates has been demonstrated before. Such lysates produce fragments from C3
and normal serum which are chemotactic (Taubman et al., 1970). They
cleave C5, producing C5a, which in turn induces further lysosomal enzyme
release (Goldstein and Weissmann, 1974). Recently data have been presented on the cleavage of C3 by leukocyte elastase into several fragments, including C3a. However, this fragment had no biologic activity (Hugli et al.,
1975). As indicated above our C3 preparation was free of C5. However, in
order to strengthen our earlier findings, we are now preparing C3 by poly-
ethylene glycol precipitation of plasma, followed by QAE-Sephadex and
hydroxyapatite chromatography (Minta et al., 1976).

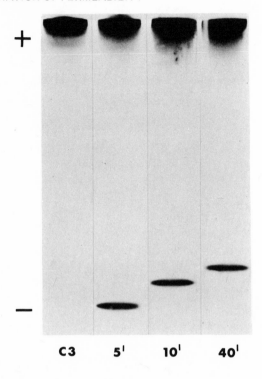

FIG. 13

Disc gel electrophoresis at pH 4.5 of C3 and of C3 (300 μg) incubated with protease (4.4 μg) for 5, 10 and for 40 minutes.

SUMMARY AND CONCLUSIONS

Human PMN-leukocytes, identified as neutrophils by electron microscopy, when interacting with immune complexes release their lysosomal enzymes. A neutral protease has been isolated and purified from the lysosomal lysate, which seems to be identical to leukocyte elastase. The protease can cleave a kinin-like peptide from kininogen, which contracts the rat uterus and enhances vascular permeability. Another lysosomal enzyme, an aminopeptidase probably converts the PMN-protease generated-kinin into bradykinin. The PMN-protease cleaves fragments from C3, some of which enhance vascular permeability and contract the guinea pig ileum.

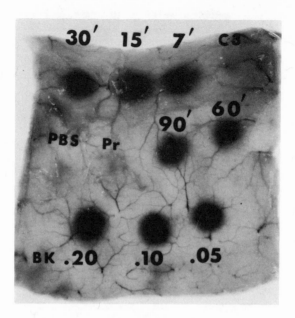

FIG. 14

Guinea pig skin. C3 (450 μg) and protease (2.2 μg)
were incubated for various lengths of time and injected (0.1 ml) intradermally into the skin of guinea
pigs which had received Evans blue and ^{125}I-label-
led HSA i.v. before the injections. Controls consisted of C3, protease (PR) and phosphate buffered
saline (PBS). Positive controls are shown in the
bottom row, represented by 0.2, 0.1, 0.05 μg of synthetic bradykinin.

ACKNOWLEDGEMENTS

The studies described in this paper were supported by the Medical
Research Council of Canada (MT-1251 and MA-5063), the Ontario Heart
Foundation and the J.P. Bickell Foundation.

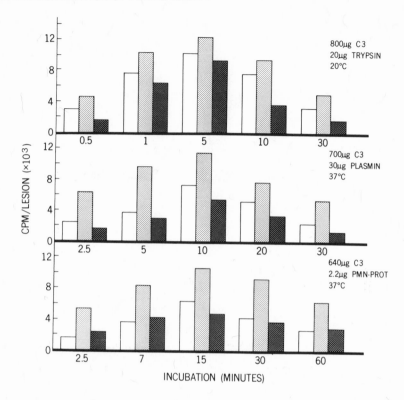

FIG. 15

Enhancement of vascular permeability induced in the
skin of 3 guinea pigs each by a mixture of C3 and
trypsin, plasmin or protease. The trypsin in the reaction mixture was inhibited with a slight excess of lima
bean trypsin inhibitor, the plasmin with soybean trypsin
inhibitor and the protease with a_1-antitrypsin.

Dr. Movat is a Research Associate of the Medical Research Council of
Canada. Dr. Minta is a Research Scholar of the Canadian Heart Foundation.
Dr. Habal was holder of a Studentship of the Medical Research Council of
Canada.

The authors wish to thank Dr. D.M. Wrobel and Mrs. I. MacDonald of the
Canadian Red Cross for generous supplies of blood and plasma.

We also wish to acknowledged the technical and secretarial assistance of
Mrs. A. Carré, Mrs. O. Freitag, Ms. M. Michael and Mr. D.R.L. Macmorine.

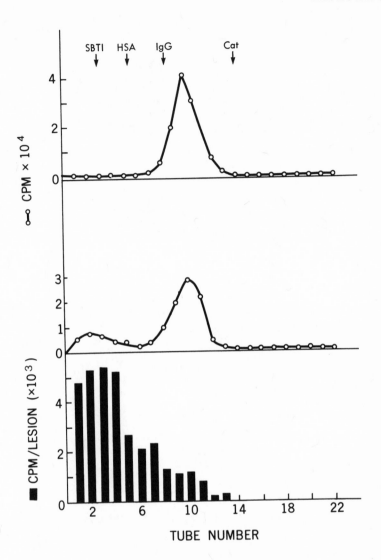

FIG. 16

Sucrose density gradient ultracentrifugation of C3 (upper
panel) and C3 incubated with protease (middle panel),
the C3 having been labelled with ^{125}I- (CPM X 10^4).
The lower panel shows the enhanced vascular permeability induced as in Figure 15 and expressed as CPM/
lesion (X 10^3) (see Table II).

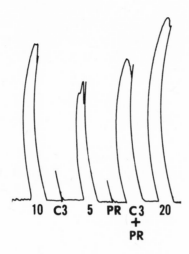

FIG. 17

Kymograph tracing of guinea pig ileum contractions. The numerals represent contractions induced by histamine in ng/ml. One hun-
dred µg of C3 induced no contraction (C3), nor did 14.3 µg of
the protease (PR), but a contraction was induced by a mixture of
the two reactants incubated for 5 minutes. The contraction was
inhibited by prior incubation with anti-C3.

REFERENCES

BEHAL, F. and FOLDS, J.D. (1967). 'Acrylamidase of neisseria cataralis.'
Arch.Biochem.Biophys., 121, 364.

ERDÖS, E.G., NAKAJIMA, T., OSHIMA, G., GECSE, A. and KATO, J.(1976).
'Kininases and their interactions with other systems.' Chemistry and
Biology of the Kallikrein-Kinin System in Health and Disease (ed. by
J.J. Pisano and K.F. Austen). Fogarty International Center Proc. No.
27, U.S. Gov. Printing Office, Washington.

FEINSTEIN, G. and JANOFF, A. (1975a). 'A rapid method for purification
of human granulocyte cation neutral proteases: purification and
further characterization of human granulocyte elastase.' Biophys.
Biochim. Acta, 403, 493.

FEINSTEIN, G. and JANOFF, A. (1975b). 'A rapid method for purification of human granulocyte cationic neutral proteases: purification and characterization of human granulocyte chymotrypsin-like enzyme.' Biophys.Biochim.Acta, 403, 477.

FOLDS, J.D., WELSH, I.R.H. and SPITZNAGEL, J.K. (1972). 'Neutral pro-teases confined to one class of lysosomes of human polymorphonuclear leukocytes.' Proc.Soc.Exp.Biol.Med., 139, 461.

GOLDSTEIN, I.M. and WEISSMANN, G. (1974). 'Generation of C5-derived lysosomal enzyme-releasing activity (C5a) by lysates of leukocyte lysosomes.' J.Immunol., 113, 1583.

HABAL, F.M., MOVAT, H.Z. and BURROWES, C.E. (1974). 'Isolation of two functionally different kininogens from human plasma: separation from proteinase inhibitors and interaction with plasma kallikrein.' Biochem. Pharmacol., 23, 2291.

HABAL, F.M., UNDERDOWN, B.J. and MOVAT, H.Z. (1975). 'Further characterization of human plasma kininogens.' Biochem.Pharmacol., 24, 1241.

HABAL, F.M. and MOVAT, H.Z. (1976). 'Rapid purification of high mole-cular weight kininogen.' Agents and Actions, in press.

HABERMANN, E. and BLENNEMANN, G. (1964). 'Über Substrate und Raktionsprodukte der kininbildenden Enzyme Trypsin, Serum-und Pankreaskallikrein sowie von Crotalusgift.' Naunyn-Schmied.Arch. Exp.Path.Pharm., 249, 357.

HEDRIK, J.L. and SMITH, A.J. (1968). 'Size and charge isomer separation and estimation of molecular weights of proteins by disc gel electro-phoresis.' Arch.Biochem.Biophys., 126, 155.

HUGLI, T.E., TAYLOR, J.C. and CRAWFORD, I.P. (1975). 'Selective cleavage of human C3 by human leukocyte elastase (HLE).' Sixth International Complement Workshop, Sarasota, Florida.

JANOFF, A. and SCHERER, J. (1968). 'Mediators of inflammation in leuko-cyte lysosomes. IX. Elastinolytic activity in granules of human poly-morphonuclear leukocytes.' J.Exp.Med., 128, 1137.

JANOFF, A. (1972). 'Neutrophil proteases in inflammation.' Ann.Rev.Med., 23, 177.

JANOFF, A. (1973). 'Purification of human granulocyte elastase by affinity chromatography.' Lab.Invest., 29, 458.

LAZARUS, G.S., DANIELS, J.R., BROWN, R.S., BLADEN, H.Z. and FULL-MER, H.M. (1968). 'Degradation of collagen by a human granulocyte collagenolytic system.' J.Clin.Invest., 47, 2622.

MALEMUD, C.J. and JANOFF,A. (1975). 'Human polymorphonuclear elastase and cathepsin G mediated the degradation of lapine articular cartilage proteoglycan.' Ann.N.Y.Acad.Sci., 256, 254.

MINTA, J.O., SAYA, M.J. and MOVAT, H.Z. (1976). 'The generation of phlogistic fragments from C3 by a protease of human neutrophil leukocytes.' To be published.

MOVAT, H.Z., STEINBERG, S.G., HABAL, F.M. and RANADIVE, N.S. (1973). 'Demonstration of a kinin-generating enzyme in the lysosomes of human polymorphonuclear leukocytes.' Lab.Invest., 29, 669.

MOVAT, H.Z. (1974). 'Release of a kinin-forming enzyme from human polymorphonuclear leukocytes following interaction with immune complexes.' Allergology, Proceedings of the VIIIth International Congress of Allergology (ed. by Y. Yamamura). Excerpta Medica, Amsterdam.

MOVAT, H.Z., HABAL, F.M., and MACMORINE, D.R.L. (1975). 'Generation of a vasoactive peptide by a neutral protease of human neutrophil leukocytes.' Agents and Actions, December, in press.

MOVAT, H.Z. (1976). 'Pathways to allergic inflammation: The sequelae of antigen-antibody formation.' Symposium on Pathways to Inflammation. Fed.Proc., 35, in press.

MOVAT, H.Z. and HABAL, F.M. (1976). 'Kininogenases of PMN-leukocyte lysosomes.' Chemistry and Biology of the Kallikrein-Kinin System in Health and Disease (ed. by J.J. Pisano and K.F. Austen), Fogarty International Center Proc. No. 27, U.S. Gov. Printing Office, Washington.

MOVAT, H.Z., HABAL, F.M. and MACMORINE, D.R.L. (1976). 'Neutral proteases of human PMN-leukocytes with kininogenase activity.' Int.Arch.Allergy, 50, 257.

OHLSSON, K. and OLSSON, I. (1973). 'The neutral proteases of human granulocytes. Isolation and partial characterization of two granulo-cyte collagenases.' Eur.J.Biochem., 36, 473.

OHLSSON, K. and OLSSON, I. (1974). 'The neutral proteases of human granulocytes. Isolation and partial characterization of granulocyte elastase.' Eur.J.Biochem., 42, 519.

PASS, E. and MOVAT, H.Z. (1976). 'An aminopeptidase of human neutro-phil leukocyte lysosomes.' To be published.

REIS, M.L., OKINO, L. and ROCHA E SILVA, M. (1971). 'Comparative pharmacological actions of bradykinin and related kinins of larger molecular weight.' Biochem.Pharmacol., 20, 2935.

RINDLER-LUDWIG, R. and BRAUNSTEINER, H. (1975). 'Cationic proteins from human neutrophil granulocytes. Evidence for their chymotrypsin-like properties.' Biophys.Biochim.Acta, 379, 606.

SAJNANI, A.N., MOVAT, H.Z. and RANADIVE, N.S. (1976). 'Redistribu-tion of immunoglobulin receptors on human neutrophils and its rela-tionship to the release of lysosomal enzymes.' Lab.Invest., in press.

SAYA, M.J. (1975). 'Studies on C3: the third component of human comple-ment.' Dissertation, University of Toronto.

SCHMIDT, W. and HAVEMANN, K. (1974). 'Isolation of elastase-like and chymotrypsin-like neutral proteases from human granulocytes.' Hoppe-Seyler's Z.Physiol.Chem., 335, 1077.

TAUBMAN, S., GOLDSCHMIDT, P.R. and LEPOW, I.H. (1970). 'Effect of lysosomal enzymes from human leukocytes on human complement components.' Fed.Proc., 29, 434.

TAYLOR, J.C. and CRAWFORD, I.P. (1975). 'Purification and preliminary characterization of human granulocyte elastase.' Arch.Biochem. Biophys., 169, 91.

DISCUSSION

GOETZL: Does you protease degrade C5 as well as C3?

MOVAT: We hope to have an answer within a few months. As you know C5 is much more difficult to isolate. However, the data of Goldstein and Weissmann with a crude lysosomal lysate would indicate (assuming that they are dealing with the same enzyme as we do)that C5 is fragmented by leukocyte lysosomal proteases.

GOETZL: What is the functional inhibiting profile of plasma α-globulins for the activity of your protease?

MOVAT: I am sorry to say that I have no answer as yet to your question.

AUSTEN: Could the 80,000 molecular weight form be a precursor of the 20,000 molecular weight protease?

MOVAT: I have no direct answer to your question, merely to say that to my knowledge all lysosomal enzymes in neutrophils are present in active form and that these cells do not contain zymogens.

VENGE (Uppsala): We have studied the effect of chymotrypsin-like cationic protein on C3 and C5 and obtained only chemo-tactically active products. Are the C3 products you obtained chemotactically active?

MOVAT: I forgot to mention that the C3 fragments we obtained are not chemotactic. However, our method of isolation would exclude the chymotrypsin-like enzyme, which according to Rindler-Ludwig and Braunsteiner are soluble only at 1.0 M NaCl concentration. We are currently working on the biological activity of this enzyme.

MÜLLER-EBERHARD: Since the polymorphonuclear enzyme you isolated is obviously not a tryptic enzyme, and since the low molecular weight C3 fragment has biological activity, is it resistant to inactivation by the serum carboxypeptidase B? It should be.

MOVAT: Certain tryptic inhibitors, such as tosyl-lysine-chloromethyl ketone do not inhibit the enzyme, whereas other alanine containing chloromethyl ketone inhibitors, which inhibit elastase inhibit also our enzyme (Movat et al. Int. Arch Allergy, Jan. 1976).

We have no inhibition studies with the C3 fragment, but pancreatic carboxypeptidase B (not the plasma carboxypeptidase N, of Erdös) inhibits the kinin-peptide.

We have studies inhibiting the generation of the C3 fragment when anti-C3 was added to the C3 prior to incubation with
the enzyme, but nothing further. As you may have noticed I was
careful not to use the term "C3a" in speaking about the fragments obtained from C3.

SPECIFICITY AND MODULATION OF THE EOSINOPHIL POLYMORPHONUCLEAR

LEUKOCYTE RESPONSE TO THE EOSINOPHIL CHEMOTACTIC FACTOR OF

ANAPHYLAXIS (ECF-A)[1]

Edward J. Goetzl[2] and K. Frank Austen

Departments of Medicine, Harvard Medical School and the

Robert B. Brigham Hospital, Boston, Mass. 02120, U.S.A.

After their generation from myeloid precursors in bone marrow, eosinophil polymorphonuclear (PMN) leukocytes circulate for a brief period in peripheral blood and then emigrate to tissue pools local-ized predominantly in the lungs, skin, intestines and genitourinary tract (Hudson, 1968; Spry, 1971; Zucker-Franklin, 1974). An increase in the level of eosinophils in peripheral blood and in involved tissues is a prominent feature of systemic immediate hypersensitivity reactions (Campbell et al, 1935). The selective influx of eosino-phils to the focus of an immediate hypersensitivity reaction is governed by the tissue levels of diverse eosinophil chemotactic factors, by the biodegradation or inhibition of the chemotactic factors, and by reversible and irreversible alterations in the chemotactic responsiveness of the target cells (Goetzl et al, 1975). The net effect of this series of interactions is the positioning of a critical number of eosinophils at the site of an immediate hyper-sensitivity reaction so that they may exercise their specific regulatory role (Goetzl et al, 1975).

Immediate hypersensitivity reactions in vitro result in the release of chemotactic activity that is uniquely preferential for eosinophils and can be attributed predominantly to the eosinophil chemotactic factor of anaphylaxis (ECF-A) (Kay et al, 1971; Kay and Austen, 1971). Of the other primary and secondary chemical mediators of immediate hypersensitivity, only histamine has been documented

[1]Supported by grants AI-07722 and AI-10356 from the National Institutes of Health.
[2]Investigator, Howard Hughes Medical Institute.

to stimulate eosinophil migration. Early in vivo studies revealed
an influx of eosinophils into pulmonary tissue, in association with
a peripheral blood eosinophilia, in response to the intraperitoneal
or intravenous injection of histamine in guinea pigs (Vaughn, 1953;
Parish, 1970). However, neither local intraperitoneal nor intradermal eosinophilia followed histamine injection in animals
(Archer, 1956; Vegad and Lancaster, 1972), and histamine chemotaxis
could not be demonstrated in vitro with guinea pig or human
eosinophils in standard Boyden chamber assays with 100-120 μm thick
cellulose nitrate filters and 2 1/2 - 3 hr incubation periods
(Kay et al, 1971; Kay and Austen, 1971).

     An in vitro eosinophilotactic activity of histamine has
recently been observed in modified Boyden chambers with 30-60 min
incubation periods and 12-15 μm thick polycarbonate filters; the
number of eosinophils migrating through the filters was assessed by
microscopic enumeration or by counting the radioactivity of
^{51}Cr-labeled eosinophils. With cellulose nitrate filters of 145 μm
thickness, the cells were assessed after these short incubation
times at a point within the filters (Clark et al, 1975). While the
eosinophilotactic activity of histamine in the modified Boyden
chambers was dependent on a concentration gradient, it differed
from other chemotactic factors with respect to the brief period in
which directed migration could be appreciated and in its very
restricted concentration range of activity. The chemotactic effect
was lost at levels only 2- to 3-fold higher than the peak chemotactic dose. In addition, 10^{-5}M histamine added to both sides of
the filter often resulted in enhanced random migration of a small
fraction of the eosinophils (Clark et al, 1975). In contrast to
ECF-A, the principal in vitro eosinophil action of histamine appears to be modulation of spontaneous migration and a brief elicitation of directed migration.

                        THE STRUCTURE OF ECF-A

     ECF-A was discovered in 1971 as a mediator released during
anaphylactic reactions in guinea pig (Kay et al, 1971) and human
(Kay and Austen, 1971) lung slices. The release of ECF-A from human
tissues by IgE-dependent mechanisms has a time-course, biochemical
requirements and responsiveness to the intracellular levels of
cyclic nucleotides similar to histamine release from the same
tissues (Wasserman et al, 1974a). ECF-A was present preformed in
purified rat mast cells in association with the granules (Wasserman
et al, 1974b), and was also extractable from human leukemic basophils (Lewis et al, 1975) and mast cell-rich tissues such as human
lung and nasal polyps (Kaliner et al, 1973; Goetzl et al, 1974b).
The sum of the activity released by immunologic mechanisms and that
in the cellular residuals of stimulated tissues was equal to that

extracted from unchallenged tissues, confirming the preformed nature
of ECF-A. Preliminary physicochemical characterization of ECF-A
obtained by extraction or immunologic activation of guinea pig and
human lung tissues and rat mast cells revealed a molecular weight
of approximately 500 by filtration on Sephadex G-25 (Kay et al,
1971; Wasserman et al, 1974b), inactivation by digestion with subtilisin or pronase but not with trypsin or chymotrypsin (Wasserman
et al, 1974c), and two anodal peaks of activity on high voltage
paper electrophoresis at pH 7 (Goetzl et al, 1974b).

The low molecular weight tetrapeptides with preferential eosinophil chemotactic activity extracted from fragments of human lung
by sonication in butanol-acetic acid or alkaline Tyrode's buffer
were isolated by sequential purification on Sephadex G-25, Dowex-1,
Sephadex G-10, and paper chromatography (Goetzl and Austen, 1975).
The ECF-A activity from IgE-mediated reactions in human lung tissues
appeared along with that in extracts of human lung during parallel
purification procedures. Fractions of the highly purified extracts
with eosinophilotactic activity contained two acidic tetrapeptides
of amino acid sequence Ala-Gly-Ser-Glu and Val-Gly-Ser-Glu. The
synthetic tetrapeptides and purified ECF-A were maximally active in
amounts from 0.1-1.0 nmole per chemotactic chamber that represent
concentrations of 10^{-7}-10^{-6}M (Goetzl and Austen, 1975). Both
purified native ECF-A and synthetic tetrapeptides were preferentially active on eosinophils as compared to neutrophils and monocytes with respect to chemotaxis and the induction of subsequent
unresponsiveness to chemotactic stimulation, termed deactivation.

REGULATION OF THE EOSINOPHIL CHEMOTACTIC RESPONSE TO ECF-A

Generation and Specificity of ECF-A

The generation of chemotactic factors during immediate and
subacute hypersensitivity reactions represents the initial pathway
in the regulation of the eosinophil chemotactic response. Whereas
immediate hypersensitivity reactions generate ECF-A and histamine,
activation of the classical or alternative (properdin) complement
pathways generate the anaphylatoxins, C3a and C5a (Vallota and
Müller-Eberhard, 1973). Further, C3a may be directly cleaved from
C3 by plasmin or specific tissue proteases (Ward, 1967 and 1971) and
C5a from C5 by a neutrophil lysosomal protease (Ward and Hill, 1970).

The second level of modulation consists of the concentration,
potency, and leukocyte specificity of each chemotactic factor which
may be determined by specific structural features. The complement-
derived factors, C3a and C5a, attract eosinophils, neutrophils and
monocytes with equivalent activity for each cell type (Ward and Hill,
1970; Snyderman et al, 1971; Kay et al, 1973; Goetzl et al, 1974b),

while natural and synthetic ECF-A preferentially attract eosinophils
when the eosinophils represent 10% or more of the target leukocyte
pool (Kay et al, 1973; Goetzl and Austen, 1975). The heterogeneity
of principles manifesting eosinophil chemotactic activity is demonstrated by Sephadex G-25 filtration of the supernatant from an
extract of isolated rat mast cells of 88% purity (Fig. 1). The
neutrophil and eosinophil chemotactic activities of each fraction
were assessed in modified Boyden chambers with leukocytes from a
hypereosinophilic patient composed of 28% eosinophils, 31% neutrophils and 41% mononuclear cells; the use of 3 μm pore filters and a
2 hr incubation period precluded mononuclear leukocytes from
progressing to the field where cells were enumerated in stained
filters. Four peaks of activity were delineated with both types of
polymorphonuclear leukocytes. The chemotactic activity appearing
in the exclusion volume was preferential for neutrophils and the
other three peaks of chemotactic activity exhibiting apparent molecular weights of 2500-3500, 300-500 and 150-200 showed progressively
greater attraction of eosinophils relative to neutrophils.

The high molecular weight peak was originally recognized in the
extracts of human leukemic basophils as a factor with predominant
chemotactic action on neutrophils (Lewis et al, 1975) and has subsequently been termed NCF-A (Austen et al, this volume). The two
smallest peaks possess selective eosinophil chemotactic activity
and correspond in size, respectively, to ECF-A tetrapeptides and a
region within the overlap of the ECF-A and histamine areas (Fig. 1).
The intermediate peak is highly chemotactic for eosinophils and
shows moderate preference for this cell type over neutrophils in
dose-response studies. Unlike ECF-A and NCF-A, the intermediate
peak is present in anaphylactic diffusates in amounts representing
only a small percent of the mast cell stores. Since it is contained
with ECF-A in mast cell-rich tissues and isolated rat mast cells in
which it is located in the granules, is inactivated by digestion with
subtilisin and is preferentially chemotactic for eosinophils, it
either is a precursor of ECF-A or a distinct but functionally
related eosinophil chemotactic factor (Boswell et al, manuscript in
preparation). A comparable peak of eosinophilotactic activity has
been recognized in tumor extracts, urine and cell culture supernatants of patients with bronchogenic carcinoma and eosinophilia
(Goetzl et al, 1976b). The availability in mast cell stores of
eosinophilotactic peptides of varying sizes which are released by
IgE-mediated reactions provides for rapid establishment of a
chemotactic gradient by the smaller factors and the maintenance of
the gradient by less diffusable larger factors, thus ensuring an
early and continuing movement of eosinophils to the focus of the
allergic reaction.

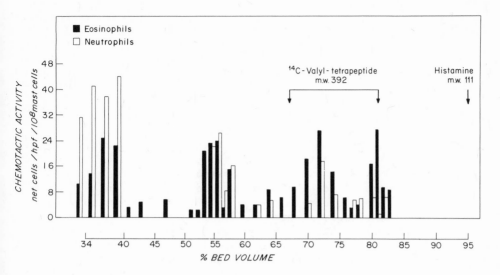

Fig. 1 Sephadex G-25 fractionation of chemotactic activity in an extract of isolated mast cells. A total of 1.1×10^8 rat peritoneal mast cells, purified to 88% mast cells by centrifugation on metrizamide cushions, were extracted in alkaline Tyrode's buffer and the supernatant applied to a 1.5 x 80 cm column with 1.42 ml fraction volumes of which 0.2 ml were assessed in duplicate for eosinophil and neutrophil chemotactic activity.

Inhibition of Eosinophil Chemotactic Factor Activity

The third level of regulation of eosinophil chemotaxis encompasses the inhibitors or inactivators of chemotactic factors. The anaphylatoxin inactivator suppresses C3a and C5a-mediated leukotaxis (Bokisch and Müller-Eberhard, 1970) and the chemotactic factor inactivator (CFI), composed of two or more exo-proteolytic enzymes present in serum and cells, irreversibly inactivates numerous chemotactic factors (Berenberg and Ward, 1973). While the in vivo

pathways of degradation of ECF-A have not yet been elucidated,
limited digestion of the valyl- and alanyl-tetrapeptides with either
aminopeptidase-M or carboxypeptidase-A reduces their eosinophil
chemotactic activity in proportion to the extent of liberation of
NH2- and COOH-terminal amino acids, respectively (Goetzl and Austen,
1975).

A special class of hydrophobic amino acid derivatives and peptides that inhibit the activity of ECF-A is exemplified by valine-
amide (Val-amide) and the NH2-terminal tripeptide, Val-Gly-Ser, that
possess neither chemotactic nor deactivating activities. Both Val-
amide and Val-Gly-Ser suppress the eosinophilotactic activity of
10^{-7}M valyl-tetrapeptide when present concomitantly in the stimulus
compartment of the Boyden chamber with 50% mean inhibition at 10^{-6}M
and 10^{-7}M, respectively (Goetzl et al, 1976a). Val-amide and Val-
Gly-Ser presumably inhibit the eosinophil chemotactic response by
competing with ECF-A for a hydrophobic site on the eosinophil
surface, and thus are without effect on eosinophil random migration.
The capacity of Val-Gly-Ser to inhibit eosinophil chemotaxis to
valyl-tetrapeptide in an equimolar relationship has been observed in
vivo as well (Wasserman et al, 1976).

Factors Which Alter Eosinophil Chemotactic Responsiveness

The fourth level of regulation of eosinophil chemotactic migration includes factors that alter chemotaxis by influencing the
responsiveness of the cells. The effects of these factors on
eosinophils are independent of the specific chemotactic stimulus,
result in enhancement or suppression of chemotaxis and generally
extend to similar actions on spontaneous migration. This group of
non-cytotoxic factors that alter eosinophil chemotactic responsiveness consist of the chemotactic factors themselves that operate
through a process termed deactivation (Ward and Becker, 1968,
1970); the neutrophil immobilizing factor (NIF) with an action
limited to suppression of migration (Goetzl et al, 1973); and
factors with multiple leukocyte-directed effects, such as Thr-
Lys-Pro-Arg, that enhances phagocytosis while diminishing random
and directed migration (Nishioka et al, 1972; Goetzl, 1975) and
ascorbate, that stimulates the hexose monophosphate shunt of eosinophils in parallel with enhancement of their random and directed
migration (Goetzl et al, 1974a).

Deactivation of eosinophils or other leukocytes is not reversible by washing the cells (Ward and Becker, 1968; Wasserman et al,
1975). The leukocyte selectivity of deactivation by chemotactic
principles parallels their chemotactic specificity (Goetzl and
Austen, 1975). Chemotactic deactivation is accompanied by a decrease
in random migration of eosinophils, as well as other leukocytes,
and by a burst of activity of the hexose monophosphate shunt (HMPS).

Stimulation of the HMPS can be elicited repetitively by serial
introduction of a chemotactic stimulus despite the maintenance of
depressed chemotactic and random migration (Goetzl and Austen,
1974). The exposure of human eosinophils to C5a or partially purified ECF-A results in their rapid deactivation in response to both
the homologous and heterologous chemotactic stimuli (Wasserman et
al, 1975). Concentrations of either chemotactic factor as low as
1/20 of the minimal chemotactic dose were capable of producing full
deactivation of eosinophils in a time-dependent manner.

Synthetic preparations of both tetrapeptides which comprise
ECF-A rapidly deactivate eosinophils in quantities as small as 0.1
picomole per 5 x 10^6 eosinophils and exhibit cross-deactivating
capacity for the other tetrapeptide and natural ECF-A (Goetzl and
Austen, 1975; Goetzl et al, 1976a). Preincubation of 8 x 10^6 eosinophils in concentrations of alanyl-tetrapeptide ranging from
10^{-8}M to 10^{-12}M, followed by extensive washing of the cells and
assessment of their chemotactic response to 10^{-7}M valyl-tetrapeptide
revealed 75-80% deactivation after a 5 min exposure to 10^{-8}M or
10^{-10}M alanyl-tetrapeptide (Fig. 2). The deactivation of eosinophils preincubated in 10^{-12}M alanyl-tetrapeptide varied with
different samples of cells from 0-40% after 1-5 min, reached
60-70% by 40 min and 80-90% at 1 1/2 to 2 hr. Thus, 1/100 of the
minimal chemotactic dose of alanyl-tetrapeptide gave brisk and
complete deactivation of eosinophils.

Cell-directed inhibitors without chemotactic activity that
irreversibly reduce eosinophil chemotactic responsiveness include
the neutrophil immobilizing factor (NIF) and the COOH-terminal tripeptide of ECF-A, Gly-Ser-Glu. NIF is generated by incubating human
peripheral blood mononuclear or polymorphonuclear leukocytes in
acid medium (ANIF), with endotoxin (ENIF), or with phagocytosable
particles (PhNIF) (Goetzl and Austen, 1972). NIF is separable from
coexistent chemotactic activity in the leukocyte supernatants by
heating and gel filtration on Sephadex G-25, exhibits an apparent
molecular weight of 4,000-5,000 and is cationic since it appears in
the effluent from diethylaminoethyl-cellulose equilibrated in 0.1M
Tris-HCl buffer at pH 8.6. Partially purified NIF suppressed the
random and chemotactic migration of eosinophil and neutrophil polymorphonuclear leukocytes but not of mononuclear leukocytes and
failed to alter PMN leukocyte viability, phagocytic capacity, adherence to surfaces, or baseline or stimulated HMPS activity (Goetzl
et al, 1973).

Although the ECF-A COOH-terminal tripeptide, Gly-Ser-Glu, has
not been studied for its other effects on eosinophil function, it
inhibits chemotaxis by a suppressive action on the cells (Goetzl et
al, 1976a). Preincubation of eosinophils with Gly-Ser-Glu, which
lacks substantial chemotactic activity, resulted in a dose- and
time-dependent suppression of their subsequent response to natural

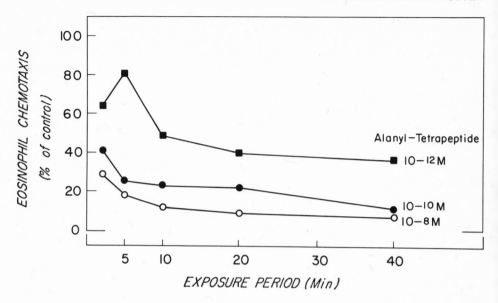

Fig. 2 Time course of eosinophil deactivation by synthetic alanyl-
tetrapeptide. Following the deactivation exposure, the eosinophils
were washed in Hanks' balanced salt solution + 0.4 g/100 ml crystalline ovalbumin three times and assessed for residual responsiveness to 10^{-7}M valyl-tetrapeptide. Suspensions of eosinophils were
of 92% purity, background migration was 4 eos/hpf with a net response to 10^{-7}M valyl-tetrapeptide of 15 eos/hpf.

or synthetic ECF-A which reached 80% inhibition after a 20 min
exposure of 9×10^6 eosinophils to 10^{-8}M tripeptide (Goetzl et al,
1976a). The action of the COOH-terminal tripeptide appears to be
on the cells themselves as evidenced by the persistence of its
effect after cell washing and the failure of the tripeptide to
inhibit significantly when present on the stimulus side of the
Boyden chamber.

A leukocyte phagocytosis-stimulating tetrapeptide, Thr-Lys-Pro-
Arg, designated "Tuftsin", was initially recognized when a cyto-

philic fraction of human γ-globulin was digested with a human PMN leukocyte-derived extract (Nishioka et al, 1972; Najjar, 1974). Nanogram quantities of the natural or synthetic peptide enhance by 2- to 2 1/2-fold the phagocytosis of latex particles or Staphy-lococcus aureus by suspensions of human, dog or guinea pig PMN leukocytes and mouse peritoneal or rabbit lung macrophages (Nishioka et al, 1972). Thr-Lys-Pro-Arg lacks in vitro leukotactic activity in micropore filter chambers, and preincubation in concen-trations ranging from 1-100 ng/ml with purified populations of human eosinophils and neutrophils suppressed their random and chemotactic migration with concomitant stimulation of their phagocytic capacity (Goetzl, 1975). Neither the baseline nor chemotactic factor-stimulated levels of HMPS activity of the leukocytes were influenced by the tetrapeptide (Goetzl, 1975).

Ascorbic acid is a non-chemotactic principle which enhances the random migration and chemotactic responsiveness of neutrophils, eosinophils and mononuclear leukocytes by 100-300% of baseline values with concomitant and equivalent stimulation of leukocyte HMPS acti-vity (Goetzl et al, 1974a). Ascorbate, at concentrations of 2 to $10 \times 10^{-3}M$, results in dose-related enhancement to maximal levels of both migration and HMPS activity of eosinophils and other leuko-cytes, but has no effect on phagocytosis.

Histamine Modulation of Eosinophil Migration

While histamine at concentrations of $3 \times 10^{-7}M$ to $1.25 \times 10^{-6}M$ (33-139 ng/ml) induces directed migration of eosinophils in some in vitro models that employ thin polycarbonate filters or brief incuba-tion periods with standard cellulose nitrate filters (Clark et al, 1975), its eosinophilotactic activity differs in several respects from that of eosinophil chemotactic factors such as ECF-A and C5a. Histamine in the stimulus compartment of a standard Boyden Millipore filter chamber, at a concentration of 80 ng/ml that stimulated maximal migration of eosinophils, did not alter the distribution of cells within the filter in a manner comparable to natural or synthe-tic ECF-A (Fig. 3). Although histamine increased the number of eosinophils migrating 20 μm or further from the cell source relative to controls, the maximum number of eosinophils remained at the top of the filter as in the buffer spontaneous migration controls. In contrast, both purified ECF-A and valyl-tetrapeptide at concentra-tions stimulating comparable movement of eosinophils to the front, produced a wave of movement such that the maximum number of eosino-phils was observed 10-20 μm into the filter at 90 minutes (Fig. 3).

Histamine-induced suppression of eosinophil chemotactic responsiveness is only observed at concentrations in the mid to upper portion of the chemotactic range for histamine (Clark et al,

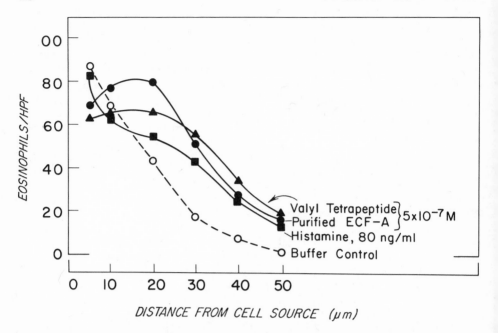

DISTANCE FROM CELL SOURCE (μm)

Fig. 3 Distribution of eosinophils in micropore filters. Eosinophils were of 88% purity and were incubated 90 min at 37°C in Hanks'
solution + ovalbumin in chambers with Millipore filters of 3 μm
pore diameter and with synthetic stimuli or ECF-A purified from
human lung and employed at a concentration of 5 x 10^{-7}M.

1975). This action again contrasts with that of the synthetic
tetrapeptides which fully deactivate at 1/100 their minimal chemotactic concentration.

     The addition of histamine to the cell compartment of Boyden
chambers at a dose of 30 ng/ml which stimulates only minimal eosinophil migration enhances the chemotactic response of eosinophils
to a low concentration of valyl-tetrapeptide in a more than additive
fashion (Fig. 4). An identical protocol utilizing a dose of 600
ng/ml histamine inhibits the spontaneous migration of eosinophils
when present on the cell side and suppresses the eosinophil response
to valyl-tetrapeptide especially when present in the cell compart-

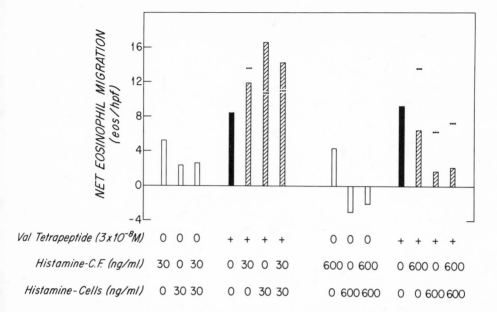

Val Tetrapeptide (3x10⁻⁸M)   0 0 0   + + + +   0 0 0   + + + +

Histamine-C.F. (ng/ml)   30 0 30   0 30 0 30   600 0 600   0 600 0 600

Histamine-Cells (ng/ml)   0 30 30   0 0 30 30   0 600 600   0 0 600 600

Fig. 4   Histamine modulation of eosinophil chemotaxis.   Eosinophil
chemotaxis was carried out in modified Boyden chambers with 3 μm
pore Millipore filters and eosinophils at a concentration of 37% in
unpurified suspensions; background migration was 6 eos/hpf.   Dashed
lines represent the response that would be obtained if both stimuli
acted on the eosinophils in a purely additive fashion.

ment.   Thus, the effects of histamine on eosinophil movement include
brief directed migration at intermediate doses, and cell-directed
modulation of random and directed migration which is stimulatory at
low and suppressive at high concentrations.   High dose suppression
of histamine-induced directed migration has been attributed to
elevation of intracellular cyclic AMP since it is prevented by the
simultaneous addition of H2-blockers (Clark et al, 1975).

CONCLUDING COMMENTS

The eosinophil leukotactic response toward a concentration gradient of a chemotactic factor is regulated at four levels (Fig. 5). Diverse pathways activated by immediate, subacute and delayed hypersensitivity reactions generate stimuli with eosinophilotactic activity (Fig. 5-1), including the following: fragments of known proteins exemplified by C5a, C3a and fibrinopeptides (McKenzie et al, 1975); products of mast cells and basophils stimulated by IgE-mediated reactions such as the ECF-A tetrapeptides and intermediate m.w. eosinophilotactic oligopeptides; lymphokines that must first interact with immune complexes (Torisu et al, 1973); and certain conversion products of arachidonic acid and other fatty acids (Turner et al, 1975; Woods et al, manuscript in preparation). The intrinsic preferential leukocyte chemotactic activity of the stimuli represents the second level of control (Fig. 5-2) with ECF-A and

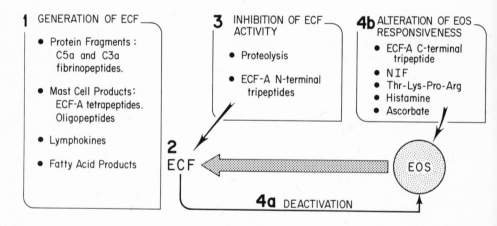

Fig. 5   Modulation of the eosinophic chemotactic response.

other mast cell-derived peptides exhibiting the most selective action on eosinophils. At the third level of control of eosinophil chemotaxis, inhibition of the activity of stimuli can result from degradation of C5a or C3a by the anaphylatoxin inactivator or chemotactic factor inactivator and of ECF-A by carboxypeptidase-A or aminopeptidases (Fig. 5-3). The activity of ECF-A is uniquely suppressed by equimolar quantities of its NH_2-terminal tripeptide substituent, presumably by eosinophil membrane receptor competition. The fourth level of regulation of eosinophil chemotaxis consists of the factors that modulate eosinophil responsiveness at the cellular level. Both chemotactic factors themselves, by way of a process termed deactivation (Fig. 5-4a) and non-chemotactic principles (Fig. 5-4b) can inhibit the responsiveness of eosinophils. The COOH-terminal tripeptide substituent of ECF-A and the neutrophil-immobilizing factor (NIF) suppress eosinophil chemotactic migration to ECF-A without influencing other functions while the basic peptide, Thr-Lys-Pro-Arg, inhibits eosinophil chemotaxis and concomitantly stimulates phagocytosis. Other cell-directed factors that modulate eosinophil chemotaxis by enhancing their response include ascorbate, which also stimulates eosinophil metabolism, and histamine, which enhances the response to ECF-A at low concentrations, stimulates directed migration at intermediate levels of 30-140 ng/ml, and suppresses the response to ECF-A at higher concentrations.

The inhibition of eosinophil migration to ECF-A by both NH_2-terminal and COOH-terminal tripeptide substituents provides evidence for multiple interaction sites in an eosinophil receptor for chemotactic factors (Fig. 6). Neither tripeptide substituent is chemotactic, indicating that both the hydrophobic NH_2-terminal residue and the negatively-charged COOH-terminal residue are required to produce maximal directed migration. Stabilization of the COOH-terminal residue at an activation site in an ionic domain could possibly be facilitated by hydrogen bonding of the serine hydroxyl-group. The NH_2-terminal tripeptide blocks ECF-A activity at equimolar concentrations by competing with the tetrapeptide for a recognition site in the hydrophobic domain. The COOH-terminal tripeptide substituent suppresses the eosinophil chemotactic response by interacting weakly or briefly with the activation site in the ionic domain. The inability of the COOH-terminal tripeptide to bind to the hydrophobic domain prevents it from inducing chemotaxis and limits deactivation to concentrations well in excess of those required for deactivation by the complete tetrapeptide.

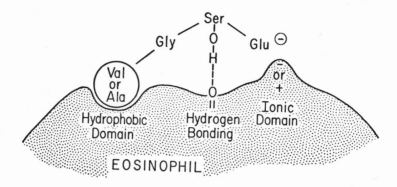

Fig. 6 Hypothetical model of the eosinophil surface receptor for
ECF-A tetrapeptides.

REFERENCES

Archer, R.K. 1956. The eosinophilic response in the horse to
    intramedullary and intradermal injections of histamine,
    ACTH, and cortisone. J. Pathol. Bact. 72:87.

Berenberg, J.A., and Ward, P.A. 1973. Chemotactic factor inac-
    tivator in normal human serum. J. Clin. Invest. 52:1200.

Bokisch, V.A., and Müller-Eberhard, H.J. 1970. Anaphylatoxin
    inactivator of human plasma: its isolation and characteri-
    zation as a carboxypeptidase. J. Clin. Invest. 49:2427.

Campbell, A.C.P., Drennan, A.M., and Rettie, R. 1935. The re-
    lationship of the eosinophile leukocyte to allergy and ana-
    phylaxis. J. Path. Bact. <u>40</u>:537.

Clark, R.A.F., Gallin, J.I., and Kaplan, A.P. 1975. The selec-
    tive eosinophil chemotactic activity of histamine. J. Exp.
    Med. <u>142</u>:1462.

Goetzl, E.J. 1975. Plasma and cell-derived inhibitors of human
    neutrophil chemotaxis. Ann. N.Y. Acad. Sci. <u>256</u>:210.

Goetzl, E.J., and Austen, K.F. 1972. A neutrophil immobilizing
    factor derived from human leukocytes. I. Generation and par-
    tial characterization. J. Exp. Med. <u>136</u>:1564.

Goetzl, E.J., and Austen, K.F. 1974. Stimulation of human neu-
    trophil leukocyte aerobic glucose metabolism by purified
    chemotactic factors. J. Clin. Invest. <u>53</u>:591.

Goetzl, E.J., and Austen, K.F. 1975. Purification and synthesis
    of eosinophilotactic tetrapeptides of human lung tissue:
    Identification as eosinophil chemotactic factor of anaphy-
    laxis. Proc. Natl. Acad. Sci. USA <u>72</u>:4123.

Goetzl, E.J., Gigli, I., Wasserman, S.I., and Austen, K.F. 1973.
    A neutrophil immobilizing factor derived from human leuko-
    cytes. II. Specificity of action on polymorphonuclear
    leukocyte mobility. J. Immunol. <u>111</u>:938.

Goetzl, E.J., Wasserman, S.I., Gigli, I., and Austen, K.F. 1974a.
    Enhancement of random migration and chemotactic response of
    human leukocytes by ascorbic acid. J. Clin. Invest. <u>53</u>:813.

Goetzl, E.J., Wasserman, S.I., and Austen, K.F. 1974b. Modula-
    tion of the eosinophil chemotactic response in immediate
    hypersensitivity. In: PROGRESS IN IMMUNOLOGY II, L. Brent
    and J. Holborow, eds., vol. 4, North-Holland Publishing Co.,
    Amsterdam, p. 41.

Goetzl, E.J., Wasserman, S.I., and Austen, K.F. 1975. Eosino-
    phil polymorphonuclear leukocyte function in immediate
    hypersensitivity. Arch. Pathol. <u>99</u>:1.

Goetzl, E.J., Boswell, R.N., and Austen, K.F. 1976a. The
    tetrapeptides comprising eosinophil chemotactic factor of
    anaphylaxis (ECF-A): Structural determinants of chemotactic
    activity. Fed. Proc. (abstract), in press.

Goetzl, E.J., Rubin, R.H., McDonough, J., Tashjian, A.H., Jr., Austen, K.F. 1976b. Production of eosinophilotactic peptides by bronchogenic carcinoma in situ and in vitro. Clin. Res. (abstract), in press.

Hudson, G. 1968. Quantitative study of the eosinophil granulocytes. Semin. Hematol. 5:166.

Kaliner, M.A., Wasserman, S.I., and Austen, K.F. 1973. The immunologic release of chemical mediators from human nasal polyps. N. Engl. J. Med. 289:277.

Kay, A.B., and Austen, K.F. 1971. The IgE-mediated release of an eosinophil leukocyte chemotactic factor from human lung. J. Immunol. 107:899.

Kay, A.B., Shin, H.S., and Austen, K.F. 1973. Selective attraction of eosinophils and synergism between eosinophil chemotactic factor of anaphylaxis (ECF-A) and a fragment cleaved from the fifth component of complement (C5a). Immunology 24:969.

Kay, A.B., Stechschulte, D.J., and Austen, K.F. 1971. An eosinophil leukocyte chemotactic factor of anaphylaxis. J. Exp. Med. 133:602.

Lewis, R.A., Goetzl, E.J., Wasserman, S.I., Valone, F.H., Rubin, R.H., and Austen, K.F.: The release of four mediators of immediate hypersensitivity from human leukemic basophils. J. Immunol. 114:87.

McKenzie, R., Pepper, D.S., and Kay, A.B. 1975. The generation of chemotactic activity for human leukocytes by the action of plasmin on human fibrinogen. Thrombosis Res. 6:1.

Najjar, V.A. 1974. The physiological role of γ-globulin. Advan. Enzymol. 41:129.

Nishioka, K., Constantopoulos, A., Satoh, P.S., and Najjar, V.A. 1972. The characteristics, isolation and synthesis of the phagocytosis stimulating peptide Tuftsin. Biochem. Biophys. Res. Commun. 47:172.

Parish, W.E. 1970. Investigations on eosinophilia. The influence of histamine, antigen-antibody complexes containing γ1 or γ2 globulins, foreign bodies (phagocytosis) and disrupted mast cells. Brit. J. Dermatol. 82:42.

Snyderman, R., Shin, H.S., and Hausman, M.H.   1971.   A chemotactic factor for mononuclear leukocytes.   Proc. Soc. Exp. Biol. Med. 138:387.

Spry, C.J.F.   1971.   Mechanism of eosinophilia: V. Kinetics of normal and accelerated eosinopoiesis.   Cell Tissue Kinet. 4:351.

Torisu, M., Yoshida, T., Ward, P.A., and Cohen, S.   1973.   Lymphocyte-derived eosinophil chemotactic factor: II. Studies on the mechanism of activation of the precursor substance by immune complexes.   J. Immunol. 111:1450.

Turner, S.R., Campbell, J.A., and Lynn, W.S.   1975.   Polymorphonuclear leukocyte chemotaxis toward oxidized lipid components of cell membranes.   J. Exp. Med. 141:1437.

Vallota, E.H., and Müller-Eberhard, H.J.   1973.   Formation of C3a and C5a anaphylatoxins in whole human serum after inhibition of the anaphylatoxin inactivator.   J. Exp. Med. 137:1109.

Vaughn, J.   1953.   The function of the eosinophile leukocyte. Blood 8:1.

Vegad, J.L. and Lancaster, M.C.   1972.   Eosinophil leukocyte-attracting effect of histamine in the sheep skin.   Indian J. Exp. Biol. 10:147.

Ward. P.A.   1967.   A plasmin-split fragment of C3 as a new chemotactic factor.   J. Exp. Med. 126:189.

Ward, P.A.   1971.   Complement-derived leukotactic factors in pathological fluids.   J. Exp. Med. 134:1095.

Ward, P.A., and Becker, E.L.   1968.   The deactivation of rabbit neutrophils by chemotactic factor and the nature of the activatable esterase.   J. Exp. Med. 127:693.

Ward, P.A., and Becker, E.L.   1970.   Biochemical demonstration of the activatable esterase of the rabbit neutrophil involved in the chemotactic response.   J. Immunol. 105:1057.

Ward, P.A., and Hill, J.H.   1970.   C5 chemotactic fragments produced by an enzyme in lysosomal granules of neutrophils. J. Immunol. 104:535.

Wasserman, S.I., Goetzl, E.J., Kaliner, M.A., and Austen, K.F.
    1974a. Modulation of the immunologic release of the eosin-
    ophil chemotactic factor of anaphylaxis from human lung.
    Immunology 26:677.

Wasserman, S.I., Goetzl, E.J., and Austen, K.F. 1974b. Pre-
    formed eosinophil chemotactic factor of anaphylaxis. J.
    Immunol. 112:351.

Wasserman, S.I., Goetzl, E.J., Ellman, L., and Austen, K.F.
    1974c. Tumor-associated eosinophilotactic factor. N. Engl.
    J. Med. 290:420.

Wasserman, S.I., Whitmer, D., Goetzl, E.J., and Austen, K.F.
    1975. Chemotactic deactivation of human eosinophils by the
    eosinophil chemotactic factor of anaphylaxis. Proc. Soc.
    Exp. Biol. Med. 148:301.

Wasserman, S.I., Boswell, R.N., Drazen, J.M., Goetzl, E.J., and
    Austen, K.F. 1976. Functional specificity of the human
    lung acidic tetrapeptides constituting eosinophil chemotactic
    factor of anaphylaxis (ECF-A). J. Allergy Clin. Immunol.,
    in press.

Zucker-Franklin, D. 1974. Eosinophil function and disorders.
    Adv. Intern. Med. 19:1.

DISCUSSION

BECKER: These two effects of histamine on eosinophils are
they inhibitable by antihistamines and if so which ones?

GOETZEL: Gallin et al. have shown that the loss of histamine enhancement of directed migration when histamine is employed at high concentrations as the chemotactic stimulus is blocked by H2 inhibitors but not by H1 inhibitors.

We have not studied the effects of inhibitors on high dose
histamine inhibition of ECF-A stimulated eosinophil chemotaxis.

LICHTENSTEIN: Regarding the nature of the high molecular
weight ECF-A, is it the parent molecule?

GOETZL: The higher molecular weight peptide eosinophil
chemotactic factors are preferentially chemotactic for eosinophils and reside with the tetrapeptides in mast cell granules
as has been shown by Dr. Neil Boswell in our laboratory. Their
precise relationship to ECF-A is not known.

MÜLLER-EBERHARD: Since you have synthesised the tetrapeptide, did you attempt to make a few derivatives or analogues
which might have greater biological activity than the natural
factors?

GOETZL: Are any active analogues of ECF-A available?

A Leu-tetrapeptide is chemotactic for eosinophils at 10^{-6}-10^{-8}M concentrations. A Phe-tetrapeptide analogue of ECF-A is only active at concentrations of 10^{-3}- 10^{-4}M.

LICHTENSTEIN: I wonder what is the mechanism of the inhibition by higher concentration of ECF-A. I am especially surprised at the steepness of the curve, maximum stimulation at 10^{-6}M and distinct inhibition at 3-5 x 10^{-6}M.

GOETZL: The inhibition may represent a deactivation of the eosinophils which occurs within 5 minutes at concentrations of tetrapeptide as low as 10^{-10}M.

LYMPHOCYTE MEDIATORS, ACTIVATED MACROPHAGES, AND TUMOR IMMUNITY

John R. David

Harvard Medical School, Robert B. Brigham Hospital

Boston, Massachusetts 02120

In the introduction to the paper concerned with lymphocyte
mediators which appeared in the Proceedings of the 2nd International Symposium on the Biochemistry of Acute Allergic Reactions,
an explanation was given to justify the inclusion of this topic in
such a meeting (1). Five years later, such an apologia seems unnecessary. Despite the many differences in the mechanisms of
acute and delayed immunologic reactions, there are now known interactions and some similarities between the two, and more will
undoubtedly be found in the future. For instance, among the many
mediators produced by lymphocytes when stimulated by antigen are
substances which regulate the production of antibody. More specifically, antigen-triggered T lymphocytes can produce both helper
and suppressor substances which affect the production of IgE by
B cells (2-4). The relationship of these regulatory lymphocyte
mediators to those which influence cell-mediated immunity is not
yet known. However, in this context it is of note that one murine
T-lymphocyte mediator which suppresses in vitro antibody formation,
soluble immune response suppressor (SIRS) is indistinguishable from
a mediator thought to play a major role in cell-mediated immune
reactions, namely migration inhibitory factor (MIF)(5,6). Further,
both SIRS and MIF produce their effects via their action on macrophages. Another interesting relationship between immediate and
delayed reactions is the finding that histamine suppresses delayed skin reactions (7). Recent studies have shown that,
in vitro, sensitive lymphocytes do not produce MIF when histamine
is present (7).

At first, I hoped to review the progress in the field of
lymphocyte mediators since the last Symposium; however, this task
is too big for the allotted space. The number of mediators has

437

greatly increased, and a partial list is shown on Table I.

TABLE I.   LYMPHOCYTE MEDIATORS

   I. Mediators Affecting Macrophages
       a) migration inhibitory factor (MIF)
       b) macrophage activating factor (MAF) indis-
          tinguishable from MIF)
       c) macrophage aggregation factor (? same as
          MIF)
       d) factor which causes disappearance of
          macrophages from the peritoneum
          (? same as MIF)
       e) chemotactic factors for macrophages
       f) factor which alters surface tension of
          macrophages
       g) antigen-dependent MIF

  II. Mediators Affecting Neutrophil Leukocytes
       a) chemotactic factor
       b) leukocyte inhibitory factor (LIF)

 III. Mediators Affecting Lymphocytes
       a) factors enhancing antibody formation
          (antigen-dependent and antigen-inde-
          pendent)
       b) factors suppressing antibody formation
       c) mitogenic factors

  IV. Mediators Affecting Eosinophils
       a) chemotactic factor *
       b) eosinophil stimulation promoter

   V. Mediators Affecting Basophils
       a) chemotactic factor
       b) chemotactic augmenting factor

  VI. Mediators Affecting Other Cells
       a) cytotoxic factors - lymphotoxin (LT)
       b) growth inhibitory factors (? same as LT)
       c) osteoclastic factor (OAF)
       d) collagen producing factor

 VII. Skin Reactive Factor

VIII. Interferon

  IX. Immunoglobulin-Binding Factor (IBF)

       *Requires antigen-antibody complexes.

It can be seen that several of these mediators have biological
properties which make them ideal candidates for a role in various
immunologically-induced inflammatory processes. Others, of special

interest, are the substances which regulate antibody production. Some of these are antigen specific (but nonimmunoglobulin) molecules and products of Ir genes (8). This paper will focus on the interaction of lymphocyte mediators with macrophages and the subsequent alteration of that cell's function.

There are numerous studies which demonstrate that macrophages play a crucial role both in the induction of the immune response and as a powerful effector cell. In the latter capacity, macrophages ingest and dispose of a variety of microorganisms, kill tumor cells and participate in a number of immunopathologic processes. It has been known for some time that macrophages obtained from immunized animals have altered morphology and metabolism and exhibit an enhanced ability to deal with a number of microorganisms (9-12). Such macrophages have been called activated. More recent studies suggest that in vivo activation of macrophages requires the interaction of specifically sensitized T lymphocytes with appropriate antigen (13,14).

How does the interaction of lymphocytes with antigen lead to activation of macrophages? Ever since the discovery that sensitized lymphocytes produced a soluble material, migration inhibitory factor (MIF) which affects the behavior of macrophages (15,16), we have considered the possibility that lymphocyte mediators might also activate macrophages. In the last Symposium, we presented preliminary evidence to support this hypothesis. Since then, our laboratory and others have accumulated considerable further evidence. The following will be a brief review of these studies, and will describe experiments which demonstrate that macrophages activated by lymphocyte mediators have an enhanced ability to kill syngeneic tumor cells.

Most of the experiments described below have been carried out using guinea pig peritoneal exudate macrophages. The macrophages were incubated as monolayers for varying periods of time with tissue culture media containing lymphocyte mediators; more recently, macrophages have been activated in suspension culture (17). The mediators were produced by incubating lymph node lymphocytes from guinea pigs sensitized to o-chlorobenzoyl bovine gamma globulin (OCB-BGG) with that antigen for 24 hours (18). Control cultures were not stimulated by antigen; after incubation, the cells were removed by centrifugation, and antigen was added to the control supernatant. In some studies, lymphocytes were stimulated by the lectin concanavalin A (Con A) instead of antigen (19). In most experiments, the supernatants were chromatographed on Sephadex G-100 columns, and fractions rich in mediators and their control counterparts were used (19). In some experiments, human monocytes and human lymphocyte mediators were used (20).

For the sake of convenience, the mediator(s) involved will be referred to as macrophage activating factor (MAF); this does not imply that there is necessarily only one factor that activates macrophages nor that MAF is different from MIF. Indeed, evidence will be presented that suggests that MIF and MAF are the same.

MACROPHAGE ACTIVATION BY LYMPHOCYTE MEDIATORS

Macrophages which have been incubated with MAF-rich lymphocyte supernatants or MAF-rich Sephadex fractions exhibit a number of changes which appear to reflect alterations in the macrophage membrane. They stick better to culture vessels (21,22) and show a marked increase in ruffled membrane movement after three days of culture using time lapse cinematography (22). Such macrophages also spread out more than controls; similar spreading was observed when the periphery of a fan of cells inhibited from migrating from capillary tubes was examined (23). Increased ameboid movement has been reported (21). On the other hand, early after incubation with mediators, it has been found that cells may spread less (24, 25).

Enhancement of both the rate and extent of phagocytosis of dead mycobacteria and starch has been observed (22). However, it should be noted that this is not seen with all particles. For example, Remold and Mednis (26) found a decrease in the phagocytosis of denatured aggregated hemoglobin by macrophages preincubated in MAF-rich Sephadex fractions compared to controls, and that the amount of denatured hemoglobin sticking to the macrophages was also less on activated than control cells. Decrease in phagocytosis of Candida albicans by mediator activated macrophages has been reported by Neta and Salvin (27). Hoff noted that mouse macrophages which have been activated in vivo by injection of mice with BCG or Trypanosoma cruzi showed a decreased ability to take up Trypanosoma cruzi compared to control macrophages (28). These results suggest that the membrane of the activated macrophage is altered leading to increased or decreased phagocytosis depending on the surface properties of the particle ingested.

Alterations of macrophages incubated with MAF which also appear to reflect membrane changes include the enhanced pinocytosis of radioactive gold (29), increase in levels of the membrane enzyme adenylate cyclase (30), increase in glucosamine incorporation(31) and decrease in electron-dense surface material (32).

Other metabolic changes in mediator activated macrophages include increased glucose oxidation through the hexose monophosphate shunt (22), increased cytoplasmic enzyme lactic dehydrogenase (33), production of collagenase (34), and a decrease in several lysosomal enzymes (33) despite an increase in the number of cytoplasmic granules (David and Remold, unpublished observation).

In addition to the morphologic and metabolic changes described above, mediator activated macrophages show important functional changes. They exhibit enhanced bacteriostasis for a number of organisms (35-39) and enhanced tumoricidal capacity. This latter function will now be dealt with in more detail. The alterations seen when macrophages are activated by lymphocyte mediators are summarized on Table II.

TABLE II. ACTIVATION OF MACROPHAGES BY LYMPHOCYTE MEDIATORS

1) Increase in adherence to glass

2) Increase in ruffled membrane activity

3) Increase in phagocytosis of some particles (dead mycobacteria) but decrease in others (aggregated hemoglobin)

4) Increase in membrane enzyme adenylate cyclase

5) Increase in incorporation of glucosamine

6) Decrease in electron-dense surface material

7) Increase in pinocytosis of colloidal gold

8) Increase in glucose oxidation through hexose monophosphate shunt

9) Increase in cytoplasmic enzyme lactic dehydrogenase

10) Decrease in lysosomal enzyme acid phosphatase, cathepsin D, β-glucuronidase

11) Increase in number cytoplasmic granules

12) Production of collagenase

13) Enhanced bacteriostasis to Listeria

14) Enhanced tumoricidal activity

TUMOR KILLING BY MACROPHAGES ACTIVATED BY LYMPHOCYTE MEDIATORS

The tumoricidal capacity of macrophages activated by MAF was studied by Piessens et al. using a syngeneic strain 2 guinea pig tumor system (40,41). Monolayers of normal strain 2 macrophages were incubated for three days in unfractionated MAF-rich and control supernatants from OCB-BGG stimulated guinea pig lymphocytes. Tumor cells labelled with ^{3}H-thymidine were then added, and, after 24 hours of cocultivation, cytotoxicity was determined by comparing the numbers of adherent tumor cells remaining in dishes containing similar numbers of activated and control macrophages. This is a

true reflection of cytotoxicity as 90% of the radioactivity which
is released from the monolayers is noncell associated, and thus,
must have come from dead cells.

The macrophages which were incubated with MAF-rich supernatants
were toxic for Line 1 hepatoma cells in 23 of 29 experiments. The
cytotoxicity ranged from 13-72% with a mean of 38% (p for each pair
<0.05)(41). Such macrophages were also cytotoxic to MCA-25 fibro-
sarcoma in 5 of 5 experiments; the degree of cytotoxicity ranged from
14-74% (mean 28% with p <0.05). On the other hand, such activated
macrophages did not kill either syngeneic fibroblasts or kidney
cells (41). Tumor cells adhered equally well to both activated and
control macrophages when measured after just two hours of cocultivation (see Figure 1).

It should be noted that macrophages could be activated by supernatants devoid of lymphotoxin activity suggesting that the effect
was not due to this mediator adsorbed to macrophages.

The observation that macrophages activated by MAF kill syngeneic tumor cells but not normal cells is consistent with the previous
findings of Hibbs et al. who reported that activated macrophages obtained from mice immunized with a number of different microorganisms
kill transformed cells but not their normal counterparts, whereas
macrophages from nonimmunized mice kill neither cell type (42,43).
Since activated macrophages exhibit certain membrane changes discussed above, it is tempting to speculate that membrane alterations
possibly analogous to those found between normal and transformed
cells might be present between normal and activated macrophages.
Such surface changes might lead activated macrophages to recognize
or have a greater affinity for altered tumor cell membranes leading
to interaction and subsequent killing of the tumor cell.

In more recent studies, it was shown that macrophages incubated for 24 hours with MAF in suspension culture also showed an
enhanced capacity to kill syngeneic tumor cells (17)(see Figure 2).
MAF-rich Sephadex G-100 fractions free of antigen were capable of
enhancing macrophage cytotoxicity. MAF was not cytophilic for
macrophages. Further, trypsinization of the activated macrophages
did not diminish cytotoxic potential (17).

What is known about the physicochemical characteristics of
MAF? When assessed in terms of enhancing macrophage ability to
kill tumors, or of macrophage sticking, or of enhancement of
glucose oxidation, MAF elutes in the same fractions which contain
MIF and several other mediators in the range between 68,000-25,000
daltons (17). When MAF is assessed in terms of enhanced adherence
or glucose oxidation, it is destroyed by neuraminidase, which also
destroys MIF but not chemotactic factor or lymphotoxin, and is recovered after isopycnic centrifugation on CsCl in a band with a

FIGURE 1

INITIAL ADHERENCE OF LABELLED LINE 1 HEPATOMA CELLS
TO MONOLAYERS OF CONTROL AND ACTIVATED MACROPHAGES

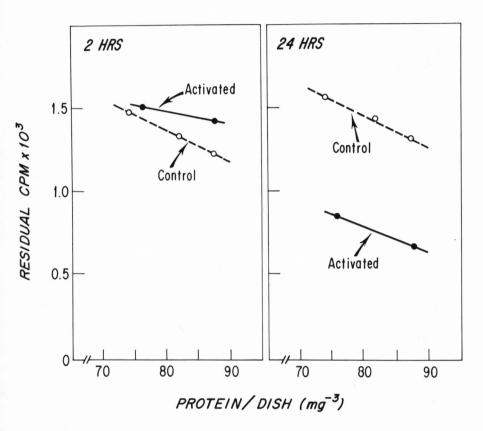

Fig. 1. Residual radioactivity adhering to macrophage monolayers
is plotted as a function of the number of macrophages (as micrograms of protein/dish) present at the time of addition of tumor
cells. Macrophages were preincubated for three days with MAF-
rich ("activated") and control lymphocyte supernatants. After 2
hours the tumor cells adhered equally well to both types of monolayers. At 24 hours the activated macrophages are cytotoxic for
the tumor cells. Each point represents the mean of triplicate
determinations (with permission of the Williams & Wilkins Co.)
(41).

FIGURE 2

CYTOTOXICITY OF PERITONEAL EXUDATE CELLS ACTIVATED IN
SUSPENSION CULTURE IN MEDIATOR-RICH LYMPHOCYTE SUPERNATANTS
FOR VARIABLE PERIODS OF TIME

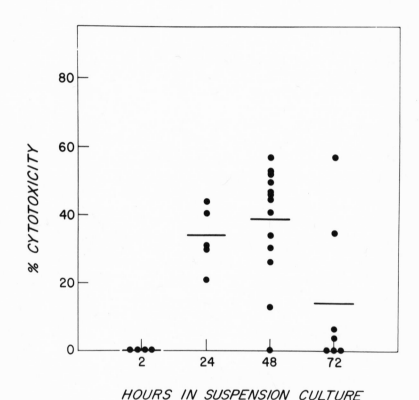

HOURS IN SUSPENSION CULTURE

Fig. 2. A:T ratio in these experiments was 25:1. The percentage
of cytotoxicity is calculated by comparing the residual adherent
radioactivity in plates containing activated macrophages with the
residual adherent radioactivity in plates containing an equal number of control macrophages. Macrophages were activated by prior
incubation in mediator-rich supernatants. Control macrophages
were incubated for the same interval in control supernatants prior
to assay (with permission of the Williams & Wilkins Co.)(17).

buoyant density slightly greater than albumin, as in MIF but not
the other two mediators (44). In preliminary studies in collaboration with H. Remold, MAF, as assessed by its ability to enhance
macrophage tumor cytotoxicity, has the same pI as MIF on isoelectric focussing. Human MAF as assessed by ability to enhance cell
adherence and glucose oxidation has the same size as human MIF, and
differs from human chemotactic factor, lymphotoxin and leukocyte
inhibitory factor (LIF) in this respect (20,45-47).

In this context, it is of note that the interaction of MIF
with macrophages leading to inhibition of migration and that of
MAF with this cell leading to activation have other features in
common. Remold has shown that macrophages which have been preincubated with esterase inhibitors will subsequently exhibit enhanced responsiveness to MIF (48,49); these studies suggest the
presence of a macrophage surface esterase which can modulate the
cells' response to the mediator. Remold also found that altering
the macrophage surface by treatment with diazotized sulfanilic
acid (DSA) had a similar effect: such macrophages were also more
responsive to MIF (50). Recently, Piessens et al. extended these
findings to the activation of macrophages by MAF (51). Macrophages
were pretreated with either a plasma esterase inhibitor (antithrombin heparin-cofactor) or DSA. When such macrophages were incubated with subthreshold concentrations of MAF (concentrations
which did not activate control macrophages) they became activated
and exhibited enhanced tumor cytotoxicity. These studies suggest
that macrophage surface esterase, and possibly other surface enzymes are capable of modulating the cells' reaction to both MIF
and MAF. The data is consistent with the hypothesis that MIF and
MAF are the same material and that inhibition of migration and
activation are triggered by similar mechanisms.

It is of interest at this juncture to compare tumor killing by
activated macrophages with killing by "armed macrophages". Evans
and Alexander described cytotoxicity by macrophages armed with a
product of activated lymphocytes called "specific macrophage arming
factor" or SMAF (52). SMAF has the following characteristics: it
is a product of thymus-dependent lymphocytes stimulated by antigen (53,54). SMAF produced by stimulating specifically immune lymphocytes with one tumor specifically arms macrophages to kill that
tumor but not others. SMAF produced by stimulating sensitive lymphocytes with antigen unrelated to the tumor target usually requires
the presence of that specific antigen to arm the macrophage for
cytotoxicity (55). The arming factor is cytophilic, i.e., it can
render macrophages cytotoxic after short periods of incubation and
is absorbed out by the macrophages. It can also be absorbed out by
the specific tumor used to produce it. It has been postulated that
it may be a cytotoxic receptor shed into the culture medium by activated lymphocytes (50) or a cytophilic antibody (56). Trypsinization
of armed macrophages abolishes their cytotoxic capacity (56,57).

It is clear from the above that the mechanism of SMAF is different from that involved in macrophage activation by MAF. In the latter, mediators induced by antigens non-cross-reacting with the tumor antigen are effective and the antigen need not be present. MAF is not cytophilic, and, further, trypsinization of activated macrophages does not alter their cytotoxic capabilities. There must exist at least two different mechanisms by which normal macrophages can be rendered cytotoxic for tumor cells, one by "arming" and one by "activation".

In addition to specific killing by armed macrophages, direct T cell mediated cytotoxicity is also specific (58,59). In vivo, both specific killing and nonspecific immunity have been reported. A classical requirement for specificity is seen in the studies of Klein and his coworkers who showed that an immune mouse would reject a lymphoma to which it was immune but not an antigenically different lymphoma mixed in the inoculum (60,61). On the other hand, with the hepatoma system, nonspecific immunity can be demonstrated: when two antigenically unrelated hepatomas are injected together into an animal immune to only one, both tumors fail to grow (62). Thus, it would appear that the degree of specificity or nonspecificity of tumor killing will depend on the type of tumor and on the predominant type of cellular immune mechanisms that are operating.

ACKNOWLEDGMENTS

This work was supported by USPHS grants AI-07685, AI-10921, and Contract NIH-NO1-CB-33896.

REFERENCES

1. David, J.R., in Biochemistry of the Acute Allergic Reactions, K.F. Austen and E.L. Becker, eds., Blackwell Scientific Publications, Oxford, England, 1971, p. 127.

2. Kishimoto, T. and Ishizaka, K., J. Immunol. 111:1194, 1973.

3. Kishimoto, T. and Ishizaka, K., J. Immunol. 114:1177, 1975.

4. Tada, T., Okumura, K., and Taniguchi, M., J. Immunol. 111:952, 1973.

5. Tadakuma, T., Kühner, A., David, J., and Pierce, C., Fed. Proc. Abstr. 34:838, 1975.

6. Kühner, A.L. and David, J.R., J. Immunol. 116:140, 1976.

7. Rocklin, R.E., J. Clin. Invest. 57, April, 1976.

8. Taussig, M. and Munro, A.J., Nature 251:63, 1974.

9. Metchnikoff, E., Immunity in Infective Disease, Cambride Univ. Press, London and New York, 1905.

10. Lurie, M.B., Resistance to Tuberculosis: Experimental Studies in Native and Acquired Defensive Mechanisms, Harvard Univ. Press, Cambridge, MA, 1964.

11. Suter, E. and Ramseier, H., Adv. Immunol. 4:117, 1964.

12. Mackaness, G.B., J. Exp. Med. 120:105, 1964.

13. Mackaness, G.B., J. Exp. Med. 129:973, 1969.

14. Lane, F.C. and Unanue, E.R., J. Exp. Med. 135:1104, 1972.

15. David, J.R., Proc. Nat. Acad. Sci. 56:72, 1966.

16. Bloom, B.R. and Bennett, B., Science 153:80, 1966.

17. Churchill, W.H., Jr., Piessens, W.F., Sulis, C.A., and David, J.R., J. Immunol. 115:781, 1975.

18. Remold, H.G., Katz, A.B., Haber, E., and David, J.R., Cell. Immunol. 1:133, 1970.

19. Remold, H.G., David, R.A., and David, J.R., J. Immunol. 109: 578, 1972.

20. Rocklin, R.E., Winston, C.T., and David, J.R., J. Clin. Invest. 53:559, 1974.

21. Mooney, J.J. and Waksman, B.H., J. Immunol. 105:1138, 1970.

22. Nathan, C.F., Karnovsky, M.L., and David, J.R., J. Exp. Med. 133:1356, 1971.

23. David, J.R. and Haber, E., in Cellular Recognition, R.T. Smith and R.A. Good, eds., Appleton-Century-Crofts, New York, 1969, p. 221.

24. Fauve, R.M. and Dekaris, D., Science 160:795, 1968.

25. Salvin, S.B., Sell, S., and Nishio, J., J. Immunol. 107:655, 1971.

26. Remold, H.G. and Mednis, A., Fed. Proc. 31:753, 1972.

27. Neta, R. and Salvin, S.B., Infec. Immunity 4:697, 1971.

28. Hoff, R., J. Exp. Med. 142:299, 1975.

29. Meade, C.J., Lachmann, P.J., and Brenner, S., Immunology 27:
     227, 1974.

30. Remold-O'Donnell, E. and Remold, H.G., J. Biol. Chem. 249:
     3622, 1974.

31. Hammond, M.E. and Dvorak, H.F., J. Exp. Med. 136:1518, 1972.

32. Dvorak, A.M., Hammond, H.F., Dvorak, and Karnovsky, M.J.,
     Lab. Invest. 27:561, 1972.

33. Remold, H.G. and Mednis, A., Inflammation, in press.

34. Wahl, L., Wahl, S.M., Mergenhagen, S.E., and Martin, G.R.,
     Science 187:261, 1975.

35. Fowles, R.E., Fajardo, I.M., Leibowitch, J.L., and David,
     J.R., J. Exp. Med. 138:952, 1973.

36. Patterson, R.J. and Youman, G.P., Infec. Immunity 1:600, 1970.

37. Godal, T., Rees, R.J.W., and Lamvik, J.O., Clin. Exp. Immunol.
     8:625, 1971.

38. Krahenbuhl, J.L. and Remington, J.S., Infec. Immunity 4:337,
     1971.

39. Anderson, S.E. and Remington, J.S., J. Exp. Med. 139:1154,
     1974.

40. Rapp, H., Churchill, W.H., Kronman, B.S., Rolley, R.T.,
     Hammond, W.G., and Borsos, T., J. Natl. Cancer Inst. 41:1,
     1968.

41. Piessens, W.F., Churchill, W.H., and David, J.R., J. Immunol.
     114:293, 1975.

42. Hibbs, J.B., Science 180:868, 1972.

43. Hibbs, J.B., Lambert, L.H., and Remington, J.S., Science 177:
     998, 1972.

44. Nathan, C.F., Remold, H.G., and David, J.R., J. Exp. Med. 137:
     275, 1973.

45. Kolb, W.P. and Granger, G.A., Proc. Nat. Acad. Sci. 61:1250, 1968.

46. Altman, L.C., Snyderman, R., and Oppenheim, J.J., J. Immunol. 110:801, 1973.

47. Rocklin, R.E., J. Immunol. 112:1461, 1974.

48. Remold, H.G., J. Immunol. 112:1571, 1974.

49. Remold, H.G. and Rosenberg, R.D., J. Biol. Chem. 250:6608, 1975.

50. Remold, H.G., Unpublished observations.

51. Piessens, W.F., Herz, S.K., David, J.R., and Remold, H.G., Fed. Proc., 1976, in press.

52. Evans, R. and Alexander, P., Nature 228:620, 1970.

53. Evans, R., Grant, C.K., Cox, H., Steele, K., and Alexander, P., J. Exp. Med. 136:1318, 1972.

54. Lohmann-Matthes, M.L., Zigler, F.G., and Fischer, H., Eur. J. Immunol. 3:56, 1973.

55. Evans, R., Cox, H., and Alexander, P., Proc. Soc. Exp. Biol. Med. 143:256, 1973.

56. Pels, E. and Den Otter, W., Cancer Res. 34:3089, 1974.

57. Lohmann-Matthes, M.L., Schipper, H., and Fischer, H., Eur. J. Immunol. 2:45, 1972.

58. Cerottini, J.C., Nordin, A.A., and Brunner, K.T., Nature 228: 1308, 1970.

59. Henney, C.S., Progr. Exp. Tumor Res., S. Karger, Basel, 1974, p. 203.

60. Klein, G. and Klein E., Nature, 178:1389, 1956.

61. Klein, E. and Klein, G., Cell. Immunol. 5:201, 1972.

62. Zbar, B., Wepsic, T., Borsos, T., and Rapp, H.J., J. Natl. Cancer Inst. 44:473, 1970.

DISCUSSION

ISHIZAKA, K.: Do you need macrophages or other accessory cells to obtain lymphokines such as MIF and MAF from antigen-primed lymphocytes?

DAVID: Although we have usually found it difficult to depleat lymphocyte preparations of macrophages so that they would no longer produce MIF or MAF, there are now two reports in the literature that macrophages are required for the production of MIF by antigen primed lymphocytes.

AUSTEN: What types of lymphocytes respond to antigen to make mediators and what cell types will make mediators of "alternative" pathways?

DAVID: The cell responsible for making antigen induced MIF differs in the various species so far studied. In studies being carried out by Alice Kuhner with Harvey Cantor, using anti-theta antibody, it looks as if it is the T cell in the mouse which makes antigen induced MIF. In man in studies with Rocklin, Chess and Schlossman, both cells which passed through Sephadex columns which took out Ig coated cells, and those eluted from the columns made MIF, suggesting that at least two types of cells make MIF, one T and the other which elutes with B cells. However, there are clinical states where B cells will make excellent antibody to an antigen but not MIF indicating that not any B cell will make MIF.

Several other workers have shown that both E forming cells and E depleted populations will make a variety of lymphocyte mediators. In the guinea pig, Yoshida and Cohen showed that T cells made antigen induced MIF but that B cells could make mitogen induced MIF too.

Concerning my comment on a "classical" and "alternate" pathway of activation, I referred to the fact that in addition to producing mediators by stimulating specific sensitive cells with antigen, one can also make them by non specific stimulation by mitogens and what may have more in vivo relevance, stimulation of B cells via the complement receptor. This "alternate pathway" would also include the induction of lymphocyte like mediators by non lymphoid cells induced for instance by viruses as reported by Cohen.

MÜLLER-EBERHARD: Could you elaborate on what is known about the mechanism of tumor cell killing by the macrophage?

DAVID: We do not know the mechanism by which activated

macrophages kill tumor cells. It is usually described as non-phagocytic killing, and I do not know of evidence that phago-cytosis plays a part. Hibbs has suggested that there is an in-jection of lysosomal enzymes from the macrophage into the tumor, a process which he is able to inhibit by trypan blue, which pre-sumably block lysosomal release in the system.

It is quite possible that parts of the activated macrophage membrane can interclate with the tumorcell membrane and shoot toxic substances into the cell. To understand the mechanisms of this killing process is an important subject for future investigation and should prove very interesting.

DIAMANT: In one slide you had an esterase as a regulator of the MIF effect. Now, suppose you had a similar metabolic effect of DFP as I showed yesterday on the rat mast cells, you would actually have the same effect, but the inhibition of migration would be due to inhibition of energy in the cells.

DAVID: Concerning the esterase on the macrophage, its existence is implied by the fact that incubating the macrophage with a number of esterase inhibitors increases its subsequent response to subthreshold amounts of MIF. It should be noted that such esterase inhibitor treated macrophages. migrate perfectly normally in the absence of MIF.

However, it is not impossible for DFP for instance to lead to certain metabolic alterations inside the cell which do alter normal migration itself but might potentiate a change caused by MIF which would be manifest by increased inhibition of migration or activation.

PERLMANN (Stockholm): Activation by mitogen, does it induce killing of tumor cell in the same way as activation by antigen?

DAVID: Yes, incubation of lymphocytes with ConA produces supernatants which, after filtration over Sephadex G 100 to remove the ConA produces a MAF which acts like antigen induced MAF to activate macrophages for tumor cytoxicity.

PERLMANN (Stockholm): In the lymphocyte induced killing of target cells the effector cell can be killed within minutes but the destruction of the target cells proceeds. Can one do the same with activated macrophages?

DAVID: The kinetics of macrophage killing of tumor is slo-wer than that by killer T cells and this question is more diffi-cult to answer. Meltzer has taken movies which show macrophages contacting tumor cells which then seem to die. Whether there is the same "kiss of death" with macrophages that has been descri-bed by Martz and Benacerraf for T lymphocyte killing we do not yet know.

PERLMANN (Stockholm): What is the recognition process which is involved in the tumor cell killing by activated macrophages?

DAVID: We do not know the recognition process of an activa-ted macrophage for a tumor cell. Certainly, the observation that macrophages seem to kill tumor cells better than normal cells, as described by Hibbs et al. also with BCG activated mouse

macrophages requires further study. I would have thought it may
well have to do with alterations of the membrane of both tumor
cells and activated macrophages, which may lead to closer contact.

BIBERFELD (Stockholm): You found a decrease in lysosomal
enzyme activity of activated macrophages, but an increase in
cytoplasmic granules. Have you any idea what these granules
represent?

DAVID: We have no explanation for the finding by Remold
and Mednis that three lysosomal enzymes are lower in guinea
pig activated macrophages than controls. Nor do we know the
make up of the granules which are increased in the guinea pig
activated macrophages.

It should be pointed out however that mouse activated macrophages have an increase in certain lysosomal enzymes and that
a lowering of these should not be considered as a sin qua non
of an activated macrophage.

BIBERFELD (Stockholm): Have you tried to abrogate the cytotoxic activity with enzyme inhibitors? Is the supernatant or
cell homogenates of cultured macrophages cytotoxic?

DAVID: Dr Willy Piessens is in the middle of carrying out
experiments to answer some of these questions. So far a supernatant factor from activated macrophages responsible for cell
killing has not been found. It should be noted that a number of
such factor have been described. A note of caution is in order.
Many times, the macrophage supernatant is compared to normal
medium. Piessens has found that simply dialyzing the normal medium may make it cytotoxic. Thus rigorous controls are necessary when studing such toxic supernatants, and supernatants from
control macrophage cultures should also be used.

TADA: I think Drs. Tadakuma, Pierce and you have shown
that conA activated mouse T cells release a factor which suppresses the antibody response, and that his factor is indistinguishable from MIF by physiocochemical means.

Is it also true for the MIF of guinea pigs, and more spe-
cially, does guinea pig MIF suppress antibody response?

DAVID: We have not carried out studies with guinea pig
MIF to see if it or a similar mediator inhibits antibody formation. Alice Kuhner is presently carrying out studies with
Harvey Cantor using anti Ly 1 and anti Ly 2,3 sera to see which
murine lymphocyte is making MIF. This may help in distinguishing
between soluble immune responce suppressor (SIRS) and MIF, but
experiments to date are too early for a definitive answer.

BECKER: I cannot bring this meeting to a close without expressing the gratitude to Dr. Uvnäs, Dr. Strandberg, Dr. Anderson, and the more graceful and less drab members of their staff for really producing a very smooth-running, highly productive symposium which contributed I think a great deal to the success of this meeting. In addition I wish to express more personally the feelings of gratitude of the foreign members and foreign participants for the tender loving care with which we were treated which we shall always remember and always cherish. Thank you.

PARTICIPANTS

K. Aas   Pediatric Department & Research Insti-
                          tute, Allergy Unit, Rikshospitalet,
                          National Hospital of Norway, University
                          Hospital, Oslo 1, Norway

K.F. Austen   Harvard Medical School, Robert B. Brig-
                          ham Hospital, 125 Parker Hill Avenue,
                          Boston, Massachussetts 02120, USA

H. Bazin   University of Louvain, Experimental
                          Immunology Unit, Clos Chapelle aux
                          Champs 30, B-1200 Brussels, Belgium

E.L. Becker   University of Connecticut, Health Center,
                          School of Medicine, Farmington, Connec-
                          ticut 06032, USA

H. Bennich   Biomedical Centre, Department of Medical
                          and Physiological Chemistry, Box 575,
                          S-751 23 Uppsala, Sweden

A. Capron   Université du Droit et de la Santé, U.E.
                          R. de Médecine, Service d'Immunologie et
                          de Biologie Parasitaire, Place de Verdun,
                          59000 Lille, France

C.G. Cochrane   Scripps Clinic and Research Foundation,
                          Department of Immunopathology, 476 Pros-
                          pect Street, La Jolla, California 92037
                          USA.

J.R. David   Harvard Medical School, Department of
                          Medicine, Robert B. Brigham Hospital,
                          125 Parker Hill Avenue, Boston, Massa-
                          chussetts 02120, USA

B. Diamant   University of Copenhagen, Department of
                                Pharmacology, Juliane Maries vej 20,
                                DK-2100 Copenhagen Ø, Denmark

E.J. Goetzl   Harvard Medical School, Department of
                                Medicine, Robert B. Brigham Hospital,
                                125 Parker Hill Avenue, Boston Massa-
                                chussetts 02120, USA

B. Gomperts   The Department of Experimental Pathology,
                                University College Hospital, Medical
                                School, London WC1E 6JJ, England

K. Ishizaka   The Johns Hopkins University, School of
                                Medicine, The Good Samaritan Hospital,
                                5601 Loch Raven Boulevard, Baltimore,
                                Maryland 21239, USA

T. Ishizaka   The Johns Hopkins University, School of
                                Medicine, The Good Samaritan Hospital,
                                5601 Loch Raven Boulevard, Baltimore,
                                Maryland 21239, USA

E. Jarrett   The Wellcome Laboratories for Experimen-
                                tal Parasitology, University of Glasgow,
                                Bearsden Road, Bearsden, Glasgow G61 1QH
                                Scotland

S.G.O. Johansson   The Blood Center, University Hospital,
                                S-750 14 Uppsala 14, Sweden

L. Lichtenstein   The Johns Hopkins University, School of
                                Medicine, Clinical Immunology Division,
                                The Good Samaritan Hospital, 5601 Loch
                                Raven Boulevard, Baltimore, Maryland
                                21239, USA

D.G. Marsh   National Institute for Medical Research,
                                The Ridgeway, Mill Hill, London NW7 1AA,
                                England

H.Z. Movat   University of Toronto, Division of Gene-
                                ral and Experimental Pathology, Depart-
                                ment of Pathology, Toronto 5, Canada

H.J. Müller-Eberhard   Scripps Clinic and Research Foundation,
                                Department of Molecular Immunology, 476
                                Prospect Street, La Jolla, California
                                92037, USA

K. Strandberg   Department of Pharmacology, Karolinska
                       institutet, S-104 01 Stockholm 60,
                       Sweden

T. Tada   Laboratories for Immunology, School of
                       Medicine, Chiba University, 1-8-1 Ino-
                       hana Chibacity, Chiba, Japan 280

B. Uvnäs   Department of Pharmacology, Karolinska
                       institutet, S-104 01 Stockholm 60,
                       Sweden

SUBJECT INDEX

Active Hageman factor, increased vascular permeability, 372
Allergen
    allergenicity, 12
    antigenicity, 9-10, 56
    and RAST, 12
    charge, 5
    denatured, 7, 65
    fluorescence, 10
    immunogenicity, 21, 27, 65, 101
    iso-, 6
    major, 4
    minor, 4
    mol. weight, 5
    N-glycosidic linkages, 10
    stability, 7
    structure, 7, 14
Allergic reactions, classification, 233
Aminopeptidase, 399
Anaphylatoxins, precursors, 340
    formation, 340, 341
    structure and function, 345, 347
Antigen-antibody reaction, and histamine release, 217
Anti-Thymocyte Serum (ATS) and IgE response, 82
Atopy, 20
ATP, and histamine release, 255

B-cells, and IgE response, 59
Bradykinin, 239, 372

Calcium, and mast cell response, 217, 220, 255, 257, 262,
    266, 307
Capping, of IgE on basophils, 202
Chemotaxis, effect of synthetic peptides, 354, 356
Coagulation, influence by IgE, 239